Informatics in Oral Medicine:
Advanced Techniques in Clinical and Diagnostic Technologies

Andriani Daskalaki
Max Planck Institute for Molecular Genetics, Germany

Medical Information Science
REFERENCE

MEDICAL INFORMATION SCIENCE REFERENCE
Hershey · New York

Director of Editorial Content: Kristin Klinger
Director of Book Publications: Julia Mosemann
Development Editor: Julia Mosemann
Publishing Assistant: Kurt Smith
Typesetter: Kurt Smith
Quality control: Jamie Snavely
Cover Design: Lisa Tosheff
Printed at: Yurchak Printing Inc.

Published in the United States of America by
Medical Information Science Reference (an imprint of IGI Global)
701 E. Chocolate Avenue
Hershey PA 17033
Tel: 717-533-8845
Fax: 717-533-8661
E-mail: cust@igi-global.com
Web site: http://www.igi-global.com/reference

Library of Congress Cataloging-in-Publication Data

Informatics in oral medicine : advanced techniques in clinical and diagnostic technologies / Andriani Daskalaki, editor.
p. ; cm.
Includes bibliographical references and index.
Summary: "This book covers a wide range of applications in oral medicine and describes through applied research projects, important methods like 3D radiographic imaging, 2D and 3D finite element analysis, proteomic analysis, genomic analysis, oral human microbiom, computational biomodeling, molecular modeling, and computational biochemistry and biophysics"--Provided by publisher.
ISBN 978-1-60566-733-1 (hardcover)
1. Dental informatics. I. Daskalaki, Andriani, 1966-
[DNLM: 1. Dental Informatics. 2. Computational Biology. 3. Computer Simulation. 4. Diagnosis, Computer-Assisted. 5. Medical Informatics. WU 26.5 I43 2010]
RK240.I54 2010
617'.075--dc22

2009023503

British Cataloguing in Publication Data
A Cataloguing in Publication record for this book is available from the British Library.

Table of Contents

Section 2
Informatic Tools in Oral Diagnostic Technologies

Section 3
3D-Visualization in Oral Diagnosis

Detailed Table of Contents

Section 1
Informatic Tools in Oral Medical Research

This chapter deals with the development of "artificial mouths" in food aroma research. After a brief outline on how aroma is perceived in vivo, the need to develop instrumental techniques that reproduce mouth conditions is explained. The devices described in the literature are then presented, and the difficulties and advances in reproducing oral functions, such as mouth temperature, saliva, breathing and mastication, are discussed. Finally, the artificial mouth designed by the authors is presented as well as the improvements it will bring in food aroma research. In particular, this is the first device enabling the aroma of especially hard food to be studied. By means of this technique, volatile compounds contributing to the aroma perception of all kinds of foodstuffs can be identified and a better understanding of the release of aroma during mastication will be possible.

Proteomics is the large-scale analysis and study of proteins, particularly their structures and functions. The focus of this book chapter is to summarize recent advances in proteome analysis using mass spectrometry and protein microarrays. Critical applications of proteomics in oral medicine will be discussed. With the rapid development of proteomics tools, this novel molecular technology may significantly accelerate oral disease research, including discovery of protein biomarkers for disease diagnosis and prognosis, elucidation of molecular determinants and key signal pathways underlying the disease mechanism, identification of novel therapeutic targets and assessment of drug efficacy and toxicity.

This chapter/manuscript will review the application of computational biology methods (bioinformatics, computational biomodeling, genomics, proteomics, oral human microbiome, molecular modeling, systems biology, protein structure prediction, structural genomics, computational biochemistry and computational biophysics methods and projects) that have been applied to oral diseases research. The emphasis of the manuscript will be on concepts from molecular biology, genetics, and traditional pathology to provide new insights into oral diseases, and the associated technologies to provide new diagnostic and prognostic information. Another goal of the manuscript will be to serve as a central reference to access of information about computational biology resources oral diseases

Growth factors are critical for normal development of craniofacial innervation. Recent evidence indicates that neuronal growth factors, and particularly members of the neurotrophin family, are also involved in activity-dependent synaptic plasticity, with wide-ranging implications for chronic pain syndromes. This chapter will present our advances in stimulation of dissociated neurons with physiological patterns of activity, and detection of endogenous peptides that are released from neurons in low abundance. ELISA in situ and the "rapid capture" ELISA methodology will be presented using Brain-Derived Neurotrophic Factor (BDNF) and Endomorphin-2 as examples.

The goal of identifying and quantifying defined oral microbial populations has gained increasing importance in clinical dentistry. Standard laboratory culture-based procedures–despite their importance for the generation of resistance profiles–are unfortunately inadequate to grow the majority of mainly anaerobic species that predominate at pathological sites, such as periodontal pockets or infected root canals. In this chapter molecular tools based on real-time quantitative polymerase chain reaction (RTQ-PCR) will be described along with ways showing the computation and analysis of the datasets. RTQ-PCR allows the determination of the amount of almost any given bacterial species or the total bacterial load in oral clinical sample in a sensitive and highly reproducible way. This chapter will be complemented by discussing potential pitfalls that should be taken into consideration for producing proper results along with referring the reader to pertinent literature that will allow an individual deepening into the concept of molecular-based diagnosis in clinical dentistry.

The Human Papillomavirus (HPV) is playing an important role in oral cancer. The molecular detection of HPV is based on the fact that the viral DNA is present in all the epithelial layers of the affected tissue and it can be detected easily with PCR or Real-Time PCR. The major disadvantage of PCR is that it cannot provide genotype information and the Real-Time PCR can only detect very few types in a multiplex assay. Although the HPV typing assays are capable of typing a relatively large spectrum of HPV genotypes, they cannot be automated or deployed in a high-throughput platform. The bead-based technology (Luminex suspension array technology) provides a rapid and cost-effective method to simultaneously detect different HPV genotypes.

Computerized Occlusal Analysis technology records, and quickly displays for clinical interpretation, tooth contact timing sequences of .003 second increments, and each tooth contacts' fluctuating force levels which occur during functional jaw movements. These measurements are recorded intraorally with an ultra-thin, mylar-encased sensor that is connected to a computer via a USB interface. This sensor is placed between a patients' teeth during functional jaw movements to record changing tooth-tooth interactions. The displayed occlusal data aids in the examination and treatment of occlusal abnormalities on natural teeth, dental prostheses, and dental implant prostheses. The software can be linked to an Electromyography software program that simultaneously records the electromyographic potential of 8 head and neck muscles. This combination of dynamic tooth contact force and time data, and functional muscular data, affords a dentist detailed, precise, and unparalleled diagnostic and treatment information, with which to address many differing clinical occlusal pathologies

Although casting is currently the first choice to produce metallic frame work selective laser melting (SLM) has established. Based on a CAD/CAM system the digital data of the frame work are transferred to the production machine. The three dimensional data set of the transferred in to numerous quasi 2-dimensional data. Each of this data sets represents a single slice, which is then produced. Due to the production process complex geometries and outstanding mechanical and chemical properites can be realised. Advantageously is also the large number of simultaniously fabricated parts, which makes this method very economic.

The Finite Element Method (FEM) is probably the most used technique to model the mechanic properties of a body. The method needs a subdivision of the body (or domain) to be simulated in simpler geometrical structures. This subdivision is known as a mesh. This chapter gives a short introduction to the FEM, then continues with the most important aspects to consider for choosing a mesh like, element type, quality and node density. Finally this chapter reviews several meshing techniques currently used in the medical-field simulations. The techniques are classified and compared.

The Finite Element Method (FEM) is a widely applied mathematical model that permit us to know the biomechanical behaviour of the human mandible in various clinical situations under physiological and standardized trauma conditions. The 3D FEM provides to simulate force systems applied and allows analysis of the response of the jawbone to the loads in 3D space. Clinical extrapolations from FEM may not give absolute values but they will provide detailed description of biomechanical pattern and a prediction of regional stresses distribution. This virtual modeling are useful to choose the most efficient localization and design of miniplate osteosynthesis and to test new biomaterials.

Numerous efforts have been made towards three-dimensional (3D) radiographic imaging in all fields of dentistry, ranging from oral surgery to orthodontics. Although computrized tomography (CT) has been available for quite some time now, its use in dentistry has always been limited because of cost, access, and dose considerations. In orthodontics, diagnosis and treatment planning has been based traditionally on 2D imaging (cephalometric and panoramic radiographs). The introduction of cone-beam computed tomography (CBCT) represented a true revolution in dento-maxillofacial radiology, and a shift from 2D to 3D data acquisition, image reconstruction, and visualization. Therefore, CBCT has now been introduced in different areas of orthodontic treatment planning and diagnostic procedures: The present book chapter will give an overview of the current literature regrading the present use of CBCT in the localization of impacted teeth for othodontic purposes. The potential, advantages, disadvantages, and also future developments in orthodontic treatment planning for impacted teeth will be discussed, also using case examples from daily clinical practice.

Computer-assisted surgery (CAS) systems comprise different technologies for 3D visualization of the patient´s anatomy, visualization software capable of virtual dental implant position planning, as well as distinct approaches for transferring the virtually planned implant positions to the corresponding patient´s anatomical sites. The aim of this chapter is to give a complete survey of CAS systems in dental implantology from the different 3D visualization technologies to the different available approaches for implant planning data transfer to the corresponding anatomical patient´s sites. Focus will be on the illumination of advantages and disadvantages for the different systems components. In this context also the diagnostic value, radiation dosages to the patient, availability and costs and latest results for the achieved transfer accuracy from planning data to the final implant positions will be discussed.

Periodontal disease is the most common oral disorder in the elderly population. Early detection of bony and soft tissue support changes is therefore crucial in relation to the prevention of tooth loss and/or the patient's general health. Unfortunately, the current diagnostic tools for accurate assessment of this periodontal status have shown several limitations. Most image analysis tools are based on 2D images, while bone remodelling is a 3D process. At present, Cone Beam Computed Tomography (CBCT) has become a powerful diagnostic tool in dentistry. This chapter will bring an overview of 2D and 3D visualization methods of the periodontal tissues and their pathologic manifestations like infrabony craters and furcation involvements. The diagnostic use of 2D radiographic projections, image filtering and subtraction will be compared to the use of 3D cross-sections and the image analysis tools for 3D visualization and/or follow-up of bony changes. For the latter, the influence of several parameters in the segmentation and/or registration process of 3D periodontal datasets will be discussed.

Section 4
Bioinformatic Applications in Bacterial Identification

Understanding how host cells have adapted to pathogens, and how barrier cells respond to limit their impact, provides a mechanistic biological interpretation of microbial disease in the mixed bacterial-human ecosystem of the oral cavity. Transcriptional profiling, statistical and ontology tools are used to uncover and dissect genes and pathways of human gingival epithelial cells that are modulated upon interaction with the periodontal pathogens. Affymetrix microarrays are applied to search the gene expression underlying infection with P. gingivalis or A. actinomycetemcomitans and identify distinct classes of up- and down-regulated genes during this process. The developed meta-analysis approach helps to extract sets of genes related to infections of the oral cavity and interaction networks by integrating and combining qualitative as well as quantitative data using statistical approaches.

The oral cavity is inhabited by more than 500 species of commensal bacteria. Some of them have been focused as pathogens of oral diseases, dental caries and periodontal diseases. However, the lack of information concerning interaction between pathogens and the rest of commensal bacteria made it difficult to understand precise etiologies of oral diseases. The authors need to explore how to know comprehensive species composing individual oral flora and to compare the results with corresponding oral health condition. In this chapter, the authors would like to trace the previous attempts to clarify

Foreword

It is really an honour and a great pleasure for me to write a foreword to this book on "Informatics in Oral Medicine". Although, my specialty is not in the field of oral medicine, dental informatics has always been my primary interest along with clinical operative dentistry and research. My involvement in dental informatics, for almost 3 decades, made me realize that oral medicine, clinical dentistry and dental research, are best served by informatics especially when public oral health and care is the target. Informatics has unlimited ways to support and assist all branches of dentistry and many are still unknown to the majority of the dental clinicians or even researchers. However, I must say that many applications have not yet been transformed from a valuable research tool to a practical tool for the everyday clinical practice.

This book covers a wide range of applications in oral medicine and describes through applied research projects, important methods like, 3D radiographic imaging, 2D and 3D finite element analysis, proteomic analysis, genomic analysis, oral human microbiom, computational biomodeling, molecular modeling, and computational biochemistry and biophysics. All the above methods and many others are today's most advanced applications in clinical and diagnostic technologies, and for this reason, this book will stimulate the curiosity and interest of scientists in informatics to work in collaboration with oral medicine scientists for the benefit of public's health care.

The editor of this book, Dr. Andriani Daskalaki is well known to me as a persistent, hard working and knowledgeable researcher, expert in the field of bioinformatics with a mind wide open to foresee the importance and necessity of books in dental and oral informatics. This alone, guarantees that this book will become soon a reference and its interesting chapters will offer valuable assistance to those who are seeking answers on how to use applications of informatics in oral medicine and dentistry for solving similar practical problems.

Most of the writers are experienced researchers and clinicians with a unique involvement in applied informatics for oral medicine, oral surgery, dentofacial orthopaedics, molecular biology, periodontology or cariology. Their knowledge has been transformed into a valuable text in this book for all readers, clinicians or researchers, not only in the field of dental sciences but in medical and basic sciences as well. For these reasons I do recommend this book as a valuable tool in oral informatics and I hope all contributors to this publication to continue to publicize their expert knowledge in this fast growing and evolving science that affect us all.

P. E. Lagouvardos
Associate Professor
Course Director in Dental Informatics
Dental School, University of Athens, Greece

Panagiotis E. Lagouvardos *graduated in 1974 from the dental school of Athens, and received his Doctor degree from the same school in 1985. Is an Associate Professor in Operative Dentistry at the dental school of the University of Athens, director of the preclinical education for undergraduate students in Operative Dentistry, and course director in Dental Informatics for dental students. Is the author of a book in "Dental Informatics", the editor in chief of the "Hellenic Dental Journal" and advisor to the Hellenic Dental Association in issues related to Dental Informatics.*

Preface

Informatics tools offer solutions to many problems in oral health clinic and research, but also face significant challenges, linking of data from the clinical diagnostic technologies.

The field of bioinformatics will have several main areas of interest in oral medicine including the development of software and analysis tools for genomics and proteomics data related to oral tissues, in particular for the analysis of data from DNA arrays, mass spectrometry, and protein-protein and protein-DNA interactions in the analysis and interpretation of these data.

Methodologies shall focus on methods from multivariate statistics, for example testing statistical hypotheses, cluster analysis and classification, and networks as well as functional annotation of sequence data.

The in silico analysis of complex biological processes, such as gene regulatory motifs, metabolic networks, and signal transduction pathways, will play an important role in the development of diseases, infections as well as oral tissue malformations. Specific efforts have to be made for the integration of databases and experimental data into the kinetic models, for example in order to test mutations or to validate drug targets for oral cancer. The aim of the book is to gain insight into technological advances in the field of oral health informatics. We aimed this book for the clinician, and the researcher in this evolving field.

ORGANIZATION OF THE BOOK

The book is roughly divided into 5 sections:

Section One, "**Informatics Tools in Oral Medical Research**" introduces the basic concepts in the use of computational tools in oral medical research. Chapter 1 deals with the development of "artificial mouths". The need to develop instrumental techniques that reproduce mouth conditions is explained. In this chapter are presented the difficulties and advances in reproducing oral functions, such as mouth temperature, saliva, breathing and mastication. Chapter 2 is focused on proteomics applications by using mass spectrometry and protein microarrays in oral medicine. The emphasis of chapter 3 is on concepts from molecular biology, genetics, and traditional pathology to provide new insights into oral diseases, and the associated technologies to provide new diagnostic and prognostic information. Chapter 4 describes novel approaches to study regulation of neurotrophin expression and release from neurons by activity.

Section Two, "**Informatics Tools in Oral Diagnostic Technologies**" serves as a comprehensive introduction to computational methods supporting oral diagnosis. Chapter 5 discusses the methods for assessing the complexity of oral plaque biofilms. Chapter 6 describes Human Papilloma Virus (HPV) detection and genotyping using the Luminex xMAP technology. Chapter 7 provides information related to Time Sequencing and Force Mapping with Integrated Electromyography to measure occlusal parameters.

Section Three, "**3D-Visualization in Oral Medicine**" includes 6 chapters. Chapter 8 deals with the description of selective laser melting in dentistry .Chapter 9 introduces techniques for the generation of 3D Finite Element Meshes of human organs. In chapter 10 the author describes the Finite Element Method (FEM), a widely applied mathematical model that permit us to know the biomechanical behavior of the human mandible in various clinical situations under physiological and standardized trauma conditions. Chapter 11 gives an overview of the current literature regarding the present use of cone-beam computed tomography in the localization of impacted teeth for orthodontic purposes. Chapter 12 present different approaches for computer-assisted surgery (CAS) in dental implantology. Chapter 13 present concepts related to imaging techniques in Periodontology.

Section Four, "**Bioinformatics Applications in Bacterial Identification,**" describes informatics tools and techniques related to oral bacteria identification. Chapter 14 describes a developed meta-analysis approach which helps to extract sets of genes related to oral infections and interaction networks by integrating and combining quantitative data using statistical approaches. Chapter 15 discuss the potential capability of modern molecular genetic technologies utilizing bioinformatics.

In Section Five, "**Informatics tools in the management of dental care**", Chapter 16 presents new innovative services in dentist appointment management.

The book "**Informatics in Oral Medicine: Advanced Techniques in Clinical and Diagnostic, Technologies**" contains text information, but also a glossary of terms and definitions, contributions from international experts, in-depth analysis of issues, concepts, new trends, and advanced technologies in oral medicine. This edition focuses more directly and extensively than ever on applications of informatics in oral medicine.

The diverse and comprehensive coverage of multiple disciplines in the field of oral health informatics in this book will contribute to a better understanding all topics, research, and discoveries in this evolving, significant field of study. I hope will make this book a helpful tool-not only for the student who needs an expert source of basic knowledge in oral health informatics, but also for the advanced researcher who needs clear, concise, and balanced information on which to conduct his research.

In shaping this book, I committed myself to making the reference book as useful as possible to students and advanced researchers coping with the demands of modern medical research. Thanks to a very hard-working advisory editorial board of scientists, excellent authors who fulfilled our invitations, and a very efficient publisher providing clear procedures and practices for a quality production, readers may now enjoy chapters on some of the major ideas that have concerned computing and its applications in oral medicine.

Andriani Daskalaki
Max Planck Institute, Berlin, Germany

Acknowledgment

The editor sincerely acknowledges the help of all persons involved in the development process of this book, without whose support the project would not have been satisfactorily completed. Deep appreciation and gratitude is due to Prof. Dr. Hans Lehrach, Director of the Department of Vertebrate Genomics, Max-Planck-Institute for Molecular Genetics, for giving me the opportunity to work in the field of systems biology and bioinformatics and generating the idea of this book.

I wish to express my appreciation to my colleagues, who, as experts in their fields, have helped me with constructive criticism and helpful suggestions.

Thanks go to all those who provided constructive and comprehensive reviews. Dr. Athina Lazakidou from the University of Peloponnese, and Dr. Amit Chattopadhyay from National Institute of Dental and Craniofacial Research (NIDCR), provided the most comprehensive, critical and constructive comments.

Special thanks also go to the publishing team at IGI Global, whose contributions throughout the whole process from inception of the initial idea to final publication have been invaluable. In particular to Julia Mosemann, who continuously prodded via e-mail for keeping the project on schedule and to Mehdi Khosrow-Pour, whose enthusiasm motivated me to initially accept his invitation for taking on this project.

Last but not least, I am grateful to my father, Dimitrios Daskalakis, for his unfailing support and encouragement.

In closing, I wish to thank all of the authors for their insights and excellent contributions to this book.

Andriani Daskalaki, PhD
Max Planck Institute, Berlin, Germany
June 2009

Section 1
Informatic Tools in Oral Medical Research

Chapter 1
Development of Artificial Mouths for In Vitro Studies of Aroma from Liquid and Solid Foods

Gaëlle Arvisenet
Food Aroma Research Laboratory, ENITIAA, France

Pauline Poinot
Food Aroma Research Laboratory, ENITIAA, France

Carole Prost
Food Aroma Research Laboratory, ENITIAA, France

ABSTRACT

This chapter deals with the development of "artificial mouths" in food aroma research. After a brief outline on how aroma is perceived in vivo, the need to develop instrumental techniques that reproduce mouth conditions is explained. The devices described in the literature are then presented, and the difficulties and advances in reproducing oral functions, such as mouth temperature, saliva, breathing and mastication, are discussed. Finally, the artificial mouth designed by the authors is presented as well as the improvements it will bring in food aroma research. In particular, this is the first device enabling the aroma of especially hard food to be studied. By means of this technique, volatile compounds contributing to the aroma perception of all kinds of foodstuffs can be identified and a better understanding of the release of aroma during mastication will be possible.

INTRODUCTION

Food is composed mainly of macromolecules, vitamins and minerals, but also of small quantities of volatile molecules without nutritional value. These compounds are responsible for the perception of the odor and the aroma of food. They belong to all chemical classes and are characterised by a low molecular weight (between 30 and 300 Da) and a high saturating vapour pressure (Richard, 1992). They are distributed between the food product and the gas phase. In a gaseous state, some of these compounds

DOI: 10.4018/978-1-60566-733-1.ch001

Figure 1. Pathways of molecules generating odor and aroma perception

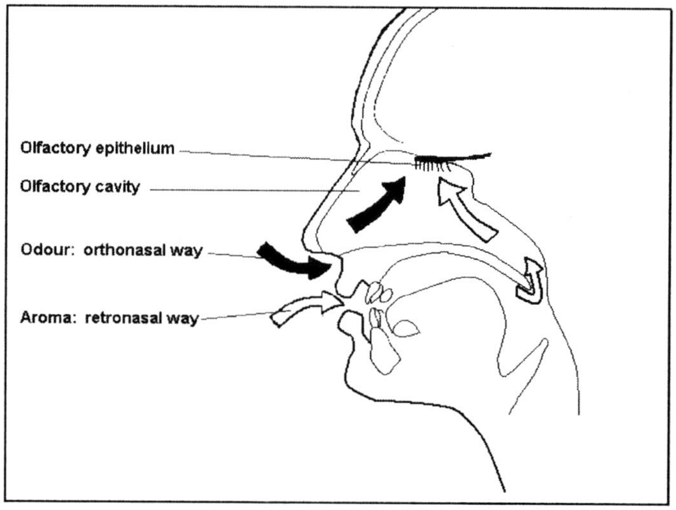

can reach the olfactory epithelium and generate a stimulus, called either odor when the product is smelt (orthonasal way) or aroma when the food is eaten (retronasal way). The overall sensation produced in the mouth by the association between taste and aroma constitutes the flavour.

Perception of aroma is a complex phenomenon, involving different steps. In the oral cavity, volatile compounds are released from the matrix into the gas phase, under the effects of mastication, mouth temperature, and saliva. Compounds are then transported via the retronasal way to the nasal cavity, where they interact with the corresponding receptors in the olfactory epithelium (Figure 1). Subsequently, sensory signals are transferred to the brain. Only those compounds released from the food in sufficiently high concentration will stimulate the olfactory receptors. Furthermore, most odorant perceptions are generated by mixtures of several aroma compounds, in well-defined proportions. A slight change in the volatile composition can modify the nature and intensity of the perception. Competition between compounds for receptors can occur. Thus, the perception is not linearly correlated with the concentration of the released volatile compounds (Stone and Sidel, 2004). Moreover, in food matrices, only a fraction of the total aroma compounds can be released, because of interactions that can occur between them and the matrix. Therefore, the perceived aroma quality and intensity cannot be predicted by the concentration of volatiles in the food.

Odor and aroma are particularly important in consumer acceptance of food. For instance, a recent survey showed that 73% of French teenagers state that the flavor of food is the main factor that influences their choice. Therefore, it is essential for food research laboratories and food companies to understand the mechanisms involved in the odor and aroma perception of a food and the link between food composition and the release of volatile compounds in mastication conditions.

INSTRUMENTAL TECHNIQUES TO STUDY VOLATILE COMPOUNDS RESPONSIBLE FOR FOOD AROMA

During the last two decades, several approaches have been developed to identify the molecules responsible for the odor and aroma of a food. Aroma perception can be studied by combining instrumental techniques and sensory analysis (Taylor, 1996).

Classical Methods

Sensory analysis consists in asking people to evaluate food aroma. For instance, they can provide information about the average sensation, by means of sensory profiles that describe product similarities and differences regardless of their complexity. The method requires a formal screening and training procedure of subjects. It involves the development and use of a sensory language, and the scoring of products in repeated trials to obtain a complete and quantitative description. It is therefore time-consuming and very expensive, and does not provide information about the reasons for the perceived characteristics. Moreover, sample palatability and safety are of particular importance when working with subjects.

Another way is to use chemical methods to analyze the compounds involved in perception. The first step is to separate volatile compounds from the other molecules of food. Instrumental techniques like capillary gas chromatography combined to mass spectrometry (GC/MS) can then identify and quantify extracted volatile compounds with increasing precision. There is a complementary method that can identify the odorant compounds among all the extracted volatile compounds. It combines their separation by gas chromatography with the detection of the separated compounds by the human nose. This method is called Gas Chromatography-Olfactometry (GC-O) (Mayol and Acree, 2001).

For a long time, chemical methods such as distillation or liquid-liquid extraction have been used to extract volatile compounds from foods (Frasse et al., 1992; Maarse, 1991; Rychlik and Grosch, 1996). These methods only provide information about the volatile composition of the food. However, it is now generally accepted that it is not the same as the composition of the volatile fraction that reaches the olfactory receptors. Therefore, compounds extracted by these methods may not closely represent the compounds that can stimulate the receptors when the food is eaten. Headspace techniques have thus been developed as they provide a measure of volatile partitioning and release. They consist in sampling the gas phase above the product and analyzing its composition. The sampling can be done in static or dynamic conditions. In static conditions, the food sample is put in a sealed container. When equilibrium is reached, a headspace sample is collected. Dynamic conditions consist in sampling the gas phase continuously thanks to an inert gas that flows through the sample. Dynamic headspace results are therefore partially determined by the kinetics of release, and the relative proportions of volatiles depend on the time for which they are purged from the food (Piggott and Schaschke, 2001). These methods have been successfully applied in many cases and can provide valuable information. However, they do not reflect accurately which compounds are transferred to the olfactory receptors. Indeed, in some cases, headspace analysis has not provided data that correspond well to the results of sensory analyses of the same products (Piggott and Schaschke, 2001). These sampling methods do not take into account the physico-chemical changes that occur in the mouth and that alter the proportions of volatiles available for transport to the olfactory epithelium (Taylor, 1996). It was thus necessary to develop alternative methods that would consider the consumer influence as well as the chemistry and physics of the food.

Novel Methods

Two innovative approaches have been recently developed to understand the mechanisms involved in aroma compound release and perception. Some are direct methods, consisting of the analysis of exhaled air. Nose-space is one of these methods. It involves the sampling, trapping and analysis of the gas flow expired by the nose by a subject while eating a food sample (Ingham et al., 1995). The collected volatile fraction is thought to have a composition very close to the compounds interacting with the receptors (Taylor and Linforth, 1994). As the perception of food aroma is not a static, unchanging experience during the course of eating, fast analysis was required to measure real-time release (van Ruth and Buhr, 2004). This led to the development of APCI/MS (Taylor et al., 2000) and PTR/MS (van Ruth and Buhr, 2004) which allow breath-by-breath analysis of volatile compounds. However, because oral physiological variables are difficult to control and can vary greatly between people, this method requires the input of several volunteers. There can be sensitivity problems for the analysis of real foods because the quantity of volatiles expired by the nose is very small. Hansson et al. (2003) reported that, in a study of model beverages, only a few compounds were above noise level and could be studied. Moreover, just a few selected compounds can be followed simultaneously by these techniques (van Ruth and Buhr, 2004). This is particularly restrictive when studying real foodstuffs, because the compounds having a higher impact on their aroma or odor are not previously known. Thus, before studying them by APCI/MS or PTR/MS, previous studies are needed to know their volatile composition and identify the compounds having a great impact on their aroma.

For these reasons, indirect techniques that simulate the process of eating have been developed. This alternative approach consists in reproducing human mouth conditions instrumentally and observing their influence on aroma release. These indirect techniques are called "artificial mouths", "model mouths" or "mastication simulators".

EVOLUTION OF MODEL MOUTH SYSTEMS

The factors affecting the release of volatile compounds from food matrices in the oral cavity are temperature, the presence of saliva, food stirring and breaking, breathing and possible adsorption by the mouth mucosa (Buettner et al., 2002; Taylor, 1996). Consequently, it is important to reproduce these conditions when studying perceived food volatile compounds.

Artificial mouth devices are derived from dynamic headspace techniques, to which successive modifications have been added in order to reproduce in-mouth conditions accurately. Several devices have been described in the literature (Lee III, 1986; Nassl et al., 1995; Roberts and Acree, 1995; van Ruth et al., 1994; van Ruth and Roozen 2000 b, Jensen et al., 2003; Rabe et al., 2002, 2004 a and b; Salles et al. 2007; Arvisenet et al. 2006 and 20082008). These models are more or less realistic but none can reproduce all the functions of the human mouth.

The different functions of these models will be presented, and the advances in reproducing their principle, the influence of saliva, the mastication movements, the swallowing step, the contact with mucosa and the respiration will be described. In the last part, the authors will present their device, which is currently the only one that has been used to extract aroma compounds from particularly hard foods.

Model Mouth Principle

Model mouths generally consist of reactors of various volumes, from 70 mL (van Ruth et al., 1995 a, 1995 b) to 5 L (Rabe et al., 2002, 2004 a), in which the food sample is placed, at a controlled temperature. As the saturation vapor pressure of aroma compounds is strongly dependent on temperature, it is particularly important to control this parameter. It is usually set at the same value as oral temperature. In model mouth devices, the temperature is thus controlled between 36°C (Nassl et al., 1995) and 37°C (Arvisenet et al., 2006 and 2008; Deibler2008 et al., 2001; van Ruth et al., 1994; van Ruth and Roozen, 2000 b) by means of a water bath (Nassl et al., 1995) or by water circulating either in the reactor double jacket (Rabe et al., 2002; Salles et al., 2007; van Ruth et al., 1994; van Ruth and Roozen, 2000,

Arvisenet et al. 2008) or in a copper coil circling the reactor (Roberts and Acree, 1996).

In all devices, except that of Nassl et al. (1995), a gas flow enters the reactor and carries volatile compounds released from the food into a system where they are either trapped before further analysis or, in some of the more recent models, analyzed on-line. In the early systems, volatiles were sampled by a syringe (Nassl et al., 1995), or trapped in Tenax (Mayr et al., 2003; Odake et al., 1998, 2000; van Ruth et al., 1995 a, 1995 b) or in silica traps (Roberts and Acree, 1995). More recently, SPME fibres have been used (Deibler et al., 2001; Hee Hong et al., 2006, Arvisenet et al. 2008). The length of chromatographic analysis has often prevented temporal release studies. The kinetic release of only one compound has been analyzed by the use of an interface between the "artificial mouth" vessel and the injection port of the chromatograph (Springett et al., 1999) or by coupling it with a membrane inlet mass spectrometer (Jensen et al., 2003). The temporal study of more compounds has been performed by the combination of several traps (Nassl et al., 1995; Rabe et al., 2002, 2004 a, 2004 b) or by the use of PTR/MS (Hansson et al., 2003; van Ruth and Buhr, 2004).

Saliva Addition

To mimic oral conditions, artificial saliva has been added to the food sample in most model mouth systems. It plays an important role in the release of volatiles from food. Firstly, hydration and dilution of food by saliva affect the partitioning of volatiles between the food, saliva and air phases. Secondly, some salivary molecules, such as proteins and salts, may modify the solubility and availability of volatile compounds, thus affecting their partitioning between food and the gaseous phase.

Numerous artificial saliva formulae have been described in the literature (Jenkins, 1978; Gal et al., 2001). Natural saliva is an extremely complex mixture with numerous constituents, and it varies according to the time of day. Thus, an exact duplication of natural saliva is impossible and artificial saliva formulae have average compositions, varying according to the studies. The artificial saliva most used in food aroma studies combines specific quantities of $NaHCO_3$, NaCl, KCl, $CaCl_2$ $2H_2O$, K_2HPO_4, NaN_3, mucin and α-amylase in distilled water (van Ruth et al., 1995 a). Comparative aroma release experiments showed no difference between the application of human saliva and the same quantity of artificial saliva (van Ruth and Roozen, 2000 b). For this reason, artificial saliva has largely been used in artificial mouth studies. While Odake et al. (1998) showed an influence of artificial saliva on the release of odorant compounds from salad dressings, Rabe et al. (2004 a) showed no significant effect of the addition of saliva on the release of volatile compounds from an aqueous solution and a starch hydrolysate. This may depend on the studied matrix and the aroma compounds it contains. The proportion of saliva also varies considerably depending on the studies. The ratios between saliva and food in the oral cavity have rarely been taken into account, probably because their measurement has been performed only recently (Pionnier et al., 2004, Arvisenet et al., 2008).

In most studies, the volume of the liquid phase remained constant throughout the experiment. The system developed by Rabe et al. (2002) contains automatic valves allowing the addition and removal of saliva during the experiment.

Attempts to Reproduce Food Crushing Instrumentally

Chewing conditions have proved more difficult to imitate in artificial mouths. Various mechanisms have been tested, depending on the device and on the texture of the foods studied. The first mouth systems described were designed to study liquid foods.

Liquid foods. Lee III (1986) placed agitated steel balls in his model mouth container to disrupt food and to stimulate chewing. At the same time, volatiles released from liquid food were removed by a gas stream, which was sent directly to a GC/MS. Later, Nassl et al. (1995) proposed a system called the "Mouth Imitation Chamber" or MIC. It consisted of a glass vessel equipped with a stirrer, two valves and septa on the top allowing the gradual addition of liquid food and saliva. Thanks to this device, they showed that stirring improved the release of volatiles from oil/water emulsions.

Rabe et al. (2002, 2004 a, 2004 b) designed a more complicated device, also based on stirring blades. They showed with this model that stirring speed had an influence on the release of aroma compounds in water. More soluble compounds were more released by vigorous stirring, probably due to an interfacial surface extension of the liquid (Rabe et al., 2004 a). Less volatile compounds showed the opposite effect, which may be explained by an improvement in the distribution of the compounds with high stirring rates. These compounds may have been in a droplet dispersion state because of their low solubility, so the vigorous stirring resulted in an improved dissolution and a decreased release. The volatiles released from a beverage in this artificial mouth were compared to those released *in vivo*, by nose-space coupled with APCI-MS. The temporal release curves obtained by the two methods were superimposable for at least three compounds (Rabe et al., 2004 b). Therefore, this artificial mouth based on stirring gives satisfactory results for the study of liquid food matrices.

Semi-solid foods. To enable the extraction of volatiles from semi-solid foods, more complex systems had to be developed. The first one, called RAS (Retronasal Aroma Simulator), was developed by Roberts and Acree (1995). It consisted of a 1 L stainless steel container designed from a modified blender. Its stirring system could be controlled to obtain shear rates similar to those occurring during eating. The stirring enabled shearing of soft foods (raspberries, peanut butter, banana, model cheese) and mixed them with artificial saliva. A gas flow flushing above the food sample was used to recover the volatile compounds released. RAS was the first system enabling the mixing of saliva and food to be studied. It gave a good approximation of time-averaged aroma release in the mouth as defined by in-mouth measurements (Deibler et al., 2001) but it was not applicable to studying the temporal dimension of release. Moreover, the stirring system, very different from the mastication process, limited the use of RAS to foods with low tear resistance. For instance, the tear resistance of chocolate was too high for the blades in the RAS to overcome (Deibler et al., 2001).

Concurrently, van Ruth et al. (1994) developed several models to study the influence of instrumental crushing by means of a plunger. Their systems were all composed of a flask with a volume similar to the human mouth (70 mL). It was kept at 37°C by water circling through a double wall and artificial saliva could be added. Two of these systems were based on improving the dynamic headspace technique, with gas flowing above the sample and artificial saliva. The first model did not contain a device to crush or stir the food sample. The other one included a plunger that moved up and down to simulate mastication.

These devices were then applied to study the aroma of semi-solid foods such as rehydrated bell peppers (van Ruth et al., 1995 a, 1995 b), French beans and leeks (van Ruth et al., 1995 b; van Ruth and Roozen, 2000 a), and cream-style dressings (Odake et al., 2000). In all these studies, the system equipped with a plunger extracted a higher proportion of volatiles compared to the dynamic headspace system.

In addition, the results obtained with these instrumental models were compared with an analysis of human breath, recovered from assessors. This demonstrated that food crushing by the plunger produced a flavor release closer to the volatile content of human breath than the other system (van Ruth et al., 1995 b; van Ruth and Roozen, 2000 a).

Following these results, van Ruth and Roozen (2000 b) improved their device by adding a screwing movement to the plunger (Fig. 2.). This system was used to study the influence of mastication on rehydrated vegetables (van Ruth and Roozen, 2000 b), oil-and-water flavored matrices (van Ruth and Roozen, 2000 b) and bananas (Mayr et al., 2003). Large differences were found in the number of odor compounds recovered, depending on the mastication rate, in all these matrices.

Solid foods. Jensen et al. (2003) developed a chamber in which two horizontal pistons compressed the food sample (chewing gum in their study), alternately with a third vertical piston. All these movements were adjustable.

Recently, Salles et al. (2007) reported the development of a chewing simulator that reproduces multidimensional movements imitating mastication. The system is a cell comprised of several mobile parts. The upper part is fixed, while the lower part moves. The latter is composed of a cylinder ending in a conical part, representing the tongue. It makes up and down movements. The third part encircles the second. It is ring-shaped, with molar patterns. It makes vertical and rotational movements. Peanuts could be successfully broken after 4 or 8 cycles of chewing in this device, and the distribution of their particle sizes was compared to peanuts chewed by 4 people. An aroma release study using this device has not yet been reported.

Swallowing Step and Contact with Mucosa

In vivo, swallowing is an important step in aroma perception, at least for liquid products, which are swallowed directly after intake. Tongue movement concurrent with swallowing opens the barrier between the tongue and the soft palate (Buettner et al., 2001) and allows volatile compounds to go to the nasal cavity where they can be in contact with olfactory receptors. After swallowing, a thin layer of the liquid remains on the surface of the larynx (Buettner et al., 2001), and is released during the exhalation following swallowing. Thus, retronasal volatile release does not originate directly from the mouth but from a displaced volume of air from the throat (Rabe et al., 2004 b). The highest *in vivo* aroma release signal for liquids is generally found in the first exhalation after swallowing (Linforth and Taylor, 2000), but the exhaled intensity of some compounds increases during on-going drinking, which proves their accumulation in the mucus layers (Rabe et al., 2004 b). This adhesion results in the aftertaste sensation. However, most model mouths described did not take the swallowing process into account. Rabe et al. (2002, 2004 a, 2004 b) simulated swallow-

Figure 2. Schematic representation of the model mouth system designed by van Ruth and Roozen (2000b). Reprinted from van Ruth, S. M., & Roozen, J. P. 2000. Influence of mastication, saliva on aroma release in a model mouth system. Food Chemistry, 71, 339-345, Copyright 2000, with permission from Elsevier.

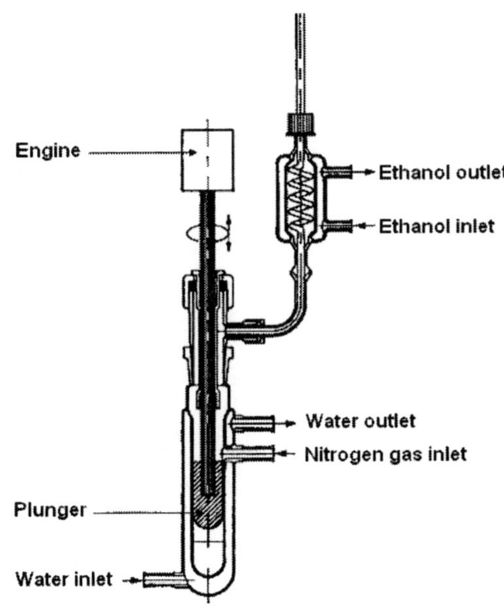

ing in their artificial mouth by filling the reactor with a flavored solution and partially emptying it within 3 s, to create a defined headspace. Boelrijk and co-workers (Weel et al., 2004; Boelrijk et al., 2006) developed an "artificial throat" to simulate the swallowing of liquid foods. It consists of a glass tube that can be opened or closed by a clamp. Liquids are loaded above the closed clamp and, after a contact time of 10 s, the clamp is opened. The liquid pours down the glass tubing and a layer remains on the surface. Volatiles contained in this layer are carried away by a stream of air flowing upward into the tube. The air is sampled at the end of the tube and analysed by APCI/MS. This system can be maintained at a controlled temperature, and the liquid can be mixed with artificial saliva. However, mouth movements are not simulated in this model.

Rabe et al. (2004 a) cultivated cells to create an artificial oral mucosa. A cylindrical layer of cells was immersed in artificial saliva and placed in the reactor. The reactor was then filled with a flavoured solution and the extraction was performed in controlled conditions of temperature and stirring. The same experiment was performed in the same conditions without cells in order to determine the role of cells by comparison. They showed no difference between the release rates of molecules from water with and without the application of artificial mucosa.

Gas Flow

The nature of the gas used to collect the volatiles released in artificial mouth devices varies greatly in the literature. Air can be used but an inert gas, like nitrogen or helium, is more often chosen. The gas flow rate above a liquid influences the quantity of released volatiles: the faster the flow, the greater the quantity of released compounds (Rabe et al., 2004 a).

The course of the gas in the device was also studied by van Ruth and co-workers (van Ruth et al., 1995 b; van Ruth and Roozen 2000 a). In one of the models they developed, the sample was purged by nitrogen, which was introduced into the bottom of the device while the gas recovery was situated at the top. The volatile release in this device was compared with that in improved dynamic headspace models, with gas flowing above the sample. All other parameters were identical. The qualitative compositions of the volatile compounds isolated in these artificial mouths were similar but the quantity extracted was greater in the system in which gas purged the sample. This has to be compared to the enhancing effect of the plunger in the third model designed by van Ruth: gas bubbling through the sample, as well as the movement of the plunger, creates mixing conditions, and a larger interface area is created (Odake et al., 2000).

Remaining Problems

None of the reported model mouths can fully simulate the complexity of the eating process. However, each of these devices mimics at least one of the mechanisms occurring in the oral cavity.

In particular, it is now necessary to develop models enabling the study of more realistic foods, with a complex structure and a hard texture, in order to understand perception in real conditions. The only real food products that have been studied in artificial mouths are soft products like some fruits and vegetables (*i.e.* raspberries, bananas, bell peppers) (Van Ruth et al., 1995 a, 1995 b) or cooked beef (Machiels et al., 2003) that can be easily mashed. To our knowledge, very hard foodstuffs have not yet been studied.

Nevertheless, such an improvement cannot just consist in grouping all the reported functions. For instance, on-line analysis, which is possible with some model foods, is a real advantage but its use for the study of complex foods would involve improvements in the fields of extraction and analysis. We have thus focused on the extraction step, and have developed an artificial mouth in which food volatiles are recovered simultaneously with crushing.

THE "MUNCH-O-MATIC": AN ARTIFICIAL MOUTH TO STUDY AROMA RELEASE FROM HARD FOOD

Our artificial mouth has thus been designed to study the release of volatiles from solid food samples. Our aim was to reproduce neither the human mouth shape nor the exact crushing conditions, but to obtain instrumentally the crushing of a hard food that gave results similar to mastication. The principal objective was to study volatile compounds released under these conditions. We had to overcome many technical difficulties to build this device.

The existing models rarely take into account *in vivo* volume ratios between the mouth, the food, artificial saliva and gas. Indeed, except for the device developed by Salles et al. (2007), the volume of the container remains constant throughout the experiment. However, *in vivo*, the lower jaw movements induce a change in the mouth volume.

Moreover, only three devices attempted to reproduce the complex process of mastication, with movements in three dimensions (Arvisenet et al. 2008, Jensen et al., 2003; Salles et al., 2007). The combination of several parts is necessary to replicate this movement. Although complex movements can be created by complicated devices (Jensen et al., 2003; Salles et al., 2007), the association of too many parts often generates a lack of airtightness. Combined with overpressure due to the gas flow into the device, this lack can lead to significant leaks of volatile compounds. These reduce the efficiency of volatile recovery and cause low reproducibility between experiments. Moreover, neither the use of ball bearings nor the greasing of the moving parts (like that joining the piston and the container) were possible. Indeed, greasing can generate undesirable volatile compounds that lead to headspace pollution. The materials of the artificial mouths must also be inert. To overcome these problems, we chose to minimise the number of parts responsible for the movements. The "munch-o-matic" is thus composed of a cylindrical sample container (600 mL), with a plunger that moves up and down at variable speeds. We have used a flexible material to allow changes in the headspace volume. In addition, this avoids greasing the parts that can be in contact with the food or the headspace. The container is maintained at 37°C by means of a laboratory thermostat *via* an outer layer. It is sealed with a cap maintained by a circlip. All the parts of the artificial mouth that can be in contact with the analyzed food are made of inert materials (treated stainless steel and PEEK).

Crushing device. As it was required for studying hard foods, the plunger used for crushing could not be smooth. It was thus notched to break down samples, like they are by teeth *in vivo*. The shape of the notches was more or less inspired by that of human teeth. Because of the cylindrical shape of the artificial mouth, it would have been difficult to copy all teeth shapes. Indeed, their arrangement is important for their function. It was thus decided to use only one shape of notch. Notches shaped like canines and molars were designed and tested separately for their ability to crush apple slices, 0.8 cm thick and 2 cm long (Arvisenet et al., 2008). Molar-shaped notches only divided apple slices into four or five pieces, still separated. In contrast, with canine-shaped notches, apples were reduced to very small particles, smaller than those obtained in the human mouth. However, small pieces remained, which could be explained by the sharpness of the tested canine notches. Indeed, highly shaped notches could stay clogged with apple pieces, which were then carried away with the piston and could not be crushed any further. The use of two notched plates, to imitate upper and lower jaws, had the same effect. We thus decided to notch only the upper plate, which makes up and down movements. Pointed notches were designed, with a shape optimised to crush samples. This shape was successfully tested on crunchy and sticky products like apples, French bread, cheese and fruit jelly. It is suitable for all food studies.

Even with a notched plunger, a one-dimensional up and down movement was not convenient to crush hard products rapidly and satisfactorily. Indeed, with each movement, notches were in contact with the same sample site they had already crushed. Therefore, only the first bite was efficient. We then decided to make another prototype, which combines a compression and a rotation movement (Figure 3). To avoid airtightness problems, the rotation is provided by the lower plate, on which the samples are placed. The speeds of compression and rotation movements are precisely controlled by motors.

Gas flow. While food is broken down, a inert gas flows through the device at a sequential rate to reproduce breathing. It carries away volatile compounds, released by the breakdown of the food, to an opening in the cap, where a Solid-Phase MicroExtraction (SPME) fibre coated with carboxen/polydimethylsiloxane (CAR/PDMS, 75 μm thickness) is located. Flowing sequences are concomitant with volume variations. The gas flows in when the headspace volume increases. It stops when the headspace volume decreases. This has two advantages. First, volatile compounds in the headspace are concentrated when the volume decreases and the following gas flow sends volatiles to the SPME fibre. This could be compared to the breathing that follows swallowing. Indeed, when the velum closes the oral cavity, the volatile compound concentration increases in the mouth. Then, after swallowing, the opening of the epiglottis and the following exhalation send compounds to the olfactory zone.

Validation Tests

Crushing of the food sample. To validate our artificial mouth, we first evaluated its food crunching ability. The crushed state of the food matrix after artificial mastication had never been described in flavour studies even though it can influence aroma release. Our study was carried out on *Golden* apples, chosen as an example of a real foodstuff with a complex structure and hard to chew. Ratios between the oral cavity and the apple quantity naturally put in the mouth were measured with 19 people, as well as the apple / saliva ratio. The means of the two ratios were calculated and used to determine the quantities of apple and artificial saliva to introduce into the model mouth for one experiment (Arvisenet et al., 2008). Apples were then "chewed" in the artificial mouth.

Figure 3. Schematic representation of the artificial mouth to study aroma release from hard food

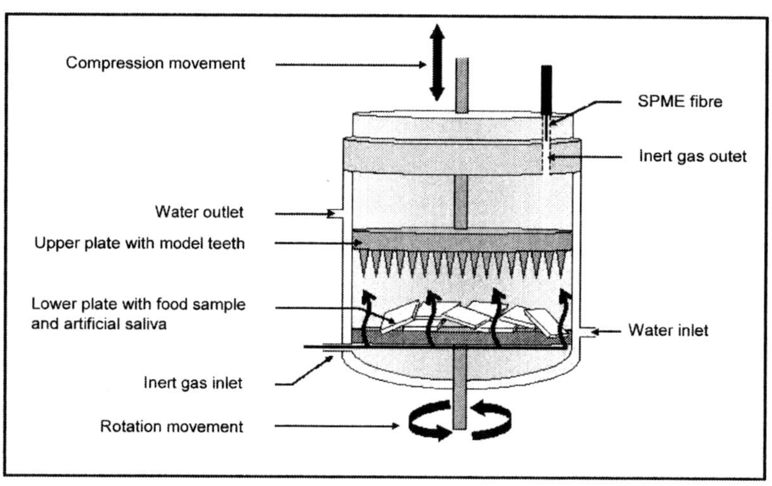

Six people were asked to peel an apple, crunch a piece of it, chew it normally and then spit out the bolus at the point when swallowing would normally have been triggered. Four randomly selected apples were used and two apple pieces from each of them were crunched by each person. After *in vivo* or *in vitro* crushing, apples were spread out in a Petri dish and digitised images were acquired. The two series of images were compared by an image analysis method described by Arvisenet et al. (2008). Images from the artificial mouth, obtained with different values for the control parameters, and images from the human mouth were superimposed to a certain extent. The degree of overlap depended on the actual values of the control parameters. Some artificial mouth conditions were therefore more relevant to mimic the chewing performed in the human mouth. These conditions were then applied to study volatile release.

Influence on volatile release. To evaluate the improvements brought by this chewing device for aroma analysis of hard food, we investigated the influence of the crushing in the artificial mouth on the extraction of *Golden* apples volatile compounds. We thus compared the volatile compounds extracted during a normal run of the artificial mouth and during a run without mastication. All the other parameters (rotation, gas flow, temperature, artificial saliva quantity) were strictly identical. We had previously shown that the amounts of extracted volatile compounds greatly depended on apple piece size (Arvisenet et al., 2006). Indeed, the smaller the pieces, the greater the surface area exposed to the headspace. Therefore, in the present study, the apples for the "no chewing" experiment were previously grated in order to obtain a surface area similar to that obtained by crushing in the artificial mouth. The results are presented in Figure 4.

Most of the compounds extracted from apples were at higher concentrations in the experiment in which crushing was applied simultaneously with aroma compound recovery. The mean quantities of 2-methylbutan-1-ol, butyl 2-methylbutanoate, nonanal, hexyl 2-methylbutanoate, hexanal, and 4-methyl-2,6-ditert-butyl-phenol seem different with the two experimental procedures but these differences are not significant. The heterogeneity of apples could explain the differences between the

Figure 4. Compounds extracted from ***Golden*** *apples by the artificial mouth with and without crushing movements. Not significant: NS; Significant at 5% risk: *; Significant at 1% risk: **; Significant at 0.1% risk: ***.*

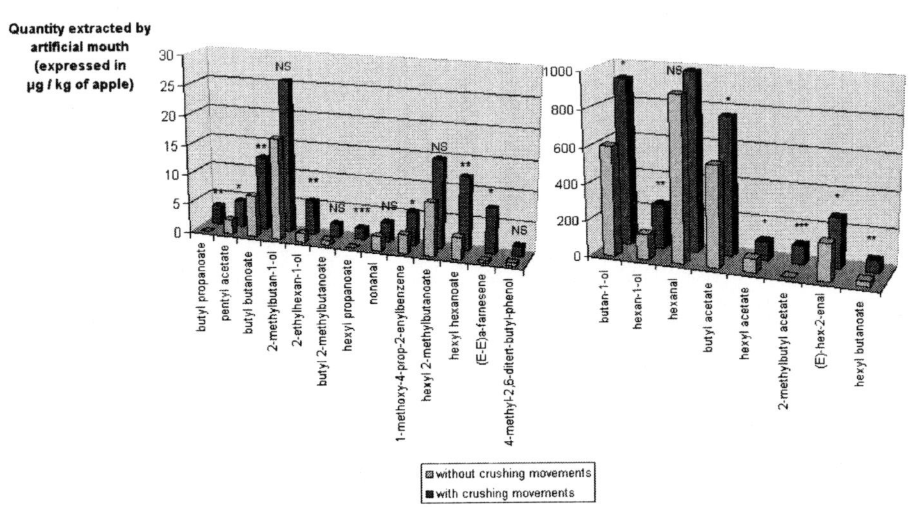

means. For all other compounds, the differences were significant. The enhancement of extraction by the crushing movements is not surprising since the movement of the plunger not only ensured the crushing, but also shook up the apple and the saliva.

A more interesting result is shown in Figure 4: some compounds like butyl propanoate, hexyl propanoate and 2-methyl-1-butylacetate are only extracted with the crushing movement. For other compounds, the ratios between the quantities obtained with crushing and without crushing strongly depend on the compounds. Therefore, the aroma resulting from the extraction with and without plunger movements may differ not only in intensity but also in quality. Indeed, in a mixture of odorant compounds, the proportions of the compounds are very important. A change in one compound concentration can modify the resulting aroma. It would be interesting to ensure that the aromatic extracts obtained with this device are more similar to what a subject perceives when eating an apple, than to the extract obtained by methods without crushing.

CONCLUSION

Artificial mouths have been developed and progressively optimised with the aim of mimicking human mouth conditions. Thanks to the most innovative devices, it is now possible to study the impact of mouth parameters on aroma perception, without taking into account inter-individual variability. We have developed an artificial mouth that can crush real food samples in a similar way to the human mouth. Moreover, we have shown that apple volatiles are released differently under the action of the artificial mastication. These results have to be confirmed with other food products. Such devices could also have applications in the simulation of the forces that chewing exerts on a pair of teeth and their surrounding tissues.

REFERENCES

Arvisenet, G., Billy, L., Poinot, P., Vigneau, E., Bertrand, D., & Prost, C. (2008). Effect of apple particle state on the release of volatile compounds in a new artificial mouth device. *Journal of Agricultural and Food Chemistry, 56*, 3245–3253. doi:10.1021/jf073145z

Arvisenet, G., Billy, L., Royer, G., & Prost, C. (2006). Role of mastication on the release of apple volatile compounds in a model mouth system. In: Flavour Science. Recent advances and trends. Eds. Bredie W. L. P. and Petersen M. A., Elsevier, 465-468.

Boelrijk, A. E. M., Weel, K. G. C., Burger, J. J., Verschueren, M., Gruppen, H., Voragen, A. G. J., & Smit, G. (2006). The artificial throat: a new device to simulate swallowing and *in vivo* aroma release in the throat. The effect of emulsion properties on release in relation to sensory intensity. In: Flavour Science. Recent advances and trends. Eds. Bredie W. L. P. and Petersen M. A., Elsevier, 565-568.

Buettner, A., Beer, A., Hannig, C., & Settles, M. (2001). Observation of the Swallowing Process by Application of Videofluoroscopy and Real-time Magnetic Resonance Imaging-Consequences for Retronasal Aroma Stimulation. *Chemical Senses, 26*, 1211–1219. doi:10.1093/chemse/26.9.1211

Buettner, A., Beer, A., Hannig, C., Settles, M., & Schieberle, P. (2002). Physiological and analytical studies on flavor perception dynamics as induced by the eating and swallowing process. *Food Quality and Preference, 13*, 497–504. doi:10.1016/S0950-3293(02)00052-6

Deibler, K. D., Lavin, E. H., Linforth, R. S. T., Taylor, A. J., & Acree, T. E. (2001). Verification of a mouth simulator by in-vivo measurement. *Journal of Agricultural and Food Chemistry, 49*, 1388–1393. doi:10.1021/jf0012401

Frasse, P., Lambert, S., Levesque, C., Melcion, D., Richard-Molard, D., & Chiron, H. (1992). The influence of fermentation on volatile compounds in French bread crumb. *Lebensmittel Wisstercraft und Technologie*, *25*, 66–70.

Gal, J. Y., Fovet, Y., & Adib-Yadzi, M. (2001). About a synthetic saliva for in vitro studies. *Talanta*, *53*, 1103–1115. doi:10.1016/S0039-9140(00)00618-4

Hansson, A., Giannouli, P., & van Ruth, S. M. (2003). The influence of gel strength on aroma release from pectin gels in a model mouth and in vivo, monitored with proton-transfer-reaction mass spectrometry. *Journal of Agricultural and Food Chemistry*, *51*, 4732–4740. doi:10.1021/jf030050y

Hong, J. H., Duncan, S. E., Dietrich, A. M., & O'Keefe, S. F. (2006). Effect of copper on the volatility of aroma compounds in a model mouth system. *Journal of Agricultural and Food Chemistry*, *54*, 9168–9175. doi:10.1021/jf061229m

Ingham, K. E., Linforth, R. S. T., & Taylor, A. J. (1995). The effect of eating on aroma release from strawberries. *Food Chemistry*, *54*, 283–288. doi:10.1016/0308-8146(95)00048-N

Jenkins, G. N. (1978). The physiology and biochemistry of the mouth. 4th ed. Blackwell Scientific, Oxford.

Jensen, K. D., Beck, H. C., Jeppesen, L., Norrelykke, M. R., & Hansen, A. M. (2003). A new system for dynamic measurements of flavour release: A combined artificial mouth and membrane inlet mass spectrometer. In: Flavour research at the dawn of the twenty-first century. Eds. Le Quéré J. L. and Etievant P., Lavoisier, London, Paris, New York, 228-231.

Lee, W. E. III. (1986). A suggested instrumental technique for studying dynamic flavour release from food products. *Journal of Food Science*, *51*, 249–250. doi:10.1111/j.1365-2621.1986.tb10888.x

Linforth, R., & Taylor, A. J. (2000). Persistence of volatile compounds in the breath after their consumption in aqueous solutions. *Journal of Agricultural and Food Chemistry*, *48*, 5419–5423. doi:10.1021/jf000488n

Maarse, H. (1991). Volatile compounds in foods and beverages. Eds. Maarse H., Dekker Inc.: New York, Basel, Hong Kong.

Machiels, D., van Ruth, S. M., Posthumus, M. A., & Istasse, L. (2003). Gas chromatography-olfactometry analysis of the volatile compounds of two commercial Irish beef meats. *Talanta*, *60*, 755–764. doi:10.1016/S0039-9140(03)00133-4

Mayol, A. R., & Acree, T. E. (2001). Advances in Gas Chromatography-Olfactometry. In: Gas-Chromatography-Olfactometry. The state of the art. Eds. Leland J.V., Schieberle P., Buettner A. and Acree T.E., Oxford University Press, 1-10.

Mayr, D., van Ruth, S. M., & Märk, T. D. (2003). Evaluation of the influence of mastication on temporal aroma release of ripe and unripe bananas, using a model mouth system and gas chromatography-olfactometry. *European Food Research and Technology*, *217*, 291–295. doi:10.1007/s00217-003-0777-1

Nassl, K., Kropf, F., & Klostermeyer, H. (1995). A method to mimic and to study the release of compounds from chewed food. *Lebensmittel Untersuchung und Forshung*, *201*, 62–68. doi:10.1007/BF01193202

Odake, S., Roozen, J. P., & Burger, J. J. (1998). Effect of saliva dilution on the release of diacetyl and 2-heptanone from cream style dressings. *Die Nahrung*, *42*, 385–391. doi:10.1002/(SICI)1521-3803(199812)42:06<385::AID-FOOD385>3.0.CO;2-B

Odake, S., Roozen, J. P., & Burger, J. J. (2000). Flavor release of diacetyl and 2-heptanone from cream style dressings in three model mouth systems. *Bioscience, Biotechnology, and Biochemistry*, *64*, 2523–2529. doi:10.1271/bbb.64.2523

Piggott, J. R., & Schaschke, C. J. (2001). Release cells, breath analysis and in-mouth analysis in flavour research. *Biomolecular Engineering*, *17*, 129–136. doi:10.1016/S1389-0344(01)00071-5

Pionnier, E., Chabanet, C., Mioche, L., Le Quéré, J. L., & Salles, C. (2004). 1. In vivo aroma release during eating of a model cheese: relationships with oral parameters. *Journal of Agricultural and Food Chemistry*, *52*, 557–564. doi:10.1021/jf030544v

Rabe, S., Krings, U., Banavara, D. S., & Berger, R. G. (2002). Computerized apparatus for measuring dynamic flavor release from liquid food matrices. *Journal of Agricultural and Food Chemistry*, *50*, 6440–6447. doi:10.1021/jf020231k

Rabe, S., Krings, U., & Berger, R. G. (2004 a). In vitro study of the influence of physiological parameters on dynamic in-mouth flavour release from liquids. *Chemical Senses*, *29*, 153–162. doi:10.1093/chemse/bjh020

Rabe, S., Linforth, R. S. T., Krings, U., Taylor, A. J., & Berger, R. G. (2004 b). Volatile release from liquids: Comparison of in vivo APCI-MS, in mouth headspace trapping and in vitro Mouth Model Data. *Chemical Senses*, *29*, 263–173.

Richard, H. (1992). Connaissance de la nature des arômes alimentaires. In: Les Arômes Alimentaires. Eds. Richard H., Multon J.L., Tec & Doc, Lavoisier, Paris, 22-40.

Roberts, D. D., & Acree, T. E. (1995). Simulation of retronasal aroma using a modified headspace technique: investigating the effects of saliva, temperature, shearing and oil on flavour release. *Journal of Agricultural and Food Chemistry*, *43*, 2179–2186. doi:10.1021/jf00056a041

Roberts, D. D., & Acree, T. E. (1996). Effects of heating and cream addition on fresh raspberry aroma using a retronasal aroma simulator and gas chromatography olfactometry. *Journal of Agricultural and Food Chemistry*, *44*, 3919–3925. doi:10.1021/jf950701t

Rychlik, M., & Grosch, W. (1996). Identification and quantification of potent odorants formed by toasting of wheat bread. *Lebensmittel Wisstercraft und Technologie*, *29*, 515–525. doi:10.1006/fstl.1996.0079

Salles, C., Tarrega, A., Mielle, P., Maratray, J., Gorria, P., Liaboeuf, J., & Liodenot, J. J. (2007). Development of a chewing simulator for food breakdown and the analysis of in vitro flavor compounds release in a mouth environment. *Journal of Food Engineering*, *82*, 189–198. doi:10.1016/j.jfoodeng.2007.02.008

Springett, M. B., Rozier, V., & Bakker, J. (1999). Use of fiber interface direct mass spectrometry for the determination of volatile flavor release from model food systems. *Journal of Agricultural and Food Chemistry*, *47*, 1125–1131. doi:10.1021/jf980199n

Stone, H., & Sidel, J. L. (2004). Introduction to sensory evaluation. In: Sensory evaluation practices. Eds. Stone H. and Sidel J. L., Elsevier Academic Press, 1-16.

Taylor, A. J. (1996). Volatile flavor release from foods during eating. *Critical Reviews in Food Science and Nutrition*, *36*, 765–784. doi:10.1080/10408399609527749

Taylor, A. J., & Linforth, R. S. T. (1994). Methodology for measuring volatile profiles in the mouth and nose during eating. In: Trends in Flavour Research. Eds. Maarse H. and van der Heij D. G., Elsevier Science B.V. Amsterdam, 3-14.

Taylor, A. J., Linforth, R. S. T., Harvey, B. A., & Blake, A. (2000). Atmospheric pressure chemical ionisation mass spectrometry for in vivo analysis of volatile flavour release. *Food Chemistry, 71*, 327–338. doi:10.1016/S0308-8146(00)00182-5

van Ruth, S. M., & Buhr, K. (2004). Influence of mastication rate on dynamic flavour release analysed by combined model mouth/proton transfer reaction–mass spectrometry. *International Journal of Mass Spectrometry, 239*, 187–192. doi:10.1016/j.ijms.2004.08.009

van Ruth, S. M., & Roozen, J. P. (2000 a). Gas chromatography / sniffing port analysis of aroma compounds released under mouth conditions. *Talanta, 52*, 253–259. doi:10.1016/S0039-9140(00)00325-8

van Ruth, S. M., & Roozen, J. P. (2000 b). Influence of mastication, saliva on aroma release in a model mouth system. *Food Chemistry, 71*, 339–345. doi:10.1016/S0308-8146(00)00186-2

van Ruth, S. M., Roozen, J. P., & Cozijnsen, J. L. (1994). Comparison of dynamic headspace mouth model systems for flavour release from rehydrated bell pepper cuttings. In: Trends in Flavour Research. Eds. Maarse H. and van der Heij D. G., Elsevier Science B.V. Amsterdam, 59-64.

van Ruth, S. M., Roozen, J. P., & Cozijnsen, J. L. (1995 a). Changes in flavour release from rehydrated diced bell peppers (*Capsicum annuum*) by artificial saliva components in three model mouth systems. *Journal of the Science of Food and Agriculture, 37*, 189–196. doi:10.1002/jsfa.2740670208

van Ruth, S. M., Roozen, J. P., & Cozijnsen, J. L. (1995 b). Volatile compounds of rehydrated French beans, bell peppers and leeks. Part 1. Flavour release in the mouth and in three mouth model systems. *Food Chemistry, 53*, 15–22. doi:10.1016/0308-8146(95)95780-A

Weel, K. G. C., Boelrijk, A. E. M., Burger, J. J., Verschueren, M., Gruppen, H., Voragen, A. G. J., & Smit, G. (2004). New Device To Simulate Swallowing and in Vivo Aroma Release in the Throat from Liquid and Semiliquid Food Systems. *Journal of the Science of Food and Agriculture, 52*, 6564–6571. doi:10.1021/jf049499x

KEY TERMS AND DEFINITIONS

APCI-MS or Atmospheric Pressure Chemical Ionisation/Mass Spectrometry: This is mass spectrometry technique coupled to a detector that directly identifies some of the volatile molecules present in the air exhaled by assessors during the consumption of a foodstuff. The molecules present in the sampled air are then ionised under atmospheric pressure. Molecule ionisation occurs thanks to the transfer of the positive charge of H_3O^+ ions. These ions come from the ionisation of water molecules present in the exhaled air. After their ionisation, the molecules present in the air are detected by a mass spectrometer. This technique identifies only some of the molecules present in the air exhaled, depending on their nature and their mass.

Flavor: This is all the stimuli perceived when a food sample is eaten. It includes the perception of the taste, the aroma, and the trigeminal sensation in the mouth.

GC or Gas Chromatography: This technique can separate volatile compounds that are present in a gaseous mix or trapped on an absorbent. After being injected into the chromatograph, the volatiles are transported via a carrier gas to a capillary column where they are retained. Then the temperature of the column is gradually increased so that the volatiles are successively desorbed from the column and separated from each other. The retention time of compounds depends on both their affinity for the capillary column and their molecular weight.

Headspace Technique: This extraction technique involves the trapping of the gas phase above a sample that is placed in a sealed container.

MS or Mass Spectrometry: This technique can detect and identify volatile molecules according to their constitutive ion masses. It also enables their chemical structure to be characterized. It is generally placed after a GC apparatus. When a molecule leaves the GC column, it goes to the ionisation chamber of the spectrometer. Here, the molecule is split up into several ions that are specific to it. By comparison with a database, the molecule can then be identified.

Nose-Space: This technique analyses volatile compounds that are released from a food sample during its consumption by assessors. This is done by placing two inlets in both nostrils of assessors. Subjects are then asked to eat a food product. During swallowing, the air exhaled through their nostrils is collected and analyzed.

Orthonasal Way: This route corresponds to the transport of volatiles directly from a sample to the olfactory receptors present in the nose. It is thus linked to the perception of the odor of a sample when it is smelt.

PTR-MS or Proton Transfer Reaction/Mass Spectrometry: This is similar to the APCI-MS technique, except that the H_3O^+ ions, which are used to ionise the volatile molecules, are formed independently from the exhaled air. The water molecules from which the H_3O^+ ions are formed are thus separated from the reaction chamber into which the air is exhaled. H_3O^+ ions are then transferred into this reaction chamber to ionise the volatile molecules present in the air. Like with APCI-MS, this technique identifies only some of the molecules present in the air, depending on their nature and their mass.

Retronasal Way: This route corresponds to the transport of volatiles from a sample in the mouth cavity to the pharynx and then to the olfactory receptors present in the nose. It is thus linked to the perception of the aroma of a sample when it is eaten.

SPME or Solid-Phase Microextraction: The SPME device is made of a silica fibre, coated with a phase in which aroma compounds are trapped.

Chapter 2
Proteomics and Related Applications in Oral Cancer and Sjögren's Syndrome

Shen Hu
University of California, USA

ABSTRACT

Proteomics is the study of a complete set of proteins present in a biological system using the technologies of large-scale protein separation and identification. It is a powerful approach for biomedical research because it aims for a comprehensive, quantitative analysis of protein expression and its changes under biological perturbations such as disease or drug treatment. The purpose of this book chapter is to give an overview of proteomics using mass spectrometry and protein microarrays and to discuss related applications of proteomics in oral cancer and Sjögren's syndrome. Proteomics may significantly accelerate the oral disease research by providing a novel molecular technology to discover protein biomarkers for disease diagnosis/prognosis, to elucidate the molecular determinants underlying the disease mechanism, and to identify novel targets for therapeutic intervention.

MASS SPECTROMETRY-BASED PROTEOMICS

Modern proteomics is primarily driven by mass spectrometry (MS), an exquisite analytical technology which measures the mass-to-charge ratio of ionized molecules. A commonly used approach for proteomic studies is based on 2-D gel electrophoresis (2-DE) with MS. In this approach, proteins are initially mapped out by 2-DE or 2-D differential gel electrophoresis (DIGE). To identify a proteins of interest, the protein spot is excised for in-gel digestion and the resulting peptides are analyzed using matrix-assisted laser desorption/ionization (MALDI) or electrospray (ESI) with time-of-flight MS (TOF MS) or more sophisticated tandem MS. The obtained masses are then *in silico* compared to either a proteome or genome database to find the best matched protein. This is achieved by using a computer program for database searching (e.g., MASCOT or SEQUEST), which calculates the absolute masses of theoretical peptides from

DOI: 10.4018/978-1-60566-733-1.ch002

each protein in the database and then compares the peptide masses of the unknown protein to the theoretical peptide masses of each protein in the database. The protein identification method based on MALDI-TOF MS or ESI-TOF MS with database searching is also known as peptide mass fingerprinting (PMF) (Pappin, 1993; Mann, 1993, Yates, 1993). Typically PMF is for the identification of an isolated protein. The presence of a protein mixture can significantly complicate the analysis and potentially compromise the results. Therefore, a mixture of 2 or more proteins typically requires the use of tandem MS to achieve confident identification of the proteins.

Tandem MS, also known as MS/MS, involves multiple stages of MS analysis, with some form of fragmentation occurring in between the stages (Aebersold & Mann, 2003). Tandem MS can be done in space by using physically separated mass analyzers with a collision cell between these elements for molecule fragmentation. For example, one mass analyzer can isolate a peptide ion from many entering a mass spectrometer. The peptide is then broken into smaller fragments in the collision cell by collision-induced dissociation (CID) and a second mass analyzer measures the fragment ions produced from the peptide. Tandem MS can also be done in time. Ions are trapped in a single mass analyzer with multiple MS steps taking place over time, as in a quadruple ion trap or Fourier transform MS (FT-MS) instrument.

Shotgun proteomics refers to the direct analysis of complex protein mixtures to rapidly generate a global profile of the protein complement. It mainly relies on tandem MS and database-searching algorithms for peptide and protein identification. The shotgun approach has been facilitated by the use of multidimensional protein identification technology (MudPIT), which incorporates 2-D liquid chromatography (2-D LC), ESI-MS/MS, with SEQUEST database searching (Washburn, 2001; Wolters, 2001). Due to its high resolving power and compatibility with ESI-MS, 2-D LC represents a primary separation method for peptides in proteomics. To realize an in-depth proteome analysis, other liquid separation techniques such as capillary electrophoresis, zoom isoelectric focusing, free-flow electrophoresis, can be used for prefractionation of proteins prior to 2-D LC-MS/MS to achieve a more comprehensive proteomic analysis (Guo, 2006; Zuo, 2006; Xie, 2006).

QUANTITATIVE PROTEOMICS

Rather than just providing a list of identified proteins, quantitative proteomics aims for global, quantitative measurement of protein levels in biological samples. Most of the quantitative proteomics methods are based on the use of stable isotope labeling of proteins or peptides, and tandem MS to compare the relative abundance of the proteins in different samples. Once protein samples are differentially labeled with stable isotopes, they can be distinguished during MS analysis by a characteristic mass shift. In addition, the relative abundance of isotope-labeled peptide pairs can be determined by comparing the ion signal intensities of the peptides. Stable isotope labeling with amino acids in cell culture (SILAC) is a straightforward approach for *in vivo* incorporation of isotope tags into proteins for MS-based quantitative proteomics. The method relies on metabolic incorporation of amino acids with substituted stable isotopes (e.g. 13C, 15N), and is particularly useful when studying cell line models (Ong et al., 2002). For clinical samples such as tissue or body fluids from disease patients, quantitative proteomics can be performed using tandem MS coupled with stable isotope labeling techniques such as isotope-coded affinity tagging (ICAT) (Gygi et al., 1999), cleavable ICAT (Hansen et al., 2003), isotope tagging for relative and absolute quantitation (iTRAQ) (Ross et al., 2004), isotope coded protein labeling (ICPL) (Schmidt et al., 2005) or proteolytic 18O labeling (Miyagi & Rao, 2007). If the isotope labeling (e.g., ICAT) occurs to intact proteins, the labeled samples are subsequently combined, digested with trypsin, and then analyzed with LC-MS/MS. Because isotope-labeled peptide pairs are virtually chemically identical, they co-elute during LC separation. The relative quantitation can be determined by the ratio of ion intensities from co-eluting isotope-labeled peptides in the MS survey scan, which defines the ratio between parent proteins in the starting samples. Subsequent MS/MS analysis generates a spectrum that can be used to search a protein sequence database to identify the protein. If the labeling reaction is performed on the proteolytic peptides using tandem mass tags, then both quantitation and identification rely on MS/MS spectra. For instance, iTRAQ utilizes isobaric tags that can be cleaved during CID to yield an isotope series (reporter ions) representing the quantity of a peptide from different samples. Since the peptide remains attached to the isobaric tags until CID is conducted, the resulted MS/MS spectrum allows for simultaneous identification (based on fragment ions) and quantitation (based on reporter ions) of the peptide. iTRAQ reagents can label peptides in up to 8 different biological samples, enabling simultaneous analysis of those samples in a single analytical run (Ross et al., 2004).

LC-MS profiling represents one of the label-free methods for relative quantification of proteins (Chelius, 2002; Wang, 2003). The method requires comparison of identical proteolytic peptides in each of the two experiments to accurately determine relative ratios of the proteins. This relies on the accuracy of mass measurement and reproducibility of chromatographic separation. Similarly, CE-MS can be used for quantitative profiling of peptides (Kaiser, 2004; Kolch, 2005). The high resolving power of CE-MS allows more than 1000 polypeptides displayed within a single analytical run. Both LC-MS and CE-MS are envisioned as promising methods for quantitative profiling provided that the ongoing technological developments are successful in improving accuracy and reproducibility. Data analysis strategies are also needed for peak alignment, normalization and accurately extracting quantitative information from the MS spectra.

Besides the discovery-based proteomics platforms described above, target-based proteomics tools are also needed for validation of proteomic findings. LC-MRM is a highly specific and sensitive method for target-based protein analysis (Anderson, 2006; Wolf-Yadlin, 2007). The method utilizes two points of selection (a peptide mass and a specific fragment mass generated by MS/MS) to eliminate background signal and noise even in very complex mixtures. Since the entire mass range is not scanned and only specific MRM transitions (combinations of peptide and fragment masses) are detected, a significant increase in sensitivity is typically observed. Careful selection and optimization of MRM transitions permits detection of multiple target proteins per LC-MS analysis. Peptide selection, to some extent, can be straightforward based on the MS/MS data obtained during the initial profiling experiments. The tryptic peptides that are most frequently detected in the LC-MS/MS analyses and exhibit high MS signal response are usually chosen as targets for MRM analysis. Multiple-charged ions with high m/z fragment ions are often chosen because favorable fragmentation is greatly improved with a multiple-charged precursor ion. In combination with stable-isotope labeled internal peptide standards, MRM can provide absolute quantitation of a target protein. This technique has been demonstrated for biomarker validation, particularly when coupled with specific enrichment of target peptides using anti-peptide antibodies (Anderson & Hunter, 2006).

The mTRAQ reagents (non-isobaric duplex form of the iTRAQ reagents) have been recently developed to enable LC-MRM analysis of amine-containing biomolecules (DeSouza et al., 2009). The mTRAQ labels come with two chemically identical versions. The heavy version is identical to the iTRAQ 117 label (mass=145 Da). However, the lighter version (mass=141 Da) is lower in mass than the iTRAQ labels by 4 Da. To quantify a target protein, one of the mTRAQ versions will be used to label known quantity of a synthetic peptide whose sequence identical to that of a selected tryptic peptide from the protein of interest, while the other version will be used to tag the tryptically digested sample homogenate. The labeled synthetic peptide is then mixed with the oppositely labeled sample at a known amount, and the combined samples are analyzed by LC-MRM for quantification of the protein.

PROTEIN MICROARRAYS

Protein microarrays are solid-phase ligand-binding assay systems using immobilized proteins on surfaces such as glass or cellulose membranes. The assays are highly sensitive and only requires minute amount of samples for analysis. The currently available protein microarrays vary markedly in the nature of their content. The most common form of protein microarrays are antibody microarrays, in which a collection of capture antibodies are spotted on a solid surface for the purpose of detecting antigens. A promising application of antibody microarray is to measure specific protein biomarkers in disease patients' samples for diagnostics/prognostics. However, due to the difficulty in expression and purification of antibodies, the arrays often contain a limited number of defined antibodies for known proteins and therefore are not a technology for global analysis of proteins. The design of antibody arrays, particularly when screening against complex samples, also needs to take into consideration the problems of cross reactivity and high cost (Spisak et al., 2007).

Antigen microarrays are composed of spotted antigens/autoantigens on a solid surface for the analysis and characterization of antibodies or autoantibodies. One of the promising applications for antigen microarray is to profile the specificity of antibody responses against autoantigens in patients with autoimmune diseases. For instance, autoantigen microarrays containing 196 distinct putative autoantigens were developed for profiling of serum autoantibodies from major autoimmune diseases including systemic lupus erythematosus (SLE) and rheumatoid arthritis (RA), and identifying disease-specific autoantibody patterns (Robinson et al., 2002). Such antibody profiling may provide insights into pathogenesis, and enable development of novel tests for diagnosis and guiding therapy in the clinic. Antigen microarray is also useful for antigen-specific assessment of immunoglobulin subclasses. An 1152-feature array composed of 140 antigens or antigen fragments to detect isotype-specific mAb has been fabricated to quantitatively monitor changes in isotype mAb concentration, and to profile antigen-specific antibody isotype production in a murine model of autoimmunity. This platform has the potential to elucidate mechanisms that govern development and evolution of antibody responses in *in vivo* systems (Graham et al., 2006). Similar to antibody microarrays, the antigen microarrays are target-based instead of discovery-based profiling technology.

Recently, a ProtoArray platform has been introduced for profiling of autoantibody responses in patients with autoimmune diseases and human cancers. The arrays contain over 8,000 proteins that are expressed in insect cells and purified under native conditions. Because the proteins present on the microarrays are full length and in their native conformation, antibodies reactive with conformational epitopes are easily recognized. This new technology platform empowers investigators with comprehensive profiling of minute amount of body fluid samples (e.g., serum or saliva) to identify autoantibody and/or autoantigen biomarkers (Hudson, et al., 2007), particularly for autoimmune diseases.

Lectins are a diverse group of proteins that have specific binding activity toward carbohydrate residues of glycoproteins and glycolipids. Recently, lectin microarray has been developed for rapid and sensitive analysis of glycans in a high-throughput fashion (Hsu, 2008; Hu, 2009). These microarrays consist of a collection of, mostly plant-derived, lectins immobilized onto a solid support at a high spatial density. Display of lectins in a microarray format enables multiple, distinct binding interactions to be observed simultaneously and therefore provide a novel method for the rapid characterization of carbohydrates on glycoproteins or glycolipids. The array can be combined with MS for profiling of glycoproteins/glycopeptides in clinical samples of disease patients (Hu & Wong, 2009).

PROTEOMIC ANALYSIS OF ORAL CANCER

Oral cancer is considered as the 6th most common human cancer, with over 350,000 new cases being diagnosed worldwide each year. Despite the treatment advances in surgery, radiotherapy and chemotherapy, the overall 5-year survival rates for oral cancer have remained low and stagnant in the past few decades. The high mortality rate of oral cancer can be attributed to factors including limited understanding of the disease mechanism, lack of clinical tools for the early detection and non-responsiveness to chemotherapy and radiation therapy. Proteomics may significantly accelerate oral cancer research by providing a novel molecular technology to discover protein biomarkers for cancer diagnosis/prognosis, to elucidate the molecular determinants of the disease, and to identify novel targets for therapeutic treatment.

Although a large number of researchers are pursuing biomarkers for different type of cancers, only a handful of protein biomarkers have been approved by the US-FDA for clinical use (Ludwig & Weinstein, 2005). These approved biomarkers are limited to a small number of cancers and only benefit a low percentage of disease patients. Up to date, there has not been any FDA-approved protein biomarker for clinical use in oral/head and neck cancer, neither for the use of early detection/screening nor for the use of monitoring and treatment selection. Since oral cancer cells are immersed in the salivary milieu, profiling of saliva proteins from oral cancer patients represents a valuable approach to finding biomarkers for the disease. We have recently demonstrated a patient-based saliva proteomics approach for oral cancer biomarker discovery (Hu, 2008; Hu, 2007). By using shotgun proteomics for profiling of saliva proteins from OSCC patients followed by immunoassay for validation, we identified a panel of 5 protein biomarkers for OSCC, including Mac-2 bind protein (M2BP), calgranulin B, profilin, catalase and CD59. M2BP is a tumor antigen whereas CD59 (protectin) is one of the complement restriction factors that are over-expressed on tumor cells, enabling tumor cells to escape from complement-dependent and antibody-mediated killing. The combination of 5 biomarkers yielded a sensitivity of 90%, and a specificity of 83% for OSCC detection (Hu et al., 2008). If successfully validated on large patient population, these candidate biomarkers can lead to a simple clinical tool for noninvasive diagnosis of oral cancer. Although many have studied the soluble fraction (proteins/peptides) of whole saliva, few have taken advantage of the diagnostic potential of the cells present in saliva. A recent study looked into the proteomic profiles of the cells contained in whole saliva from patients with OSCC and confirmed that the potential of using cells in whole saliva as a source for discovery of protein biomarkers for OSCC (Xie et al., 2008).

Proteomic analysis of OSCC has revealed a number of target proteins that may have a regulatory role in the disease development (Chen, 2004; He, 2004; Turhani, 2006; Wang, 2008; Ralhan, 2009; Patel, 2008; Weng, 2008). RACK1 (receptor for activated C-kinase) is an anchor protein for protein kinase C. This protein was found up-regulated in OSCC by 2-DE/MS and immunohistochemical examination suggested that the expression of RACK1 correlated well with the severity of the epithelial dysplasia, clinical stage and lymph node involvement. RNA interference specifically targeted to silence RACK1 could initiate apoptosis of OSCC cells. These observations indicated that RACK1 not only involves in cell proliferation and apoptosis but is also linked to clinical invasiveness and metastasis in oral carcinogenesis (Wang et al., 2008). M2BP is a tumor antigen that we found significantly elevated in saliva of patients with OSCC. This protein was also found over-expressed in secretomes of OSCC cell lines as well as in the tumor tissues and sera of patients with OSCC. Moreover, knock-down of M2BP impaired the growth, migration, and invasion of OSCC cells. These results suggested that M2BP has a potential role in regulating growth and motility of OSCC cells (Weng et al., 2008). Apart from contributing to our understanding the molecular mechanism, these proteins may also have clinical or therapeutic implications for OSCC. The extensive protein alterations from these previous studies also suggest that multiple cellular and etiological pathways are involved in oral carcinogenesis, and multiple protein molecules should be simultaneously targeted as an effective strategy to counter the disease.

We are also trying to identify protein biomarkers for metastatic oral cancer using quantitative proteomics (Zhang et al., 2008). Successful treatment of oral cancer largely depends on accurate clinical staging of lymph node metastasis. This is because oral cancer frequently metastasizes to the regional lymph nodes and this nodal involvement is the strongest determinant of patient prognosis. Unfortunately, current routine clinical and pathological staging methods are suboptimal for detecting lymph node metastasis. Clinical staging of lymph nodes is far less accurate than pathological staging. However, pathological staging also has limitations because it fails to detect micrometastasis in a subset of nodal specimens. Due to the high impact of lymph node metastasis in optimal patient management, there is a critical need for new clinical methods that can improve the detection or prediction of lymph node metastasis in patients with OSCC. Proteomic analysis of OSCC may identify protein biomarkers that can forecast the metastatic potential of primary tumor. In a recent study, Lin-7C was found down-regulated in OSCC cells based on a 2-D DIGE/MS analysis. Further testing of the protein level in primary OSCCs with node-positive or node-negative metastatic lesions suggests that Lin-7C expression status in primary tumors predicts lymph node metastasis with high accuracy. More importantly, experimental metastases in multiple organs of immunodeficient mice were inhibited in cells expressing Lin-7C. These results have established Lin-7C as a potential target of early detection, prevention, and therapy for OSCC metastasis (Onda et al., 2007).

PROTEOMIC ANALYSIS OF SJÖGREN'S SYNDROME

Sjögren's syndrome (SS) is a chronic autoimmune disorder clinically characterized by dry mouth and dry eyes symptoms. The disease primarily affects women, with a ratio of 9:1 over the occurrence in men. Primary SS occurs alone, whereas secondary SS presents in connection with another autoimmune disease, such as RA or SLE. Patients with SS have a significantly higher risk of developing lymphoma than the general population, and the most common forms are mucosa-associated lymphoid tissue (MALT) lymphomas that remain localized to the salivary glands.

SS is a complex disease that can go undiagnosed for several months to years. Although the underlying immune-mediated glandular destruction is thought to develop slowly over several years, a long delay from the start of symptoms to the final diagnosis has been frequently observed. A new international consensus for the diagnosis of SS requires objective signs and symptoms of dryness, including a characteristic appearance of a biopsy sample from a minor or major salivary gland and/or the presence of autoantibody such as anti-SSA and anti-SSB. However, establishing the diagnosis of SS has been difficult in light of its nonspecific symptoms (dry eyes and mouth) and the lack of both sensitive and specific biomarkers for detection. Although the tissue biopsy is a highly specific diagnostic procedure, it is invasive, time-consuming and requires the evaluation from an expert histopathologist.

We, along with other researchers, have discovered potential saliva protein biomarkers for SS using proteomics (Hu, 2007; Ryu, 2006; Baldini, 2008; Peluso, 2007). By using 2-DE/MS, we identified 16 down-regulated proteins and 25 up-regulated proteins in whole saliva from patients with primary SS, which reflected the damage of glandular cells and inflammation of the oral cavity system in the disease patients (42). Further validation on independent patient population suggested that alpha-enolase, cathepsin D and beta-microglobulin are robust biomarkers for SS detection. A hallmark of many autoimmune diseases is the presence of autoantibodies, which have long been used for the diagnosis and classification of these diseases. Autoantibodies may exist years before the diagnosis of an autoimmune disease, and could be used for early prediction of the disease onset (Arbuckle et al., 2003). The most widely used biomarkers of SS are IgG autoantibodies (rarely IgA) against two nuclear proteins, Ro-52/SS-A and La/SS-B. These antibodies are detected in serum and can be produced locally in the affected salivary glands. However, these two autoantibody biomarkers are not specific to SS, and their presence is not correlated with clinical severity of SS. Therefore, we are testing protein microarrays for profiling of salivary autoantibodies from patients with SS. Our aim is to identify highly specific and sensitive autoantibody biomarkers for SS, which can distinguish SS from other autoimmune diseases such as RA and SLE.

Figure 1. Systems biology analysis of primary SS and SS/MALT lymphoma. Parotid gland tissues from normal controls and patients with primary SS and SS/MALT lymphoma were analyzed using both DNA microarrays and proteomics. A novel statistical methodology, weighted gene co-expression network analysis, was then used to reveal activated signal pathways and key target genes underlying the disease pathogenesis. For details, see reference 47.

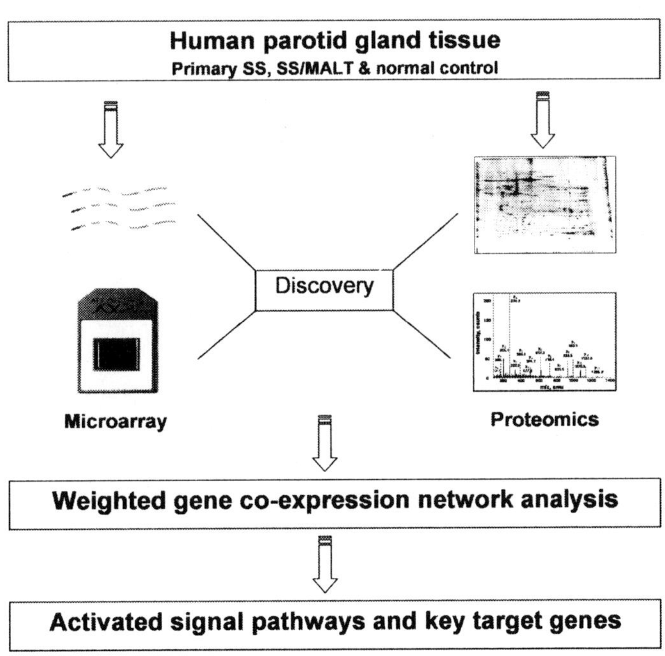

Elucidating the molecular mechanisms underlying SS and SS/MALT lymphoma also remains an important challenge. To identify key target genes and activated signaling pathways associated with the pathogenesis of SS and SS/MALT lymphoma, we conducted a systems analysis of parotid glands manifesting primary SS or SS/MALT lymphoma phenotypes. The tissue samples were assessed concurrently by gene-expression microarray profiling and proteomics analysis, followed by weighted gene-coexpression network analysis (Figure 1). We found that signal pathways including proteasome degradation, apoptosis, signal peptides of the class I major histocompatibility complex (MHC), complement activation, cell growth and death, and integrin-mediated cell adhesion are activated in primary SS, whereas in primary SS/MALT lymphoma, signal pathways such as translation, ribosome biogenesis and assembly, proteasome degradation, class I MHC signal peptides, the G13 signaling pathway, complement activation, and integrin-mediated cell adhesion are activated. Correlation analyses of gene expression and proteomics data revealed 6 highly connected target genes for primary SS and 8 target genes for MALT lymphoma (Hu et al., 2009). The identified pathways provide further insights into the molecular mechanisms of primary SS and SS/MALT lymphoma, whereas the concordantly changed genes represent promising targets for therapeutic intervention, diagnosis, and prognosis.

REFERENCES

Aebersold, R., & Mann, M. (2003). Mass spectrometry-based proteomics. *Nature, 422*, 198–207. doi:10.1038/nature01511

Anderson, L., & Hunter, C. L. (2006). Quantitative mass spectrometric multiple reaction monitoring assays for major plasma proteins. *Molecular & Cellular Proteomics, 5*, 573–588. doi:10.1074/mcp.M500331-MCP200

Arbuckle, M. R., McClain, M. T., Rubertone, M. V., Scofield, R. H., Dennis, G. J., & James, J. A. (2003). Development of autoantibodies before the clinical onset of systemic lupus erythematosus. *The New England Journal of Medicine, 349*, 1526–1533. doi:10.1056/NEJMoa021933

Baldini, C., Giusti, L., Bazzichi, L., Lucacchini, A., & Bombardieri, S. (2008). Proteomic analysis of the saliva: a clue for understanding primary from secondary Sjögren's syndrome? *Autoimmunity Reviews, 7*, 185–191. doi:10.1016/j.autrev.2007.11.002

Chelius, D., & Bondarenko, P. V. (2002). Quantitative profiling of proteins in complex mixtures using liquid chromatography and mass spectrometry. *Journal of Proteome Research, 1*, 317–323. doi:10.1021/pr025517j

Chen, J., He, Q. Y., Yuen, A. P. W., & Chiu, J. F. (2004). Proteomics of buccal squamous cell carcinoma: The involvement of multiple pathways in tumorigenesis. *Proteomics, 4*, 2465–2475. doi:10.1002/pmic.200300762

DeSouza, L. V., Romaschin, A. D., Colgan, T. J., & Siu, K. W. (2009). Absolute quantification of potential cancer markers in clinical tissue homogenates using multiple reaction monitoring on a hybrid triple quadrupole/linear ion trap tandem mass spectrometer. *Analytical Chemistry, 81*, 3462–3470. doi:10.1021/ac802726a

Graham, K. L., Vaysberg, M., Kuo, A., & Utz, P. J. (2006). Autoantigen arrays for multiplex analysis of antibody isotypes. *Proteomics, 6*, 5720–5724. doi:10.1002/pmic.200600345

Guo, T., Rudnick, P. A., Wang, W., Lee, C. S., Devoe, D. L., & Balgley, B. M. (2006). Characterization of the human salivary proteome by capillary isoelectric focusing/nanoreversed-phase liquid chromatography coupled with ESI-tandem MS. *Journal of Proteome Research, 5*, 1469–1478. doi:10.1021/pr060065m

Gygi, S. P., Rist, B., Gerber, S. A., Turecek, F., Gelb, M. H., & Aebersold, R. (1999). Quantitative analysis of complex protein mixtures using isotope-coded affinity tags. *Nature Biotechnology*, *17*, 994–999. doi:10.1038/13690

Hansen, K. C., Schmitt-Ulms, G., Chalkley, R. J., Hirsch, J., Baldwin, M. A., & Burlingame, A. L. (2003). Mass spectrometric analysis protein mixtures at low levels using cleavable 13C-isotope-coded affinity tag and multidimensional chromatography. *Molecular & Cellular Proteomics*, *2*, 299–314.

He, Q. Y., Chen, J., Kung, H. F., Yuen, A. P. W., & Chiu, J. F. (2004). Identification of tumor-associated proteins in oral tongue squamous cell carcinoma by proteomics. *Proteomics*, *4*, 271–278. doi:10.1002/pmic.200300550

Hsu, K. L., Gildersleeve, J. C., & Mahal, L. K. (2008). A simple strategy for the creation of a recombinant lectin microarray. *Molecular BioSystems*, *4*, 654–662. doi:10.1039/b800725j

Hu, S., Arellano, M., Boontheung, P., Wang, J., Zhou, H., & Jiang, J. (2008). Salivary proteomics for oral cancer biomarker discovery. *Clinical Cancer Research*, *14*, 6246–6252. doi:10.1158/1078-0432.CCR-07-5037

Hu, S., Wang, J., Meijer, J., Ieong, S., Xie, Y., & Yu, T. (2007). Salivary proteomic and genomic biomarkers for primary Sjögren's syndrome. *Arthritis and Rheumatism*, *56*, 3588–3600. doi:10.1002/art.22954

Hu, S., & Wong, D. (2009). Lectin microarray. *Proteomics Clinical Applications*, *3*, 148–154. doi:10.1002/prca.200800153

Hu, S., Yu, T., Xie, Y., Yang, Y., Li, Y., & Zhou, X. (2007). Discovery of oral fluid biomarkers for human oral cancer by mass spectrometry. *Cancer Genomics & Proteomics*, *4*, 55–64.

Hu, S., Zhou, M., Jiang, J., Wang, J., Elashoff, D., & Gorr, S. (2009). Systems biology analysis of Sjögren's syndrome and mucosa-associated lymphoid tissue lymphoma in parotid glands. *Arthritis and Rheumatism*, *60*, 81–92. doi:10.1002/art.24150

Hudson, M. E., Pozdnyakova, I., Haines, K., Mor, G., & Snyder, M. (2007). Identification of differentially expressed proteins in ovarian cancer using high-density protein microarrays. *Proceedings of the National Academy of Sciences of the United States of America*, *104*, 17494–17499. doi:10.1073/pnas.0708572104

Kaiser, T., Wittke, S., Just, I., Krebs, R., Bartel, S., & Fliser, D. (2004). Capillary electrophoresis coupled to mass spectrometer for automated and robust polypeptide determination in body fluids for clinical use. *Electrophoresis*, *25*, 2044–2055. doi:10.1002/elps.200305788

Kolch, W., Neusüss, C., Pelzing, M., & Mischak, H. (2005). Capillary electrophoresis-mass spectrometry as a powerful tool in clinical diagnosis and biomarker discovery. *Mass Spectrometry Reviews*, *24*, 959–977. doi:10.1002/mas.20051

Ludwig, J. A., & Weinstein, J. N. (2005). Biomarkers in cancer staging, prognosis and treatment selection. *Nature Reviews. Cancer*, *5*, 845–856. doi:10.1038/nrc1739

Mann, M., Højrup, P., & Roepstorff, P. (1993). Use of mass spectrometric molecular weight information to identify proteins in sequence databases. *Biological Mass Spectrometry*, *22*, 338–345. doi:10.1002/bms.1200220605

Miyagi, M., & Rao, K. C. (2007). Proteolytic 18O-labeling strategies for quantitative proteomics. *Mass Spectrometry Reviews*, *26*, 121–136. doi:10.1002/mas.20116

Onda, T., Uzawa, K., Nakashima, D., Saito, K., Iwadate, Y., & Seki, N. (2007). Lin-7C/VELI3/MALS-3: an essential component in metastasis of human squamous cell carcinoma. *Cancer Research, 67*, 9643–9648. doi:10.1158/0008-5472.CAN-07-1911

Ong, S. E., Blagoev, B., Kratchmarova, I., Kristensen, D. B., Steen, H., & Pandey, A. (2002). Stable isotope labeling by amino acids in cell culture, SILAC, as a simple and accurate approach to expression proteomics. *Molecular & Cellular Proteomics, 1*, 376–386. doi:10.1074/mcp.M200025-MCP200

Pappin, D. J., Hojrup, P., & Bleasby, A. J. (1993). Rapid identification of proteins by peptide-mass fingerprinting. *Current Biology, 3*, 327–332. doi:10.1016/0960-9822(93)90195-T

Patel, V., Hood, B. L., Molinolo, A. A., Lee, N. H., Conrads, T. P., & Braisted, J. C. (2008). Proteomic analysis of laser-captured paraffin-embedded tissues: a molecular portrait of head and neck cancer progression. *Clinical Cancer Research, 14*, 1002–1014. doi:10.1158/1078-0432.CCR-07-1497

Peluso, G., De Santis, M., Inzitari, R., Fanali, C., Cabras, T., & Messana, I. (2007). Proteomic study of salivary peptides and proteins in patients with Sjögren's syndrome before and after pilocarpine treatment. *Arthritis and Rheumatism, 56*, 2216–2222. doi:10.1002/art.22738

Ralhan, R., Desouza, L. V., Matta, A., Chandra Tripathi, S., Ghanny, S., & Dattagupta, S. (2009). iTRAQ-multidimensional liquid chromatography and tandem mass spectrometry-based identification of potential biomarkers of oral epithelial dysplasia and novel networks between inflammation and premalignancy. *Journal of Proteome Research, 8*, 300–309. doi:10.1021/pr800501j

Robinson, W. H., DiGennaro, C., Hueber, W., Haab, B. B., Kamachi, M., & Dean, E. J. (2002). Autoantigen microarrays for multiplex characterization of autoantibody responses. *Nature Medicine, 8*, 295–301. doi:10.1038/nm0302-295

Ross, P. L., Huang, Y. N., Marchese, J. N., Williamson, B., Parker, K., & Hattan, S. (2004). Multiplexed protein quantitation in saccharomyces cerevisiae using amine-reactive isobaric tagging reagents. *Molecular & Cellular Proteomics, 3*, 1154–1169. doi:10.1074/mcp.M400129-MCP200

Ryu, O. H., Atkinson, J. C., Hoehn, G. T., Illei, G. G., & Hart, T. C. (2006). Identification of parotid salivary biomarkers in Sjogren's syndrome by surface-enhanced laser desorption/ionization time-of-flight mass spectrometry and two-dimensional difference gel electrophoresis. *Rheumatology (Oxford, England), 45*, 1077–1086. doi:10.1093/rheumatology/kei212

Schmidt, A., Kellermann, J., & Lottspeich, F. (2005). A novel strategy for quantitative proteomics using isotope-coded protein labels. *Proteomics, 5*, 4–15. doi:10.1002/pmic.200400873

Spisak, S., Tulassay, Z., Molnar, B., & Guttman, A. (2007). Protein microchips in biomedicine and biomarker discovery. *Electrophoresis, 28*, 4261–4373. doi:10.1002/elps.200700539

Turhani, D., Krapfenbauer, K., Thurnher, D., Langen, H., & Fountoulakis, M. (2006). Identification of differentially expressed, tumor-associated proteins in oral squamous cell carcinoma by proteomic analysis. *Electrophoresis, 27*, 1417–1423. doi:10.1002/elps.200500510

Wang, W., Zhou, H., Lin, H., Roy, S., Shaler, T. A., & Hill, L. R. (2003). Quantification of proteins and metabolites by mass spectrometry without isotopic labeling or spiked standards. *Analytical Chemistry, 75*, 4818–4826. doi:10.1021/ac026468x

Wang, Z., Jiang, L., Huang, C., Li, Z., Chen, L., & Gou, L. (2008). Comparative proteomics approach to screening of potential diagnostic and therapeutic targets for oral squamous cell carcinoma. *Molecular & Cellular Proteomics*, *7*, 1639–1650. doi:10.1074/mcp.M700520-MCP200

Washburn, M. P., Wolters, D., & Yates, J. R. III. (2001). Large-scale analysis of the yeast proteome by multidimensional protein identification technology. *Nature Biotechnology*, *19*, 242–247. doi:10.1038/85686

Weng, L. P., Wu, C. C., Hsu, B. L., Chi, L. M., Liang, Y., & Tseng, C. P. (2008). Secretome-based identification of Mac-2 binding protein as a potential oral cancer marker involved in cell growth and motility. *Journal of Proteome Research*, *7*, 3765–3775. doi:10.1021/pr800042n

Wolf-Yadlin, A., Hautaniemi, S., Lauffenburger, D. A., & White, F. M. (2007). Multiple reaction monitoring for robust quantitative proteomic analysis of cellular signaling networks. *Proceedings of the National Academy of Sciences of the United States of America*, *104*, 5860–5865. doi:10.1073/pnas.0608638104

Wolters, D. A., Washburn, M. P., & Yates, J. R. III. (2001). An automated multidimensional protein identification technology for shotgun proteomics. *Analytical Chemistry*, *73*, 5683–5690. doi:10.1021/ac010617e

Xie, H., Onsongo, G., Popko, J., de Jong, E. P., Cao, J., & Carlis, J. V. (2008). Proteomics analysis of cells in whole saliva from oral cancer patients via value-added three-dimensional peptide fractionation and tandem mass spectrometry. *Molecular & Cellular Proteomics*, *7*, 486–498. doi:10.1074/mcp.M700146-MCP200

Xie, H., Rhodus, N. L., Griffin, R. J., Carlis, J. V., & Griffin, T. J. (2005). A catalogue of human saliva proteins identified by free flow electrophoresis-based peptide separation and tandem mass spectrometry. *Molecular & Cellular Proteomics*, *4*, 1826–1830. doi:10.1074/mcp.D500008-MCP200

Yates, J. R., Speicher, S., Griffin, P. R., & Hunkapiller, T. (1993). Peptide mass maps: a highly informative approach to protein identification. *Analytical Biochemistry*, *214*, 397–408. doi:10.1006/abio.1993.1514

Zhang, L., Jiang, J., Arellano, M., Zhang, L., Yan, X., & Wong, D. T. (2008). Quantification of serum proteins of metastatic oral cancer patients using LC-MS/MS and iTRAQ labeling. *The Open Proteomics Journal*, *1*, 72–78. doi:10.2174/1875039700801010072

Zuo, X., Lee, K., Ali-Khan, N., & Speicher, D. W. (2005). Protein profiling by microscale solution isoelectrofocusing (MicroSol-IEF). *Current Protocol in Protein Science,* Chapter 22, Unit 22.6.

KEY TERMS AND DEFINITIONS

Database Searching: The methodology that use a computer algorithm and program to compare the experimental MS data with a protein or DNA sequence database to identify peptides or proteins.

Mass Spectrometry: The analytical technology used to measure the mass to charge ratio of a molecule or particle.

Protein Microarray: The solid-phase ligand-binding assay system using immobilized proteins on surfaces (e.g., glass or cellulose membrane) to measure the level of biomolecules or assess the protein-ligand interactions.

Proteomics: The identification, characterization and quantification of all proteins present in a biological system (e.g., organelle, cell, tissue, organ or organism) to provide accurate and comprehensive data about that system.

Quantitative Proteomics: The methodology to obtain quantitative information about all proteins expressed in a biological sample.

Shotgun Proteomics: The analytical method to identify proteins in complex mixtures using a combination of high performance liquid chromatography, tandem mass spectrometry and database searching.

Tandem Mass Spectrometry: Tandem mass spectrometry (MS/MS) involves multiple steps of mass selection or analysis, usually separated by some form of fragmentation. Tandem MS can be done in space by using physically separated mass analyzers with a collision cell between these elements for molecule fragmentation. For example, one mass analyzer can isolate a peptide ion from many entering a mass spectrometer. The peptide is then broken into smaller fragments in the collision cell by collision-induced dissociation and a second mass analyzer measures the fragment ions produced from the peptide. Tandem MS can also be done in time. Ions are trapped in a single mass analyzer with multiple MS steps taking place over time.

Chapter 3
Systems Approach to Understanding Oral Diseases

Amit Chattopadhyay
NIDCR, National Institutes of Health, USA

ABSTRACT

This chapter reviews the principles of systems biology and their application through computational methods (bioinformatics, computational biomodeling, genomics, proteomics, oral human microbiome, molecular modeling, systems biology, protein structure prediction, structural genomics, computational biochemistry and computational biophysics methods and projects) that have been applied to oral diseases research. The emphasis of the chapter is on concepts from molecular biology, genetics, and traditional pathology to provide new insights into oral diseases, and the associated technologies to provide new diagnostic, therapeutic and prognostic information. Another goal of the manuscript will be to serve as a central reference to access of information about systems biology resources for research into oral diseases.

INTRODUCTION

Factors underlying biological and socio-biological states include a complex interplay of several biological, behavioral, economic, and social factors. A reductionist view usually assesses the interplay of factors using a "drill-down" approach by examining smaller parts of a system under the paradigm that these parts, when fit-together, will translate to a fully functional whole. However, often such aggregative method does not work properly. The systems dynamics approach, developed by JW Forester in the mid 1950s (Forrester, 1985) and has been since used in business, engineering, and transportation. Its use to address problems in biology and health is recent. Models developed in this way can be limited by the available information, experience and expertise at hand from a group of persons who are involved in the process and therefore is a function of the insight of the group developing these models as well as the available data.

DOI: 10.4018/978-1-60566-733-1.ch003

Table 1. Commonly used terms in context of systems biology (Adapted from Fisher & Henzinger, 2007)

Biomics	Systems analysis of the biome (climatically and geographically defined areas of ecologically similar climatic conditions such as communities of all types of life forms).
Fluxomics	Study that deals with the dynamic changes of molecules within a cell over time.
Genomics	Study of the genomes of organisms.
Glycomics	Study dealing with identification of the entirety of all carbohydrates in a cell or tissue.
Interactomics	Study dealing mostly with protein-protein interactions but is also applicable to study of interactions between all molecules within a cell.
Metabolomics	Study dealing with identification and measurement of all small-molecules metabolites within a cell or tissue.
Proteomics	Study dealing with complete identification of proteins and protein expression patterns of a cell or tissue.
Transcriptomics	Study dealing with whole cell or tissue gene expression measurements.
Closed system	A closed system is completely self-contained and is not modified by the environment.
Deterministic system	A deterministic system always has the same response to a particular stimulus under a set of conditions. Therefore, the output from such a system can always be predicted.
Distributed system	A distributed system consists of a collection of autonomous computers connected through a network of that enables them to coordinate their activities and to share the resources of the system so that users perceive the system as a single, integrated computing facility.
Nondeterministic system	A nondeterministic system has several different possible reactions to the same stimulus under the same set of conditions. Therefore, the output cannot be predicted from the input.
Non-reactive system	A non-reactive system carries on the same process irrespective of the changes in other processes.
Open system	An open system is interacts with the environment and is modified by these environmental interactions.
Reactive system	A reactive system consists of parallel processes, where each process may change in reaction to another process changing its state.

BIOLOGICAL SYSTEMS

Several types of biological systems can be described based on their inherent properties (Table 1). Biological systems are complex open systems for which four fundamental universal properties of complex biological systems have been recognized that are not are not apparent from study of the parts. These properties are: emergence, irreducibility, modularity and robustness.

- **Emergence:** This implies that the system has unique properties that occur due its existence as a system, and are not inherent in or integral to their parts and cannot be projected from the individual properties of the parts. Therefore, the system is more than the sum of its parts i.e. the system emerges as a more complex entity than a simple mix of its individual parts. For example, the life in a cell is an emergent property because it does not occur just by putting together DNA, RNA, proteins, carbohydrates and lipid along with other minerals in a soup. Emergence is a key to complex biological systems and is a result of interactions between the different composing parts in specific manners. It is seen at different levels of biological organization and a direct result of the complexity of this organization. Other examples of emerging properties include: the functional properties of proteins are not evident only in the linear chain of their constituting amino acids, but "emerge" from the secondary, tertiary and quaternary structure of the proteins – changing these complex structures also takes away the protein function.

- **Irreducibility:** Complex biological systems are irreducible into sections of component parts without loss of identity and function. Although a reductionist approach allows us to examine the components of the complex system as the emergent properties disappear thereby preventing complete complex-system analysis.
- **Modularity:** Complex biological systems are modular in nature i.e. they are a functional entity of interacting parts that exist as a unit with a common function. For example, every cell can be considered to be a unit of modular system with defined function. During wound healing (especially by primary intention), the lost/damaged modules (cells) are replaced by other modules that are manufactures by the body. Modularity is a safeguard against failure of the biological system, permits limiting and confining the damage, efficient organized mop-up and reconstruction operations; and is a key to the robustness of the system.
- **Robustness:** Overall, complex biological systems are sturdy and strong in form. They maintain their phenotypical form in the face of adverse environmental insults, genetic variations and random variability. It takes a large force of insults to alter the form of biological systems. Positive and negative feedback loops, feed forward loops and various other mechanism act as checks and balances in biological systems. An example of robustness is the effect of mutations: although mutations may occur at an appreciable rate, and be accumulated, it takes a large "volume" to effect a phenotypical change. Robustness of a biological system is easily demonstrable in would healing (especially by secondary intention) in that even if the modularity function is lost/ disables, alternative modes may be pressed into function in a way that even if modularity is not restored, and function of a part of the system is lost, the overall phenotypical robustness of the organism is maintained – for example, in the damaged epithelium, even though healing by scar formation does not replace the epithelium, it maintains robustness by maintaining the critical physical barrier function of the epithelium.

SYSTEMS BIOLOGY

Rapid development of computer technology and computer assisted medical technology has led to an explosion of overwhelming availability of data. Current scientific manpower is somewhat short for being able to analyze all the data that comes out. Most of this biological data has been and is being generated under the reductionist paradigm, but often, merely adding the components back do not result in the reconstruction of the original figure. This has caused a paradigm shift in scientific methods such that a more comprehensive understanding of the biological phenomenon now entails careful consideration of the interaction of the different parts with each other at the time of their existence, and the role of their products that feed the backward loops (feedback loop) and forward loops (feed forward loop) enmeshed in myriad mechanisms that come into being simultaneously as well as substantially later in time. One aspect of such interactions is evidences of cellular and molecular cross talk, for example the diverse modes of molecular and functional cross-talk between canonical signaling pathways in hematopoietic cells (Fraser & Germaine, 2009), which led the authors to urge "caution about overly facile interpretation of genome- and proteome-level studies".

Whereas de-construction of the biological systems to the level of understanding of molecular-level interactions has proceeded rather along lines of expectations, the re-construction of the biological system from these molecular level understanding is posing a major challenge to scientists. Biological systems are therefore now being examined as "complex systems", and a "systems" approach is being developed to describe biological systems to understand their true nature. In essence, it is increasingly being appreciated that the biological system is much more than the sum of its parts! Biological systems have been described as complex information processing systems, and the primary goal to study them is to investigate how they behave. Biological systems are adapted to unstructured environments and are able to learn from experience (Iyengar, 1998).

The quest for efficient computational approaches to self-organized data representation in modeling biological systems has undergone a significant evolution in the last few years. Specifically, the application of neural computing concepts to some of the topological properties of biological molecules requires implementation of efficient computer-based strategies with massive processing abilities. For example, the DNA molecule contains an immense amount of information in coded form. This coded information controls the growth, development and major characteristics of biological systems. Therefore the control of information stored in the DNA molecule is a major computational problem of research interest for researchers... (Iyengar, 1998).

Systems biology has been defined as "a comprehensive quantitative analysis of the manner in which all the components of a biological system interact functionally over time" (Aderem, 2005). It integrates chemistry, computer science, engineering, life sciences, mathematics, physics and other sciences to provide understanding of biological processes. Systems biology views organisms as an interacting system of genes, proteins and biochemical reactions that are key elements in organisms' life-cycle, determining its form and function. Development in technology, such as automated DNA sequencers, microarray technology and mass spectrometry have outputted large scale genomic, transcriptomics, proteomic, interactomic, Glycomics, Fluxomics, Biomics, and metabolomic data enabling high throughput biology (Table 1).

The use of systematic genomic, proteomic and metabolomic technologies to construct models of complex biological systems and diseases is becoming increasingly commonplace. These endeavors, collectively known as systems biology, establish an approach by which to interrogate and iteratively refine our knowledge of the cell. In so doing, systems biology integrates knowledge from diverse biological components and data into models of the system as a whole (Ideker, 2004).

Systems biology model development faces several challenges such as confounding by several factors, functional redundancy, biases, information errors, random errors and processes effecting examined factors.

The true test of a good system model is successful prediction of the system's behavior under targeted alterations (genetic or environmental perturbations) of experimental conditions. But the very properties that make biological systems interesting and worthwhile to study their emergent properties, robustness, stability, modularity and adaptability to change, also make their behavior hard to predict at the molecular level. Confounding factors include functional redundancy (i.e., a given process might be accomplished by several different molecular mechanisms), and the stochasticity of cell populations (what is measured, e.g., gene expression, could be an average of a wide range of discrete responses among individual cells) (Institute for Systems Biology, 2009).

MODELING PARADIGMS IN SYSTEMS BIOLOGY

Systems biology research adopts the following principles to develop a good systems model and minimize errors (Institute for Systems Biology, 2009).

1. Global approaches should be taken to data collection and analyses
2. Information derived from diverse data types should be integrated
3. Mathematical and statistical modeling is essential to the quantitative analysis of a system's properties
4. Biology should drive technology which, in turn, makes better biology possible
5. Systems biology research should create an interactive inter-disciplinary scientific culture
6. The results of research should be freely disseminated

Systems biology uses data to construct models to describe biological systems which may be time-static descriptive diagrammatic models and graphic mathematical models i.e. "those that use computer power to analyze mathematical relationships between quantities" (mathematical models); or time-dependent dynamic models as are now becoming commonly available i.e. those resembling a computer program (computational models), which is central to an emerging field that maybe called "executable" biology (Fisher & Henzinger, 2007). Mathematical models convert the biological questions to a single/ set of mathematical equations that are then solved to find a numerical solution; whereas computational modeling takes an algorithmic approach by developing a series of step-by-step sequences of instructions that a permit the models to be developed depending upon a set of conditions for each step- in the sequence which makes the models dynamic allowing assessment of outcomes depending on a variety of inputs at each step. Complex mathematical models are solved using computers requiring algorithms and computational simulations to communicate with the computer; a step that requires proofs to demonstrate that the algorithm arrives at appropriate solutions with adequate precision; whereas this step is not required in computational modeling (Fisher & Henzinger, 2007). One way of visual-

Figure 1. Computational and mathematical modeling paradigms

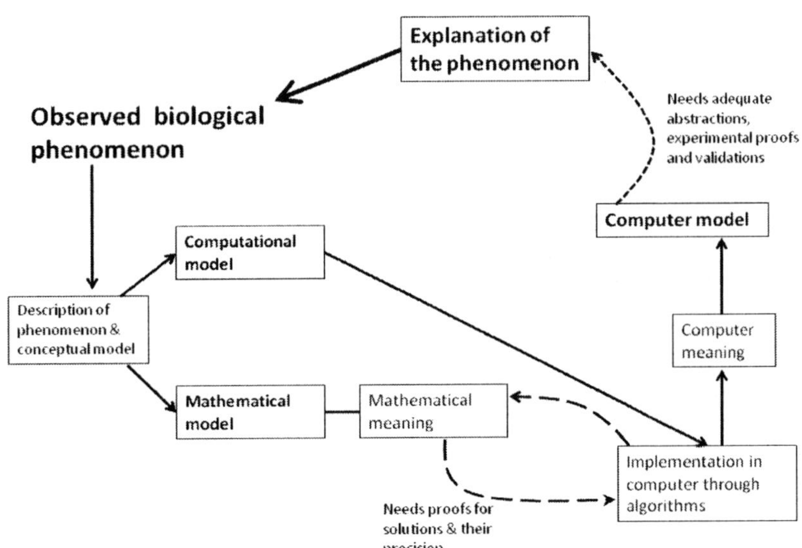

izing the fundamental difference between mathematical and computational modeling is shown in Figure 1.

Although they utilize available quantitative information, computational modeling is essentially qualitative in nature. Computational modeling allows easier incorporation of non-linear states and incorporation of causal associations to accommodate feed forward and feedback loops into the computer models without the need for constant mathematical validation of algorithms, which makes it a more efficient way to solve problems when large dynamic systems are being assessed where the number of interdependencies are vast, and easy quantification of each reaction step involved in mathematical model is not possible. These models also allow for easy validation using experimental data, and can model a variety of hypothetical situations that may be further validated with new experiments. In such a process, the results of either (i.e. experimental biology and computational models can be influenced from each other leading to their refinement and adjustment to realize better quality information and comprehensive description of the phenomenon under study. One of the major advantages of computational models is to incorporate time as a dynamic factor in the models, and assess influence of time on biological systems in ways that may not be possible in real life situations. Figure 2 describes such interactions between experimental data and computational models.

Useful Software in Systems Biology and Biological Interaction Software

Wet lab techniques for sequencing, gene expression profiling, biochemical and biophysical genetic analysis, hybrid analysis, proteome analysis are available easily. These techniques allow assessment of gene function, protein function, and protein-protein interactions. However, a key question is to understand how the genes program cellular behavior or give rise to a particular phenotype. Computational tools such as sequence analysis, mathematical analytical and numerical modeling,

Figure 2. Parallelism, interaction and differences between experimental method and computational modeling

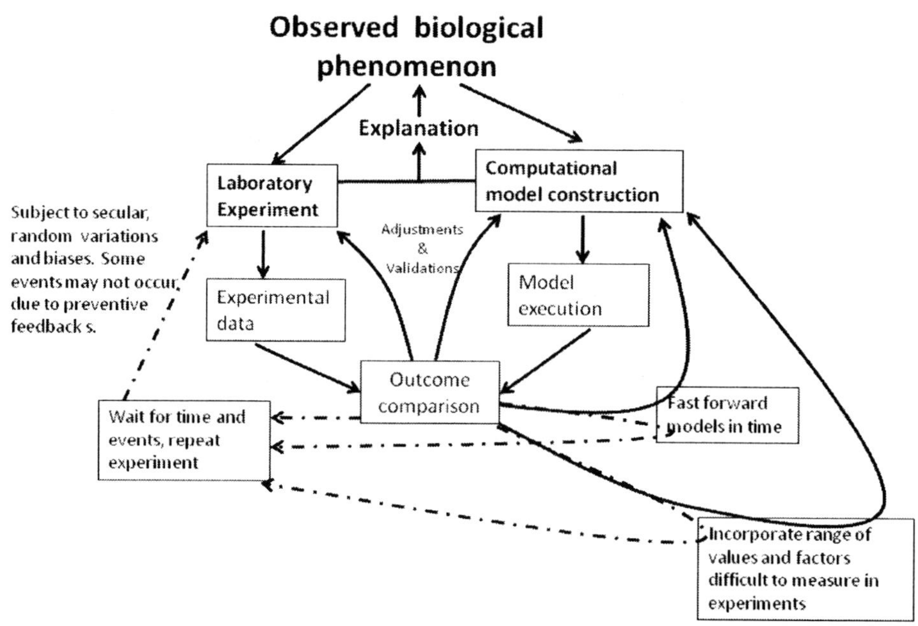

and qualitative modeling are useful in developing the complete picture. However, "mathematical modeling in biology has been hindered by the lack of software tools to build, analyze, and visualize models, particularly for researchers unfamiliar with programming and numerical methods (You, 2004). However, in the past few years, several software products have been developed that are useful in modeling cellular processes, which has also helped in development of databases of biological interactions (Table 2).

A massive body of information is accessible through various knowledge databases through the internet – Table 3 describes some of them that can be accessed freely over the internet at the web site: http://www.ncbi.nlm.nih.gov/sites/gquery?itool=toolbar through the National Center for Biotechnology Information (NCBI) which is a part of the United States National Library of Medicine (NLM) at the U.S. National Institutes of Health in Bethesda, MD, USA.

Table 2. Some examples of software, languages and biological interaction databases useful in systems biology

Software	**Web site**
Archemedes	http://archimedesmodel.com/
Cell Designer	http://systems-biology.org/software/celldesigner/
Cellerator	http://www.cellerator.org/
DBsolve	http://systems-biology.org/software/simulation/dbsolve.html
Dynetica	http://sourceforge.net/projects/dynetica/
E-Cell	http://www.e-cell.org
Gepasi	http://www.gepasi.org/
Jarnac/ Jdesigner	http://sbw.kgi.edu/software/jdesigner.htm
NetLogo	http://ccl.northwestern.edu/netlogo/
Stella	http://www.iseesystems.com/softwares/Education/StellaSoftware.aspx
StochSim	http://www.pdn.cam.ac.uk/groups/comp-cell/StochSim.html
Virtual cell	http://www.ibiblio.org/virtualcell/
Standard modeling languages	
Systems Biology markup language (SBML)	http://sbml.org/Main_Page
Cell markup Language (CellML)	http://www.cellml.org/
Systems Biology Graphical Notation (SBGN)	http://www.sbgn.org/Main_Page
Biological interaction databases	
AfCS-nature Signaling Gateway	http://www.signaling-gateway.org/
Biomolecular Object Network Databank	http://bond.unleashedinformatics.com/
The Database of Interacting Proteins	http://dip.doe-mbi.ucla.edu/dip/Main.cgi
EcoCyc	http://www.ecocyc.org/
Kyoto Encyclopedia of Genes and Genomes	http://www.ecocyc.org/
Signaling Transduction Knowledge Environment	http://stke.sciencemag.org/
NCI-Nature Pathway Interaction Database	http://pid.nci.nih.gov/
Biological Interaction database for Protein-nucleic Acid	http://www-cryst.bioc.cam.ac.uk/bipa

Table 3. Knowledge databases in biomedical research

Protein Clusters (ProtClustDB) This database contains collection of related protein sequences (clusters) consists of Reference Sequence proteins encoded by complete genomes. This database contains both curated and non-curated clusters.
PubChem This database contains descriptions of chemical samples, from a variety of sources, and links to other databases. It includes several other databases such as: Substances Database, BioAssay database, and Compound database.
Cancer Chromosomes: Cytogenic Chromosomes This database contains three integrated databases: the NCI/NCBI SKY/M-FISH & CGH Database, the NCI Mitelman Database of Chromosome Aberrations in Cancer, and the NCI Recurrent Aberrations in.
GEO DataSets This database contains curated gene expression and molecular abundance DataSets assembled from the Gene Expression Omnibus (GEO) repository.
GEO Profiles This database contains individual gene expression and molecular abundance profiles assembled from the GEO repository.
PopSet This database contains a set of DNA sequences that have been collected to analyze the evolutionary relatedness of a population.
UniSTS This database contains sequence tagged sites (STSs) derived from STS-based maps and other experiments.
3D Domains This database contains compact structural domains identified automatically in MMDB, Entrez's macromolecular three-dimensional structure database.
Conserved Domain Database (CDD) This database contains protein domain models imported from outside sources, such as Pfam and SMART, and curated at NCBI. It links over 12,000 models to other NCBI databases, including protein sequences, bibliographic citations, and taxonomy.
UniGene This database contains sets of transcript sequences that appear to come from the same transcription locus (gene or expressed pseudogene), together with information on protein similarities, gene expression, cDNA clone reagents, and genomic location
dbGap This database contains phenotype and genotype data, as well as the associations between them.
Nucleotide This database contains records for all Entrez Nucleotide sequences that are not found within the Expressed Sequence Tag (EST) or Genome Survey Sequence (GSS) divisions of GenBank.
EST (Expressed Sequence Tag) This database contains all records found within the Expressed Sequence Tag (EST) division of GenBank.
GSS (Genome Survey Sequence) This database contains all records found within the Genome Survey Sequence (GSS) division of GenBank.
Protein This database contains entries in the Entrez search and retrieval system that have been compiled from a variety of sources, including SwissProt, PIR, PRF, PDB, and translations from annotated coding regions in GenBank and RefSeq.
Genome This database contains the whole Genomes of over 1000 viruses and over 100 microbes
Structure: Molecular Modeling Database (MMDB) This database contains 3-D macromolecular structures, including proteins and polynucleotides. It includes more than 20,000 structures and is linked to the rest of the NCBI databases, including sequences, bibliographic citations, taxonomic classifications, and sequence and structure neighbors.
Taxonomy: This database contains the names of all organisms that are represented in the genetic databases with at least one nucleotide or protein sequence
SNP (single nucleotide polymorphism) This database contains all reported SNPs.
Gene This database contains information about the characteristics and defining sequences of genes from species in Genome, RefSeq, and other model organisms.
SRA (Short Read Archive) This database contains Raw sequence data from sequencing instruments.
BioSystems This database contains records that group together molecules that interact in biological systems.
HomoloGene This database contains an automated system for detecting homologs among the annotated genes of several completely sequenced eukaryotic genomes.
GENSAT This database contains maps of the expression of genes in the central nervous system of the mouse, using both in situ hybridization and transgenic mouse techniques.
Probe This database contains a public registry of sequence-specific reagents designed for use in a wide variety of biomedical research applications, together with information on reagent availability, experimental protocols, probe effectiveness, and computed sequence similarities.
Genome Project This database contains a collection of complete and incomplete large-scale sequencing, assembly, annotation, and mapping projects for cellular organisms.
OMIM (Online Mendelian Inheritance in Man) This database contains a catalog of human genes and genetic disorders, with links to literature references, sequence records, maps, and related databases.
OMIA (Online Mendelian Inheritance in Animals) This database contains a catalog of genes, inherited disorders and traits in animal species (other than human and mouse).

As described in and accessible from URL: http://www.ncbi.nlm.nih.gov/sites/
Last accessed: June 15, 2009

SYSTEMS SCIENCE IN ORAL HEALTH RESEARCH: SOME EXAMPLES

Application of systems science in general and the systems biology approach (especially computational technology) is just starting to be used in oral health research, and it is hoped that soon such methods will be used increasingly. Use of microarray technology in dental research is starting and it is expected that all areas of dentistry will be affected by developments in molecular medicine, pharmacogenomics and newer therapeutic modes. Microarrays have been used in research related to periodontal diseases, endodontic infections, dental caries, temporomandibular disorders, autoimmune disorders, developmental disorders and dental related drug development (Nazmul-Hossain et al., 2008), although not extensively. Concepts of systems biology and extensive use of associated computational methods are also filtering in.

Oral-Based Diagnostics

Medical diagnostic science may be made much easier if easily available, non-invasive genetic samples can be taken from oral mucosa and saliva. With the great emphasis in salivary proteomics and metabolomics, oral diagnostic devices can be developed. For this to happen,

[T]he three key issues are: (1) performance of measurements of multiple analytes in order to profile the status of a (group) of diseases; (2) utilization of a generic approach in the design of detection platforms that can be easily adapted for the detection of different target molecules; note that this is achievable with easily substituted specific bioreagents such as antibodies and nucleic acid probes; and (3) the need to achieve the highest possible level of sensitivity since levels of target analytes may be orders of magnitude lower in saliva than in other body fluids, and newly discovered analytes are unlikely to occur in high concentration... Lastly, diagnostics need to anticipate developments in future health care such as personalized medicine, aiming at early prediction and intervention (Tanke, 2007).

However, oral biology/ tissue/ fluid – based diagnostics will first need to develop analytical techniques with explicitly defined parameters that can be factored into models – both qualitative and quantitative. Current literature suggests that use of mathematical modeling based evidence is not yet fully entrenched in oral health research, although significant strides are being made (Chattopadhyay, 2009). However, significant development in oral epidemiological research and multi-level exposure, clustering of effect-tissues by exposure groups and "systems thinking" has already started impacting thinking of oral disease etiology. It is therefore expected that more quantitative and qualitative computational modeling based approaches would be used in oral health research.

Periodontal Inflammation

Researchers have been searching for a comprehensive understanding and explanation of periodontal disease, especially so that it can be correctly categorizes, defined and measured. It has become increasingly clear that several complex factors and mechanisms are involved in periodontal disease (or, a group of diseases that are loosely called "periodontal disease") which is an outcome of interactions between host immunology, local environment factors and microbial impacts. Therefore, the biologic phenotype of the individual is critical in development of periodontal disease (immune function is the critical phenotype that impacts periodontal disease). Epigenetic contributions may influence clinical phenotype expression of periodontal disease patients.

Biologic processes, including the characteristics of the biofilm and of the host inflammatory and immune responses, tend to vary among individu-

als, despite producing a similar clinical picture or diagnostic category. As such, disease classification should be based on clinically apparent signs and symptoms and reflect the underlying biologic phenotypes that contribute to pathogenesis in a given individual at the microbial, cellular, and molecular level. Other factors that may influence the biologic phenotype and clinical expression of disease include inter-individual variability that exists at the subject-level, such as unique environmental exposures, as well as differences in genetic and possibly epigenetic composition. By delineating the multiple factors that contribute to the clinical presentation of periodontal disease in a specific individual, it should be possible to develop more homogeneous diagnostic categories for periodontitis in which to place individuals at risk. This should allow a more accurate prognosis and provide insight into the ideal customized treatment for a given individual (Offenbacher et al., 2008).

Offering a systemic biology paradigm to approach periodontal disease, Offenbacher et al. (2008) emphasized the complex clustering of risk factors and biologic factors that may impact periodontal disease and need for different biological and mathematical modeling approach to periodontal disease. Clustering of biologic and environmental determining factors vis-à-vis periodontal disease occurs at different levels. Person level factors (e.g. biofilm, smoking, systemic diseases such as diabetes and obesity) may interact with genetic and epiegentic composition (e.g. age, gender that may contribute to diverse range of responses in inflammatory reaction observed at the molecular level). Epigenetic mechanisms involving "DNA and histone modifications, result in the heritable silencing of genes without a change in their coding sequence" (Egger et al., 2004) and may be determined by environmental factors, and may also regulate inflammatory response in individuals (Bobetsis et al., 2007). Interactive outcomes of these with biologic phenotype (e.g. cellular & molecular response factors, inflammatory biomarkers) may result in the ultimate clinical phenotype presentation (Offenbacher et al., 2008).

Streptococcus Mutans Stress Response

Computational analysis in oral microbiology research is common. For example, completed in 2001, the complete genome sequence of Streptococcus mutans, a bacterial pathogen commonly associated with human dental caries, was published in 2002 (Ajdic' et al, 2002). *S. mutans* adapts well to the rapidly changing oral biofilm environment on surfaces of teeth. However, S. mutans lacks many of the sensing systems and alternative sigma factors that bacteria often use to coordinate gene expression in response to stress and changes in their environment. However, the organism has "integrated the stress regulon and global transcriptional regulators to coordinate responses to environmental fluctuations with modulation of virulence in a way that ensures persistence in the oral cavity and capitalizes on conditions that are favorable for the development of dental caries" (Lemos & Burne, 2008). They examined the in dissection of the stress regulon of *S. mutans* and its intimate interrelationship with pathogenesis, and reviewed genomic and proteomic studies that addressed stress survival pathways utilized by S. mutans in the tooth biofilm system. Computational studies determined the role of protection, repair and quality control of macromolecules; and pH homeostasis and metabolic pathways in stress regulation of S. mutans:

- Membrane-bound F-ATPase (H+-translocating ATPase) is considered the primary determinant of acid tolerance of *S. mutans* because it allows the organism to maintain a cytoplasmic pH that is more alkaline than the extracellular environment. and that acid tolerance in oral streptococci with the pH optima and absolute level of activity of the F1FO-ATPase.

- A mechanism for acid resistance used by many oral streptococci is the production of ammonia by urease enzymes or the arginine deiminase system.
- Acid tolerance of S. mutans is malolactic fermentation (MLF), which catalyzes the conversion of dicarboxylic L-malate, a major acid in fruits such as apple, to the monocarboxylic lactic acid and CO2.
- Several molecular chaperones (GroEL and DnaK), proteases and DNA repair systems (RecA, the endonuclease Smn and the UV repair excinuclease UvrA) as up-regulated during growth at low pH.

Other mechanisms used by *S. mutans* to adapt to stress include nutritional regulators and alteration of catabolic pathways; two-component signal transduction systems; and cell envelope alterations. Therefore, strategies that "short-circuit regulatory pathways used by *S. mutans* to sense and respond to environmental signals may have a potent capacity to disrupt cariogenic biofilms and form the basis of caries prevention and therapies (Lemos & Burne, 2008).

Secretory Leukocyte Protease Inhibitor (SLPI) in Saliva

SLPI is an important innate immunty biomolecule found in several body fuids. In the oral cavity, salivary SLPI, a 12-kDa antiprotease, has been associated with anti-HIV-1 activity, oral candidiasis and periodontal diseases (Chattopadhyay et al, 2004; Cox et al., 2006; Jana et al., 2005; Moutsopoulos et al., 2006). SLPI prevents spread of microbes

Figure 3. Assumed SLPI molecule structure, a dual inhibitor of the leukocyte proteases Cathepsin G and Chymase with therapeutic efficacy in animals models of inflammation, 1T31 (de Garavilla et al. 2005)

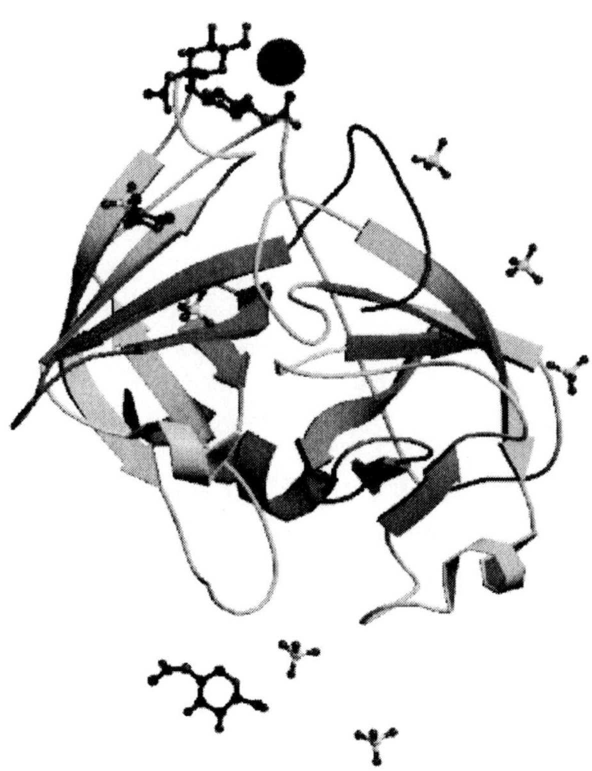

on mucocutaneous surfaces in vivo by blocking colonization of transient pathogens and/or their release of destructive proteases such as elastase in oral sites (Shugars et al.,2001) . The gene for SLPI in humans has been identified {GeneID: 6590; SLPI secretory leukocyte peptidase inhibitor [Homo sapiens]; URL: http://www.ncbi.nlm.nih.gov/sites/entrez?Db=gene&Cmd=ShowDetailView&TermToSearch=6590}. Fig 3 shows the structure of SLPI protein molecule was that was published by de Garavilla et al. (2005), as available in the protein data bank.

SLPI contains the whey acidic protein (WAP) domain which play important roles in the antimicrobial and/or antiprotease activities (Fitch et al., 2006). The WAP family includes: SLPI, WFDC2, WFDC5, and WFDC12. Idoji et al. (2007) hypothesized that genes highly expressed in the tongue, salivary glands, snout epidermis, and trachea contribute to maintenance of the levels of salivary protease inhibitors. For their in-silico study, they used the Novartis mouse expression database selected and annotated oral organspecific cDNA clones from the expression database; and conducted "PSI-BLAST homology searches using either the mouse SLPI N-WAP domain with 45 amino acid residues or its C-WAP domain with 47 amino acid residues as queries against the database at the NCBI" (Idoji et al., 2008). They then conducted multiple alignments using CLUSTAL W program; and scored levels of homology by analyzing the aligned control and test sequences using the CCResid program. Following this, they conducted phylogenetic and molecular evolutionary analyses.

[W]e found that the four WAP family members, SLPI, WFDC2, WFDC5, and WFDC12, are highly expressed in the oral organs, such as the trachea, tongue, and salivary glands. Since their WAP domains play pivotal roles in the antimicrobial and/or antiprotease activities and their application in therapeutics are expected to have practical value, we collected 98 WAP homologues and tried to predict their physiological functions by analyzing their amino acid sequence structures. From the multiple alignments of amino acid sequences, we predicted that most of the mammalian N-terminal WAP domains derived from SLPIs and the WAP domains derived from WFDC12s have antimicrobial activities, whereas most of the mammalian C-terminal WAP domains derived from SLPIs and the WAP domains derived from elafins have antiprotease activities. From the phylogenetic tree, it was revealed that an ancestral WAP protein initially diverged into the WFDC5-C WAP domain and the ancestral protein for the other WAP domains. Subsequently, the ancestral protein for the other WAP domains diverged into two ancestral proteins, one for elafin and SLPI-C WAP domains and the other, for SLPI-N, WFDC15b, WFDC12, and WFDC5-N WAP domains, respectively. Moreover, the tree indicated that the WFDC5-N and WFDC12 WAP domains share a common ancestral protein (Idoji et al., 2008).

The potential for use of recombinant SLPI to prevent oral candidiasis was discussed by Chattopadhyay et al. (2004). Furthermore, Shugars et al. (2001) demonstrated that the elderly are particularly susceptible to mucosal infections and are known to produce diminished amounts of oral SLPI. In thgis context, in-silico studies by idoji et al. (2008) these studies suggest that supplying recombinant WAPs to the saliva of elderly patients could prevent mucosal infections. Increasingly virulent strains of bacteria and antibiotic resistance mean that proteinase inhibitors have the capacity to become the next 'magic bullet' (Fitch et al., 2006). Therefore, studies using systems biology paradigm with insightful computational analysis may start to play increasingly important role in finding new olecular targets, and also providing evidence for newer diagnostics and therapies.

Oral Cancer

Oral cavity carcinoma is the sixth most common cancer and is often detected in later stages. Oral squamous cell carcinoma (OSCC), the predominant type of cancer found in the oral cavity, is a disfiguring and deadly cancer. Oral cancer survival rates in the US have remained stable at low levels for several decades. In the US, each year some 31,000 new cases of oral cancer are diagnosed and more than 7,500 people die of oral cancer. Overall age adjusted incidence rate (year 2000-2003) was 10.5 per 100,000 and age adjusted mortality rate was 2.7 per 100,000 (Ries et al., 2007). The overall average 5-year survival rate is 58.8%. There is a lot of interest in early detection and diagnosis of oral cancer to reduce its morbidity and resultant mortality. For this, to occur, one way is to establish biomarkers for those premalignant lesions that are at greater risk for developing oral cancer, which can be detected early.

Currently, histology-based methods are used for diagnosing and grading OSCC. However, for the more critical lesions that are not clearly "dysplastic" in nature, and are not clearly non-dysplastic", disagreements among pathologists are common, and the diagnostic dilemma can not only lead to great economic costs in terms of false-positive and false-negative results, but also carry great emotional costs for patients and families. Furthermore, definition of "dysplasia" is subjective. Some techniques, such as assessment of silver stainable nucleolar organizer regions (AgNORs) have been proposed as alternatives to traditional histological analysis (Chattopadhyay, 1993; Chattopadhyay et al., 1994; Chattopadhyay et al., 2002; Ray et al., 2003; Chattopadhyay & Ray, 2008). However, there still occur some premalignant lesions that may not be easily distinguishable from oral cancer in histology reports because these lesions do not form a clearly separate cluster between normal tissue and cancer, and some overlap in distribution exists (Chattopadhyay et al., 1993; Chattopadhyay et al., 1994). Reporting on applications of bioinformatics to gene expression profiles of OSCC, Kuo et al. (2003a) also found that dysplastic permalignant lesion samples did not cluster together as a group but were found in either the "normal" or "cancer" clusters (two sides of the distribution). They inferred that there are subtle changes that occur in the progression of OSCC which are not captured through histology reports. They also opined that constructing signaling pathways through the identification of the specific genes and the sequence in which they appear in the transformation of normal to cancer can be beneficial in our understanding of OSCC.

Todd et al. (2002) investigated differentially expressed genes that could discriminate among normal, dysplastic, and cancer samples by using DNA microarrays after collecting the samples were collected by laser capture microdissection. From this study, they could identify

"... several genes and expressed sequence tags (ESTs) from the normal and dysplasia comparison to be associated with cancer. For example, we found DDB2, a damage-specific DNA protein, to be a potential biomarker for the progression of OSCC. The implication of this is that DDB2 can be a potential novel therapeutic target for prevention or therapy. In another study, we applied a hierarchical clustering algorithm using average-linkage heuristic and Euclidean distance metrics to the gene expression profiles of normal, dysplastic, and cancer samples (Kuo et al., 2003a). We were able to separate the normal and cancer samples based on their expression profiles. An interesting observation was made with the "dysplasia" samples, which did not cluster together as a group."

Oral cancers, like other cancers, are complex diseases involving multi-factorial etiology and outcome determinants including personal/ group behavioral factors, infective organisms, socio-economic impacts, genetic make-up and gene-environment interactions. Changes occurring at the level of the DNA can be multiple, and may be heritable. Furthermore, oral cancer is not a homogenous disease: there may exist differences in types of cancers I the oral and craniofacial region, histological differentiation; clinical staging and grading at presentation; and molecular types and subtypes. Translational cancer research will benefit from data integration and computational analysis under a systems biology paradigm. Integration of clinical data (e.g. disease phenotypes and treatment outcomes) with laboratory data (e.g. molecular and imaging data: genomic variations, gene transcripts, protein levels and modifications, small RNAs, metabolites, and biological images) can be relatively easily achieved. However, their further integration with integration and aggregation with data associated with disease-specific regulatory and metabolic processes, molecular signatures, biomarkers and drug targets to develop computational and statistical algorithms is a major challenge for computational biology (Mathew et al., 2007). Though challenging, such computational analyses will provide evidence for rational design of drugs and therapies, and help in refining clinical trial making them more efficient in economic terms and in terms of outcomes research; and finally provide more effective treatment, substantial part of which could be directed personalized therapy.

CONCLUSION

Factors underlying biological and socio-biological states include a complex interplay of several biological, behavioral, economic, and social factors. Reductionist view of disease processes and their outcomes is useful in understanding fundamental mechanisms, but fail to explain inter-relatedness between parts and their interactions to produce disease, and limit the choices for diagnosis and therapeutic applications. Biological systems are complex open systems that are emergent, irreducible, modular and robust. Systems biology approach; as a comprehensive quantitative and qualitative analysis of the manner in which all the components of a biological system interact functionally over time, is a well suited paradigm to answer most questions related to diseases of the oral and craniofacial region as these occur due to the complex interplay of a variety of factors that are clustered at different levels.

ACKNOWLEDGMENT

Dr. Chattopadhyay contributed to this chapter in his personal capacity. The views expressed are his own and do not necessarily represent the views of the National Institutes of Health or the United States Government.

REFERENCES

Aderem, A. (2005). Systems biology: its practice and challenges. *Cell*, *121*(4), 511–513. doi:10.1016/j.cell.2005.04.020

Ahmed, S., & Nawshad, A. (2007). Complexity in interpretation of embryonic epithelial-mesenchymal transition in response to transforming growth factor-beta signaling. *Cells, Tissues, Organs*, *185*(1-3), 131–145. doi:10.1159/000101314

Ajdic, D., McShan, W. M., McLaughlin, R. E., Savic, G., Chang, J., & Carson, M. B. (2002). Genome sequence of Streptococcus mutans UA159, a cariogenic dental pathogen. *Proceedings of the National Academy of Sciences of the United States of America*, *99*(22), 14434–14439. doi:10.1073/pnas.172501299

Auf dem Keller, U., Doucet, A., & Overall, C. M. (2007). Protease research in the era of systems biology. *Biological Chemistry*, *388*(11), 1159–1162. doi:10.1515/BC.2007.146

Bobetsis, Y. A., Barros, S. P., Lin, D. M., Weidman, J. R., Dolinoy, D. C., & Jirtle, R. L. (2007). Bacterial infection promotes DNA hypermethylation. *Journal of Dental Research*, *86*(2), 169–174. doi:10.1177/154405910708600212

Bork, P., & Serrano, L. (2005). Towards cellular systems in 4D. *Cell*, *121*(4), 507–509. doi:10.1016/j.cell.2005.05.001

Boughner, J. C., & Hallgrimsson, B. (2008). Biological spacetime and the temporal integration of functional modules: a case study of dento-gnathic developmental timing. *Developmental Dynamics*, *237*(1), 1–17. doi:10.1002/dvdy.21383

Chattopadhyay, A. (1993). AgNORs in tumoral pathology. Review of literature and observations on the technic and reaction in normal oral epithelium. *Indian Journal of Dental Research*, *4*(2), 47–53.

Chattopadhyay, A. (2010). *Oral Health Epidemiology: Principles and Practice*. Sudbury, MA: Jones & Bartlett Publishers.

Chattopadhyay, A., Chawda, J. G., & Doshi, J. J. (1994). Silver-binding nucleolar organizing regions: a study of oral leukoplakia and squamous cell carcinoma. *International Journal of Oral and Maxillofacial Surgery*, *23*(6 Pt 1), 374–377. doi:10.1016/S0901-5027(05)80060-8

Chattopadhyay, A., Gray, L. R., Patton, L. L., Caplan, D. J., Slade, G. D., & Tien, H. C. (2004). Salivary secretory leukocyte protease inhibitor and oral candidiasis in human immunodeficiency virus type 1-infected persons. *Infection and Immunity*, *72*(4), 1956–1963. doi:10.1128/IAI.72.4.1956-1963.2004

Chattopadhyay, A., & Ray, J. G. (2008). AgNOR cut-point to distinguish mild and moderate epithelial dysplasia. *Journal of Oral Pathology & Medicine*, *37*(2), 78–82.

Chattopadhyay, A., Ray, J. G., & Caplan, D. J. (2002). AgNOR count as objective marker for dysplastic features in oral leukoplakia. *Journal of Oral Pathology & Medicine*, *31*(9), 512–517. doi:10.1034/j.1600-0714.2002.00153.x

Cheverud, J. M. (2007). The relationship between development and evolution through heritable variation. *Novartis Foundation Symposium*, *284*, 55–65. doi:10.1002/9780470319390.ch4

Cox, S. W., Rodriguez-Gonzalez, E. M., Booth, V., & Eley, B. M. (2006). Secretory leukocyte protease inhibitor and its potential interactions with elastase and cathepsin B in gingival crevicular fluid and saliva from patients with chronic periodontitis. *Journal of Periodontal Research*, *41*(5), 477–485. doi:10.1111/j.1600-0765.2006.00891.x

De Garavilla, L., Greco, M. N., Sukumar, N., Chen, Z. W., Pineda, A. O., & Mathews, F. S. (2005). A novel, potent dual inhibitor of the leukocyte proteases cathepsin G and chymase: molecular mechanisms and anti-inflammatory activity in vivo. *The Journal of Biological Chemistry*, *280*(18), 18001–18007. doi:10.1074/jbc.M501302200

Egger, G., Liang, G., Aparicio, A., & Jones, P. A. (2004). Epigenetics in human disease and prospects for epigenetic therapy. *Nature*, *429*(6990), 457–463. doi:10.1038/nature02625

Fisher, J., & Henzinger, T. A. (2007). Executable cell biology. *Nature Biotechnology*, *25*(11), 1239–1249. doi:10.1038/nbt1356

Fitch, P. M., Roghanian, A., Howie, S. E., & Sallenave, J. M. (2006). Human neutrophil elastase inhibitors in innate and adaptive immunity. *Biochemical Society Transactions*, *34*(Pt 2), 279–282. doi:10.1042/BST20060279

Forrester, J. W. (1985). 'The Model' Versus a Modeling 'Process'. *System Dynamics Review*, *1*(1 & 2), 133–134. doi:10.1002/sdr.4260010112

Fraser, I. D., & Germain, R. N. (2009). Navigating the network: signaling cross-talk in hematopoietic cells. *Nature Immunology, 10*(4), 327–331. doi:10.1038/ni.1711

Friboulet, A., & Thomas, D. (2005). Systems Biology-an interdisciplinary approach. *Biosensors & Bioelectronics, 20*(12), 2404–2407. doi:10.1016/j.bios.2004.11.014

Ideker, T. (2004). Systems biology 101--what you need to know. *Nature Biotechnology, 22*(4), 473–475. doi:10.1038/nbt0404-473

Idoji, Y., Watanabe, Y., Yamashita, A., Yamanishi, K., Nishiguchi, S., & Shimada, K. (2008). In silico study of whey-acidic-protein domain containing oral protease inhibitors. *International Journal of Molecular Medicine, 21*(4), 461–468.

Institute for systems biology (2009). *Premise of Systems Biology*. Last accessed June 13, 2009 from http://www.systemsbiology.org/Systems_Biology_in_Depth/Premise_of_Systems_Biology

Iyengar, S. S. (1998). Introduction. In S.S. Iyengar (Ed). *Computer modeling and simulations of complex biological systems*. Boca Raton, FL: CRC Press.

Jana, N. K., Gray, L. R., & Shugars, D. C. (2005). Human immunodeficiency virus type 1 stimulates the expression and production of secretory leukocyte protease inhibitor (SLPI) in oral epithelial cells: a role for SLPI in innate mucosal immunity. *Journal of Virology, 79*(10), 6432–6440. doi:10.1128/JVI.79.10.6432-6440.2005

Jernvall, J., & Salazar-Ciudad, I. (2007). The economy of tinkering mammalian teeth. *Novartis Foundation Symposium, 284*, 207–216. doi:10.1002/9780470319390.ch14

Jernvall, J., & Thesleff, I. (2000). Reiterative signaling and patterning during mammalian tooth morphogenesis. *Mechanisms of Development, 92*(1), 19–29. doi:10.1016/S0925-4773(99)00322-6

Kuo, W. P. (2003). Overview of bioinformatics and its application to oral genomics. *Advances in Dental Research, 17*, 89–94. doi:10.1177/154407370301700121

Kuo, W. P., Hasina, R., Ohno-Machado, L., & Lingen, M. W. (2003). Classification and identification of genes associated with oral cancer based on gene expression profiles. A preliminary study. *The New York State Dental Journal, 69*(2), 23–26.

Lemos, J. A., & Burne, R. A. (2008). A model of efficiency: stress tolerance by Streptococcus mutans. *Microbiology, 154*(Pt 11), 3247–3255. doi:10.1099/mic.0.2008/023770-0

Liu, E. T. (2005). Systems biology, integrative biology, predictive biology. *Cell, 121*(4), 505–506. doi:10.1016/j.cell.2005.04.021

Mathew, J. P., Taylor, B. S., Bader, G. D., Pyarajan, S., Antoniotti, M., & Chinnaiyan, A. M. (2007). From bytes to bedside: data integration and computational biology for translational cancer research. *PLoS Computational Biology, 3*(2), e12. doi:10.1371/journal.pcbi.0030012

Moutsopoulos, N. M., Greenwell-Wild, T., & Wahl, S. M. (2006). Differential mucosal susceptibility in HIV-1 transmission and infection. *Advances in Dental Research, 19*(1), 52–56. doi:10.1177/154407370601900111

Nazmul-Hossain, A. N., Patel, K. J., Rhodus, N. L., & Moser, K. L. (2008). Microarrays: applications in dental research. *Oral Diseases, 14*(1), 25–29.

Offenbacher, S., Barros, S. P., & Beck, J. D. (2008). Rethinking periodontal inflammation. *Journal of Periodontology, 79*(8Suppl), 1577–1584. doi:10.1902/jop.2008.080220

Priami, C., & Quaglia, P. (2004). Modelling the dynamics of biosystems. *Briefings in Bioinformatics, 5*(3), 259–269. doi:10.1093/bib/5.3.259

Ries, L. A. G., Melbert, D., Krapcho, M., Stinchcomb, D. G., Howlader, N., Horner, M. J., et al. (Eds.). (2008). *SEER Cancer Statistics Review*, 1975-2005, National Cancer Institute. Bethesda, MD, http://seer.cancer.gov/csr/1975_2005/, based on November 2007 SEER data submission, posted to the SEER website.

Shugars, D. C., Watkins, C. A., & Cowen, H. J. (2001). Salivary concentration of secretory leukocyte protease inhibitor, an antimicrobial protein, is decreased with advanced age. *Gerontology, 47*, 246–253. doi:10.1159/000052808

Stock, D. W. (2001). The genetic basis of modularity in the development and evolution of the vertebrate dentition. *Philosophical Transactions of the Royal Society of London. Series B, Biological Sciences, 356*(1414), 1633–1653. doi:10.1098/rstb.2001.0917

Tanke, H. J. (2007). Genomics and proteomics: the potential role of oral diagnostics. *Annals of the New York Academy of Sciences, 1098*, 330–334. doi:10.1196/annals.1384.042

Todd, R., Lingen, M. W., & Kuo, W. P. (2002). Gene expression profiling using laser capture microdissection. *Expert Review of Molecular Diagnostics, 2*, 497–507. doi:10.1586/14737159.2.5.497

You, L. (2004). Toward computational systems biology. *Cell Biochemistry and Biophysics, 40*(2), 167–184. doi:10.1385/CBB:40:2:167

KEY TERMS AND DEFINITIONS

Emergence: Emergent properties of biological systems occur due their existence as a system, and are not inherent in or integral to their parts. These cannot be projected from the individual properties of the parts to the system.

Irreducibility: Irreducibility of complex biological systems implies that the system cannot be broken into sections of component parts without loss of identity and function as the system.

Modeling: Modeling in systems biology is the process of developing a model that describes a pattern, or representation plan or workings of biological processes as a system. The true test of a good system model is successful prediction of the system's behavior under targeted alterations (genetic or environmental perturbations) of experimental conditions.

Modularity: Modularity of complex biological systems implies that they are a functional entity of interacting parts that exist as a unit with a common function.

Robustness: Robustness of complex biological systems implies that they are sturdy and strong in form i.e. they maintain their phenotypical form in the face of adverse environmental insults, genetic variations and random variability.

Systems Biology: Systems biology views interactions in living cells and their organized forms as complex information processing systems. Primary goal of systems biology is to study them is to investigate how they behave.

Chapter 4
Novel Approaches to Studying Activity-Dependent Regulation of Neurotrophins and Neuropeptides in Sensory Pathways from Orofacial Tissues

Agnieszka Balkowiec
Oregon Health & Science University, USA

Ewa Balkowiec-Iskra
Medical University of Warsaw, Poland

ABSTRACT

Growth factors are critical for normal development of craniofacial innervation. Recent evidence indicates that neuronal growth factors, and particularly members of the neurotrophin family, are also involved in activity-dependent synaptic plasticity, with wide-ranging implications for chronic orofacial pain syndromes. The authors' laboratory has developed novel approaches to studying regulation of neurotrophin expression and release from neurons by activity. This chapter presents their advances in preparation of neuron-enriched cultures of trigeminal ganglia followed by stimulation with physiological patterns of electrical activity alone, and in combination with neuropeptides and inflammatory mediators. It also describes the authors' modified, ultra-sensitive ELISA methods (ELISA in situ and 'rapid capture' ELISA) for detection of endogenous neurotrophic factors, and other neuropeptides that are expressed and released in quantities below the detectability thresholds of standard assays. These methodologies are presented using Brain-Derived Neurotrophic Factor (BDNF) and Endomorphin-2 as examples.

DOI: 10.4018/978-1-60566-733-1.ch004

INTRODUCTION

Primary sensory neurons with cell bodies in the trigeminal ganglion (TG) carry nociceptive information from the craniofacial region, including several structures linked to chronic pain conditions, such as the meninges (migraine headaches), temporomandibular joint (TMJ; TMJ disorder), muscles of mastication (bruxism-associated muscle soreness), and teeth (odontalgias).

TG neurons have commonly been used as a model for studies of mechanisms that govern development of mammalian primary sensory neurons during embryonic stages. The unambiguous definition and easy accessibility of the components of the trigeminal system throughout the embryonic development have given rise to investigations of many fundamental processes involved in neural development using this model (for review, see Davies, 1988, 1997). On the other hand, the mechanisms of *postnatal* maturation of TG neurons, including the role of neuronal growth factors, are largely unknown. Similarly, very little has been done to characterize activity-dependent plastic changes in trigeminal pathways in response to disease processes, such as those involving neuroinflammation.

One reason for this gap in the current understanding of the trigeminal system is the limited number of research tools to: 1) reliably mimic different levels of activity in TG neurons associated with various pathophysiological conditions, and 2) detect resulting changes in expression and release of peptide neuromodulators, such as neurotrophins. The objective of this chapter is to facilitate filling this gap by presenting new strategies developed in our laboratory to: 1) prepare neuron-enriched dissociated cultures of TG, 2) detect relatively small quantities of neurotrophins and other neuropeptides expressed and/or released from TG neurons, and 3) stimulate neurotrophin and other neuropeptide expression and release from TG neurons with patterns of electrical stimuli that closely mimic neuronal activity *in vivo*.

BACKGROUND

There is mounting evidence that neurotrophins play a critical role in mechanisms of activity-dependent plastic changes in spinal sensory pathways, including chronic pain phenomena, such as allodynia. Recent data from our and other laboratories indicate that TG neurons express the neurotrophin brain-derived neurotrophic factor (BDNF) after the time the neurons depend on growth factors for survival (Buldyrev et al., 2006, Ichikawa et al., 2006). This raises the possibility that BDNF is a mediator of postnatal maturation and plasticity in trigeminal pathways, including those carrying nociceptive signals. Given the enormous significance of the trigeminal system in etiology of several common, debilitating pain conditions, such as migraine headaches or trigeminal neuralgia (tic douloureux), a complete understanding of the role played by neurotrophins in this system seems critical.

The first step in understanding the roles of neurotrophins at trigeminal synapses is to characterize conditions under which neurotrophins are synthesized, transported to TG neuron terminals, and released from these neurons in order to exert synaptic actions. The conditions include the effects of different patterns of neuronal activity that can be associated with certain disease states, role of other neuropeptides and inflammatory mediators, etc. The approach taken by our laboratory to address these questions is based on primary cultures of dissociated rat trigeminal ganglion neurons at various postnatal ages. The neurons are activated by electrical field stimulation to closely mimic the activity of TG neurons *in vivo*. Moreover, various modulators of neuronal function are added in conjunction with the electrical activation. Changes in neurotrophin expression and release are detected and measured by customized immunoassays. The following paragraphs provide a detailed description of this approach.

DISSOCIATED CULTURES OF TRIGEMINAL GANGLION NEURONS AS A MODEL FOR STUDYING ACTIVITY-DEPENDENT PLASTICITY OF OROFACIAL SENSORY PATHWAYS

Issues, Controversies, Problems

In vitro models are commonly used in the field of neurobiology. One major reason for that is the need to take apart the complex *in vivo* network of interacting neurons in order to answer specific questions about its building blocks. Indeed, the trigeminal system is no exception, and the dissociated TG culture model has several advantages. However, one aspect of primary neuronal cultures is often underappreciated or overlooked: the role of non-neuronal cells and auto-/paracrine interactions among cultured neurons. If not considered, it can potentially lead to incorrect interpretation of data. For example, it is well established that non-neuronal cells can influence neuronal development, including expression of transmitter phenotype (Sun et al., 1994; MacPhedran and Hall, 2001) and neurite outgrowth (Bandtlow et al., 1990; De Koninck et al., 1993). Our studies show that the effect of calcitonin gene-related peptide (CGRP) on BDNF release from cultured trigeminal ganglion neurons is influenced by the presence of non-neuronal cells (Buldyrev et al., 2006). Similarly, the role of nerve growth factor (NGF) in increasing synaptophysin expression in TG neurites is obscured in the presence of non-neuronal cells (Tarsa & Balkowiec, 2009). As to the auto- and/or paracrine interactions among neurons themselves, one example would be neurotrophins released from neurons to provide trophic support. Below, we provide recommendations for both issues.

Solutions and Recommendations

In order to dissect the role of non-neuronal cells in the phenomena observed in our TG cultures, we developed a method of separating dissociated TG neurons from non-neuronal cells before plating. The method is based on the Percoll density gradient. One half of dissociated TG cells (10-12 ganglia in 0.5 ml of plating medium) is slowly layered on top of a two-layer gradient of Percoll (Sigma, St. Louis, MO, USA; 35%-60%; 1 ml each) and centrifuged for 10 minutes at 800 x *g* at 4 °C. A vast majority of non-neuronal cells and cell debris form a visible thin layer at the 'plating medium-35%' interface and, therefore, can be easily separated from neurons, which accumulate at the '35%-60%' interface. The neuron-enriched interface is collected and rinsed twice with culture medium before plating (Buldyrev et al., 2006; Tarsa & Balkowiec, 2009). The other half of dissociated TG cells is plated immediately after dissociation. The Percoll separation procedure results in the elimination of 80-90% of non-neuronal cells from TG cultures (Figure 1 A). The results of any given experimental treatment can be directly compared between the neuron-enriched and mixed cultures.

Using this approach, we showed that survival dependence of TG neurons on a specific growth factor is determined by the presence of non-neuronal cells. While NGF supports survival of neonatal TG neurons under both conditions (Figure 1 B, D), glial cell line-derived neurotrophic factor (GDNF) is effective only in neuron-enriched cultures (Figure 1 C, D). Both GDNF and NGF are known to be expressed postnatally by peripheral targets of TG neurons, including teeth (Lillesaar et al., 2001; Luukko et al., 1997; Nosrat et al., 1998).

If cultured TG neurons express neurotrophic factors, there is a possibility that these factors act in an autocrine or paracrine fashion to support neuronal survival. Thus, before moving forward with characterizing their activity-dependent expression, release

*Figure 1. (**A**) A representative example of sister cultures of dissociated postnatal day (P)0 rat TG grown in the absence (Control) or presence of 50 ng/ml NGF, and immunostained for Neurofilament 68 and 160 ($NF_{68,160}$), a pan neuronal marker, (**B**) dose-response of P0 $NF_{68,160}$-immunoreactive (IR) TG neurons grown in mixed culture to NGF, n=24 cultures per group, (**C**) total number of P0 $NF_{68,160}$-IR TG neurons grown in mixed culture in the absence (Control) or presence of 50 ng/ml of BDNF (n=23), GDNF (n=12), CNTF (n=12) or LIF (n=23), (**D**) total number of P0 $NF_{68,160}$-IR TG neurons grown in neuron-enriched culture in the absence (Control), or presence of 50 ng/ml of GDNF or NGF; n=3; * $p<0.05$, ** $p<0.01$, *** $p<0.001$*

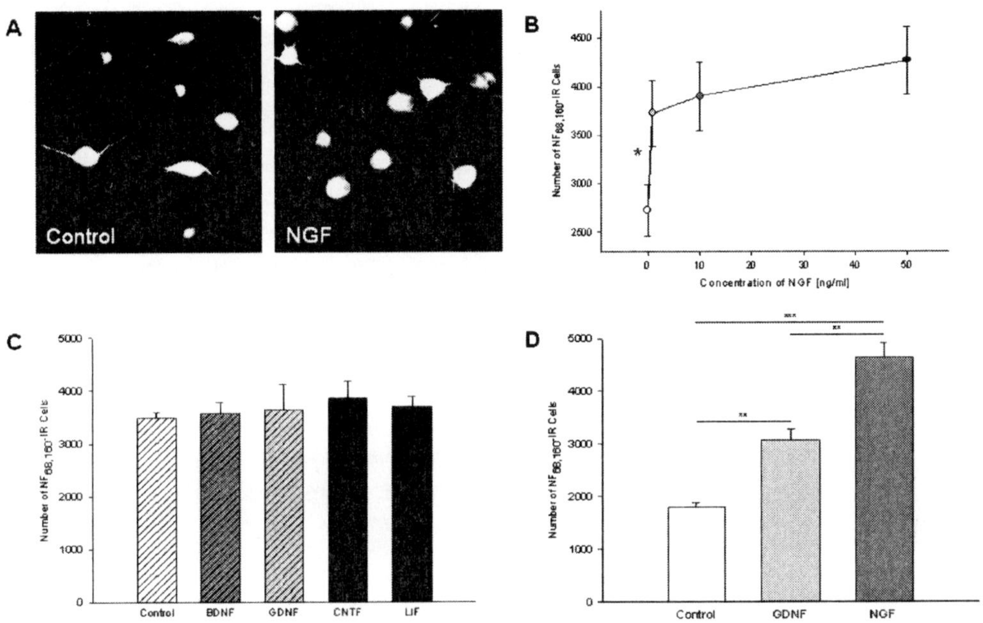

and postsynaptic effects, it is important to rule out other potential roles. The approach employed in our studies with respect to BDNF is to use TrkB-Fc, a fusion protein with BDNF scavenging properties, or anti-TrkB function-blocking antibodies (Buldyrev et al., 2006). In addition, simultaneous application of depolarizing concentrations of KCl (40-50 mM) will likely increase neuropeptide expression (through an increase in calcium influx) and, consequently, constitutive and activity-dependent release. This will enable a more pronounced cellular response to the neuropeptide under investigation. Comparing the numbers of surviving neurons (or any other cellular response) in the presence vs. absence of the scavenger or function blocking anti-receptor antibody, will determine whether the given endogenously expressed factor exerts any auto- or paracrine effect on neuronal survival.

APPLICATION OF ENZYME-LINKED IMMUNOSORBENT ASSAYS TO DETECT ACTIVITY-DEPENDENT CHANGES IN EXPRESSION AND RELEASE OF NATIVE NEUROTROPHINS AND OTHER NEUROPEPTIDES

Issues, Controversies, Problems

Analysis of release of endogenous neurotrophins from neurons has been hampered by the limited ability of conventional assays to detect the relatively small quantities of these factors released during physiological stimulation. Studies have used enzyme-linked immunosorbent assay (ELISA) to detect neurotrophin release either from tissue slices or following neurotrophin overexpression in transfected cells (Blöchl & Thoenen, 1995, 1996; Heymach et al., 1996; Krüttgen et al., 1998). It is unknown, however, if overexpressed to very high concentrations and naturally expressed, i.e. native, BDNF share the same cellular mechanisms of sorting and release. Our studies in hippocampal cultures strongly suggest that native and overexpressed BDNF do not share the same mechanisms of release. Specifically, overexpressed BDNF is shunted primarily to a potassium depolarization-sensitive release mode, which does not stimulate release of native BDNF. Therefore, to study activity-dependent expression and release of *endogenous* neurotrophin BDNF in sensory neurons, we developed ELISA *in situ*, a modification of conventional sandwich ELISA methodology. Similarly, to study activity-dependent release of the sensory neuropeptide Endomorphin-2, we made another modification to the standard ELISA protocol, termed 'rapid capture' ELISA. Both technologies are described in the following paragraphs.

Solutions and Recommendations

To study release of endogenous neurotrophins from primary sensory neurons, we use ELISA *in situ*. This technique incorporates a substrate-bound antibody against the peptide of interest into the cell culture system, so that the neurons are grown in the presence of the antibody and, as a result, the released peptide can be immediately captured for subsequent detection by colorimetric methods (Figure 2). We found that using this technique we can readily detect both constitutive and regulated release of native neurotrophins from dissociated cultures of trigeminal and other neurons (Balkowiec & Katz, 2000, 2002; Buldyrev et al., 2006; Martin et al, 2009).

For detection of the neurotrophin BDNF, a 96-well, flat-bottom ELISA plate is UV-sterilized for 10 min and coated with anti-BDNF monoclonal antibody (BDNF E_{max}™ ImmunoAssay System, Promega Corp., Madison, WI, USA) at

Figure 2. Schematic representation of the ELISA in situ methodology

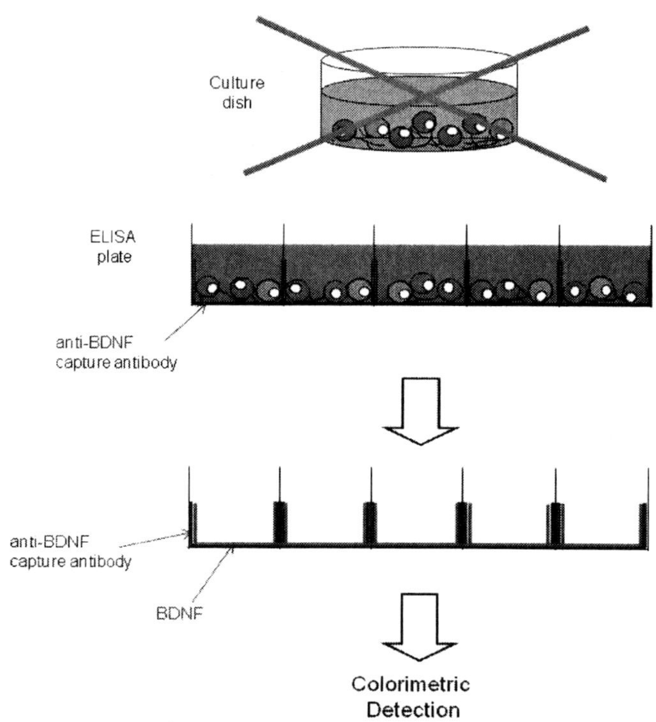

4°C for 12-18 hours. Next, the plate is washed and blocked, followed by two 1-hr incubations with culture medium to remove any residue of the ELISA washing solution. Then, neurons are plated in anti-BDNF-coated wells, and grown for 3 days, or longer (up to 14 days), under various experimental conditions in neuron-enriched or mixed cultures. Samples of recombinant BDNF at known concentrations, that are used to generate a standard curve, are diluted in the plating medium and incubated in the same plate as the cells. At the end of the culture period, the plate is extensively washed to remove all cells and cell debris, and the anti-human BDNF polyclonal antibody is applied, followed by subsequent steps according to the ELISA manufacturer's protocol (BDNF E_{max}™ ImmunoAssay System, Promega). Several modifications of the manufacturer's protocol are introduced. Namely, washing and blocking solutions used prior to cell plating are sterilized with a 0.2 μm syringe filter, and the concentrations of the anti-BDNF monoclonal, anti-human BDNF polyclonal, and anti-IgY-HRP antibodies are increased three-, two-, and twofold, respectively. Increasing the antibody concentration improves the assay's performance and compensates for losses due to prolonged incubations at 37°C. Those adjustments need to be made for each individual neuropeptide-ELISA system, and validated by linearity of the standard curve generated under the modified conditions.

Incorporation of the anti-BDNF coating antibody into the culture system dramatically increases detectability of BDNF in both naive cultures and cultures depolarized by elevated extracellular potassium (Figure 3 A). The efficacy of the *in situ* assay appears to be primarily related to rapid capture of released BDNF that prevents

*Figure 3. Incorporation of the BDNF capture antibody into the culture system dramatically increases detectability of BDNF. (**A**) Mean BDNF levels measured in sister cultures of newborn nodose ganglion primary sensory neurons grown for 72 hrs in the absence (Control, gray bars) or presence of depolarizing concentrations of potassium (40 mM; KCl, black bars); n=21; *** P<0.001, n.s., not significant, (**B**) Mean BDNF levels measured in wells containing primary sensory neurons (Cells) or culture medium without cells (Med.), to which human recombinant BDNF [500 pg/ml] was added for 72 hours (hatched bars) in the absence (Standard ELISA) or presence of anti-BDNF monoclonal capture antibody (ELISA in situ). BDNF levels were also measured in control cultures (solid gray bars), to which exogenous BDNF was not added. *** P<0.001, n.s., not significant (modified from Balkowiec & Katz, 2000).*

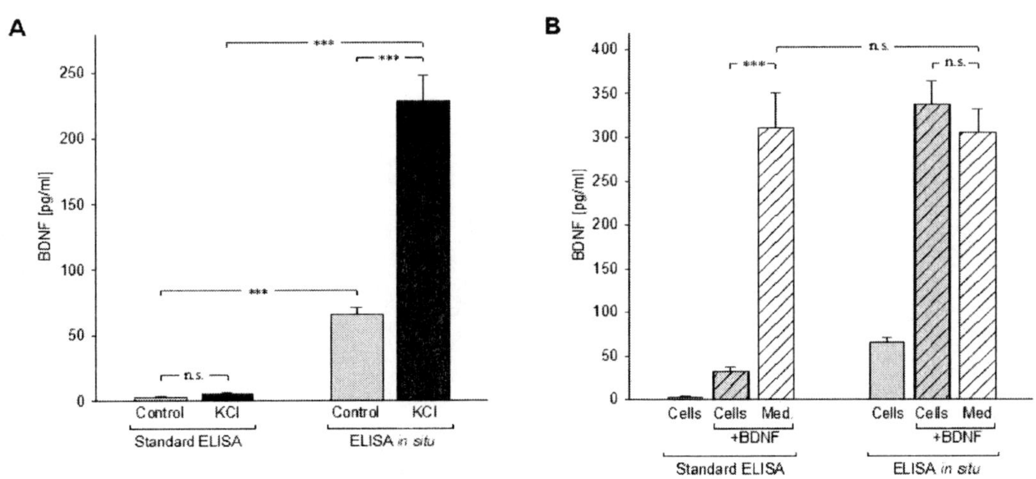

BDNF binding back to the cultured cells (Figure 3 B). The substrate-bound anti-BDNF, which is present throughout the entire culture period in the *in situ* paradigm, successfully competes with BDNF binding to TrkB on cells, thereby enhancing detectability of BDNF in culture medium. This theory is supported by our published data indicating that treatment of cultures with a function blocking anti-TrkB antibody significantly increases the ability of conventional ELISA to detect BDNF added to standard cultures, i.e. without the capture antibody (Balkowiec & Katz, 2000). However, other mechanisms of BDNF loss from standard cultures, such as binding to the culture plate, heat- and protease- mediated degradation, are also minimized under the ELISA *in situ* conditions.

Another advancement achieved in our laboratory is a parallel quantification of activity-dependent changes in expression and release of neurotrophins / neuropeptides, using ELISA *in situ*. Cells are grown in sister cultures in the presence of the neurotrophin capture antibody, as described above, and are subjected to a given experimental treatment. Following the treatment, culture wells designated for quantification of the protein cell content (expression) undergo sonication with a microprobe to disrupt cell membranes and free-up the neurotrophin. Sonication (three 5-sec rounds at 2W; Sonicator 3000, Misonix, Inc., Farmingdale, NY, USA) is performed in the presence of proteinase inhibitors (10 μM aprotinin and 100 μM leupeptin). The cell lysate is then incubated for 2 hours in the same well to allow neurotrophin binding to the capture antibody, followed by rinsing the plate and continuing with the protocol described above for release studies. This approach provides additional very useful, if not critical, data by simultaneously evaluating the cellular levels of a given protein and the rate of its release from neurons.

Particularly relevant to the field of oral medicine, and specifically orofacial pain, is our most recent application of the ELISA approach to examining effects of various inflammatory mediators on levels of BDNF expression and release in TG neurons. Using our methods, we are able to detect changes in BDNF expression levels in response to treatments with various inflammatory mediators, such as pro-inflammatory cytokines Interleukin-1β and Interleukin-6, known to play a critical role in tooth pulp inflammation (Figure 4).

Figure 4. Mean levels of cellular BDNF expression measured in newborn trigeminal ganglion neurons grown in dissociated cultures and treated for 24 hours with various concentrations of Interleukin-1β

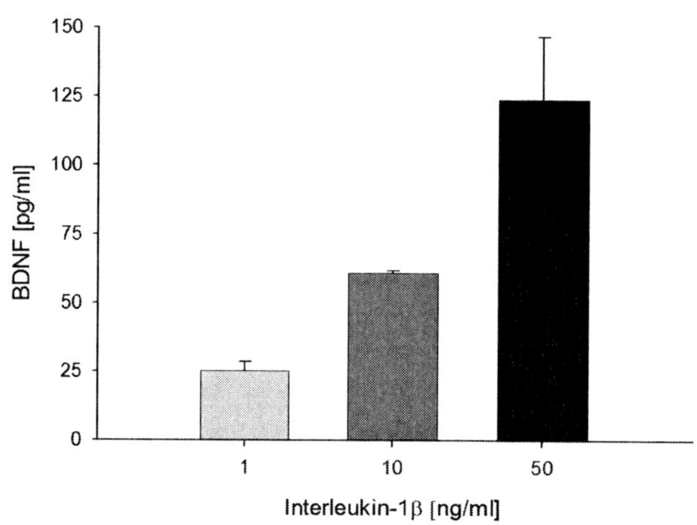

Intriguingly, we also observe interactions among different cytokines in their effects on levels of BDNF expression. Studies underway are directed towards understanding the molecular mechanisms and physiological significance of the observed interactions.

Neuroinflammation is widely considered an underlying mechanism of a range of pathologies beyond those associated with TG nociceptors. The most prominent examples include autoimmune demyelinating diseases, such as multiple sclerosis and Guillain-Barré syndrome, and neurodegenerative diseases, such as Alzheimer's and Parkinson's disease (Balkowiec-Iskra et al., 2003, 2007a, 2007b; Kurkowska-Jastrzebska et al., 2005, 2009). Thus, the methods developed in our laboratory for TG and other primary sensory neurons can be easily adopted by other fields of neuroscience.

Since the establishment of ELISA *in situ* for examining regulation of neurotrophic factors, we have developed several related approaches to studying release of other low-abundance neuropeptides. One of them is the 'rapid capture' ELISA methodology for detection of the endogenous opioid Endomorphin-2 (END-2; Scanlin et al., 2008). In this variant of a competitive sandwich ELISA, the soluble capture antibody (anti-END-2 polyclonal; at twice the concentration recommended for the conventional assay) is added directly to cultured neurons at the beginning of stimulation. END-2 standards are prepared in HEPES-buffered physiological saline containing anti-END-2 polyclonal antibody, and incubated in the same culture plate for the duration of stimulation. At the end of the stimulation period, experimental samples and standards are transferred to the ELISA plate, and anti-END-2 polyclonal antibody with biotinylated END-2 is applied, followed by subsequent detection steps of the competitive sandwich ELISA. Similar to ELISA *in situ*, the immediate access of END-2 to its antibody outcompetes receptor binding and/or degradation of this neuropeptide. In support, the conventional assay is effective at reliably detecting END-2 only when the cells are pretreated with a μ-opioid receptor antagonist (Scanlin et al., 2008).

The modified ELISA protocols are sufficiently sensitive to detect differences in neurotrophin and other neuropeptide expression and release in response to short-term electrical field stimulation with different physiologically-relevant patterns. Several examples are given in the next section.

ELECTRICAL FIELD STIMULATION AS THE METHOD OF CHOICE FOR EXAMINING ACTIVITY-DEPENDENT REGULATION OF NEUROTROPHINS AND OTHER NEUROPEPTIDES

Issues, Controversies, Problems

Most studies of activity-dependent regulation of neurotrophin expression and release have stimulated cells using agents causing continuous membrane depolarization, such as elevated extracellular potassium, veratridine or glutamate receptor agonists (Ghosh et al., 1994; Blöchl and Thoenen, 1995; Heymach et al., 1996; Griesbeck et al., 1999; Canossa et al., 2001). However, studies of other peptide transmitter systems, such as neuropeptide Y, all indicate that the pattern of nerve impulses is critical for coding peptide release (Lundberg et al., 1989; Whim and Lloyd, 1994). Moreover, Hartmann et al. (2001) found that cellular mechanisms of BDNF-GFP release from hippocampal neurons evoked by high-frequency presynaptic stimulation differ from those evoked by chronic depolarization with high potassium. In addition, there is evidence that patterned electrical stimuli and chronic depolarization induce neuronal gene expression *via* distinct signaling pathways, involving different voltage-activated calcium channel subtypes and intracellular protein kinases (Brosenitsch and Katz, 2001).

Over the past decade, we have been optimizing a setup for electrical field stimulation of dissociated primary sensory neurons for studies of neurotrophin and other neuropeptide expression and release in response to transient, repetitive stimuli that closely resemble patterns of nerve activity *in vivo*. The following paragraphs describe our progress in this area, and presents advantages of the patterned electrical stimulation approach specifically for studies of orofacial pain.

Solutions and Recommendations

To study activity-dependent changes in expression and release of endogenous neurotrophins and other neuropeptides, we use electrical field stimulation of dissociate cultures of primary sensory neurons grown in 96-well, flat bottom ELISA plates (for ELISA *in situ* studies of protein expression and release, as described in the previous section) or in 48-well tissue culture-treated plates (for quantitative RT-PCR analysis of mRNA levels).

Following an initial incubation, dissociated sensory ganglion cultures (neuron-enriched or mixed) are stimulated in culture wells fitted with paired platinum or Ag/AgCl electrodes (0.2-0.25 mm wire diameter; one pair per well), connected in parallel (four wells per set; Figure 5 A) to one of four independent outputs of the stimulator (MultiStim System; Digitimer; Welwyn Garden City, Hertfordshire, UK). The stimulation pattern delivered by each of the outputs is controlled by the 8-channel programmable pulse generator Master-8-cp (AMPI, Jerusalem, Israel). Four additional wells are also fitted with pairs of electrodes, but are not connected to the stimulator and serve as no-stimulation controls (Fig. 5B). The culture plate is returned to the incubator, and cultures are stimulated with biphasic rectangular pulses of 0.2-0.5 ms duration and amplitude of 80-120 mA applied across each well, delivered at various patterns (Buldyrev et al., 2006; Scanlin et al., 2008; Martin et al, 2009).

*Figure 5. Schematic representation of the setup for electrical field stimulation and immunodetection of activity-dependent changes in BDNF expression and release in dissociated cultures of primary sensory neurons. (**A**) Stimulating electrode fitting in four adjacent wells of a 96-well ELISA plate, (**B**) The bird eye view of the plate fitted with stimulation electrodes. Row B represents four wells of unstimulated controls, whereas each of rows C-F is connected to one channel of the stimulator. Vertically fading color intensities in columns 11 and 12 represent decreasing concentrations of BDNF in the standard curve generated for each plate.*

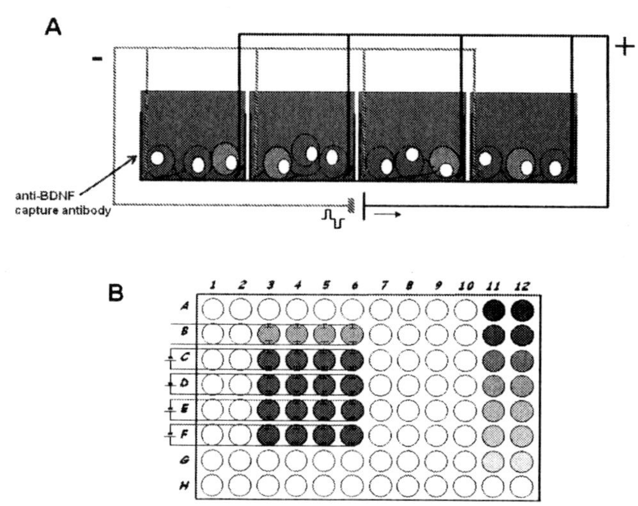

Using this approach, we previously showed that patterned electrical stimulation is strikingly more effective than continuous KCl-depolarization in releasing native BDNF from primary sensory and hippocampal neurons (Balkowiec and Katz, 2000, 2002). Moreover, the magnitude of BDNF release is regulated by frequency and pattern of stimulation (Balkowiec and Katz, 2000, 2002; Lever et al., 2001; Gärtner and Staiger, 2002; Buldyrev et al., 2006; Martin et al, 2009). These data suggest that, rather than depolarization per se, activation of specific signaling pathways by patterned stimulation is required to evoke BDNF release.

Our more recent results further underscore the importance of applying electrical stimulation, as compared to chronic depolarization, in dissecting cellular and molecular mechanisms of neuropeptide regulation in neurons. These studies reveal novel, previously undefined, mechanisms of activity-dependent regulation of neurotrophin and other neuropeptide expression and release. For example, in the area of mRNA regulation, we observe a pattern-dependent activation of specific gene promoters in primary sensory neurons. Another example comes from studies in which electrical field stimulation acts synergistically with calcitonin gene-related peptide (CGRP) to increase BDNF release from trigeminal ganglion (TG) neurons. We find that CGRP applied in the presence of patterned electrical stimulation leads to a dramatic potentiation of BDNF release from TG neurons, compared to either method of stimulating BDNF release applied separately (Figure 6). These data suggest that electrical stimulation may increase the pool of BDNF available for release, or act to bring functional CGRP receptors to the cell surface. Intriguingly, the potentiating effect is dependent on the stimulation pattern, such that the potentiation takes place in the presence of bursting (3 pulses at 5 Hz every 3 sec; average frequency of 1 Hz), but not tonic (1 Hz), stimulation.

Our recent studies related to mechanisms of orofacial pain in the context of neuroinflammation employ a simultaneous application of electrical field stimulation of dissociated TG neurons and various inflammatory mediators. Similar to the effects of CGRP, our data point to a crosstalk between the electrical and chemical stimuli that affects regulation of BDNF expression in neurons. In the presented example, electrical field stimulation with stimulus amplitudes significantly below

Figure 6. Low-frequency (1 Hz) electrical field stimulation significantly strengthens the effect of 100 nM CGRP on BDNF release from newborn rat TG neurons in vitro. Quantities of BDNF release have been normalized to the level of BDNF released in cultures treated with 100 nM CGRP alone.

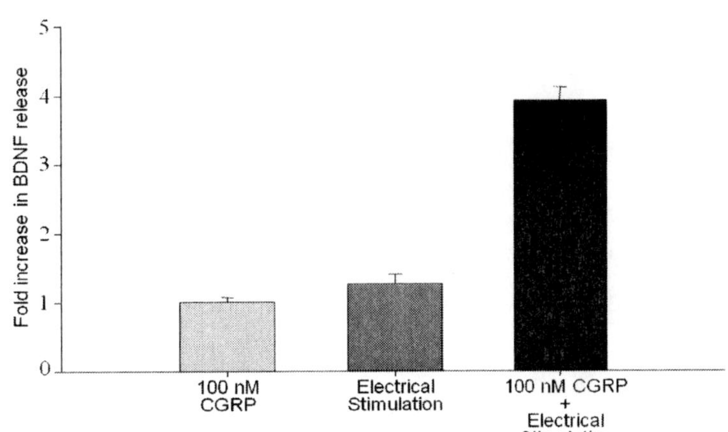

Figure 7. Low-frequency, subthreshold electrical field stimulation (1 Hz, 25 mA per well) potentiates the effect of Interleukin-1β (10 ng/ml) on BDNF expression in newborn rat TG neurons in vitro

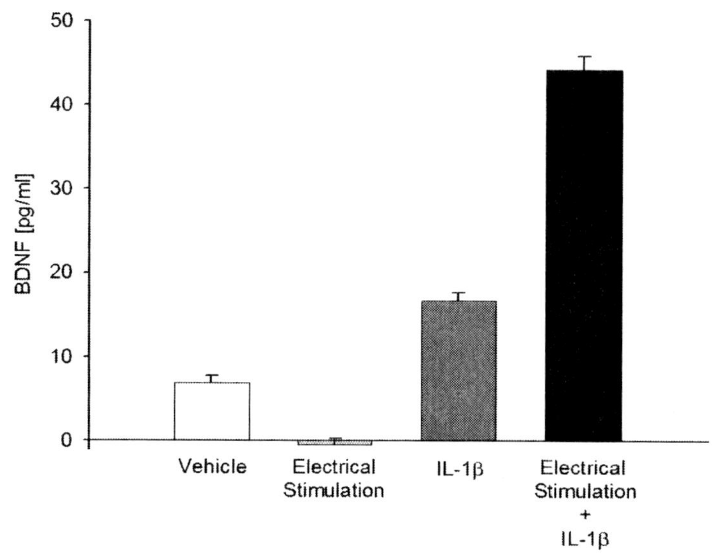

the threshold for upregulation of BDNF expression (25 mA per well) dramatically strengthens the effect of Interleukin-1β (Figure 7).

Those are potentially very important findings with implications for understanding and treatment of common orofacial pain conditions, such as trigeminal neuralgia, TMJ disorder, and migraine headaches, but also other disorders of the nervous system that involve a neuroinflammatory process.

FUTURE RESEARCH DIRECTIONS

The results presented in this chapter point to the role of neuronal activity patterns as a critical component in the final outcome of neurotrophin and other neuropeptide regulation in neurons. Many aspects of the regulation still remain to be uncovered: from currently unidentified auto- or paracrine factors acting in concert with neuronal activity to specific intracellular sites and signaling pathways. Electrical field stimulation opens up enormous opportunities for the in-depth exploration of the physiological significance behind the multitude of patterns experienced by each neuron, both in the peripheral and central nervous system. The frequency-dependence of BDNF release from TG neurons is just a tip of the iceberg of information processing in the system. As demonstrated here using Endomorphin-2 as an example, other neuropeptides and neuromodulators can also be examined using the same or similar approaches. It is the authors' hope that the methods presented in this chapter will aid diagnostic technologies employed to address current challenges of oral medicine.

CONCLUSION

We have shared here our research models that provide new opportunities for defining physiological mechanisms of neurotrophin and other neuropeptide expression and release in neuronal systems, with the overarching goal of a better understanding of their roles in synaptic development and function. We have also identified several areas of research that are likely to be advanced more swiftly with application of the described methodologies. These research areas are likely to prove most critical in understanding and solving current challenges faced by oral medicine, and specifically trigeminal pain issues. Finally, the research approaches presented in this chapter, such as neuronal stimulation combined with inflammatory mediators, will likely be applicable not only to the field of oral medicine, but also other areas of neurobiology concerned with understanding the pathophysiology of neurological disorders, such as multiple sclerosis, Alzheimer's and Parkinson's disease, for which neuroinflammation is thought to be an underlying mechanism.

REFERENCES

Balkowiec, A., & Katz, D. M. (2000). Activity-dependent release of endogenous brain-derived neurotrophic factor from primary sensory neurons detected by ELISA in situ. *The Journal of Neuroscience*, *20*, 7417–7423.

Balkowiec, A., & Katz, D. M. (2002). Cellular mechanisms regulating activity-dependent release of native brain-derived neurotrophic factor from hippocampal neurons. *The Journal of Neuroscience*, *22*, 10399–10407.

Balkowiec-Iskra, E., Kurkowska-Jastrzebska, I., Joniec, I., Ciesielska, A., Czlonkowska, A., & Czlonkowski, A. (2007a). Dopamine, serotonin and noradrenaline changes in the striatum of C57BL mice following myelin oligodendrocyte glycoprotein (MOG) 35-55 and complete Freund adjuvant (CFA) administration. *Acta Neurobiologiae Experimentalis*, *67*, 379–388.

Balkowiec-Iskra, E., Kurkowska-Jastrzebska, I., Joniec, I., Ciesielska, A., Muszynska, A., & Przybylkowski, A. (2007b). MPTP-induced central dopamine depletion exacerbates experimental autoimmune encephalomyelitis (EAE) in C57BL mice. *Inflammation Research*, *56*, 311–317. doi:10.1007/s00011-007-6128-0

Balkowiec-Iskra, E., Kurkowska-Jastrzebska, I., Joniec, I., Czlonkowska, A., & Czlonkowski, A. (2003). Post intoxicative therapeutic immunization with myelin oligodendrocyte glycoproteine (MOG 35-55) suppresses spontaneous regeneration of dopaminergic neurons injured with 1-methyl-4 phenyl-1,2,3,6-tetrahydropiridine (MPTP). *Acta Neurobiologiae Experimentalis*, *63*, 109–115.

Bandtlow, C., Zachleder, T., & Schwab, M. E. (1990). Oligodendrocytes arrest neurite growth by contact inhibition. *The Journal of Neuroscience*, *10*, 3837–3848.

Blöchl, A., & Thoenen, H. (1995). Characterization of nerve growth factor (NGF) release from hippocampal neurons: evidence for a constitutive and an unconventional sodium-dependent regulated pathway. *The European Journal of Neuroscience*, *7*, 1220–1228. doi:10.1111/j.1460-9568.1995.tb01112.x

Blöchl, A., & Thoenen, H. (1996). Localization of cellular storage compartments and sites of constitutive and activity-dependent release of nerve growth factor (NGF) in primary cultures of hippocampal neurons. *Molecular and Cellular Neurosciences*, *7*, 173–190. doi:10.1006/mcne.1996.0014

Brosenitsch, T. A., & Katz, D. M. (2001). Physiological patterns of electrical stimulation can induce neuronal gene expression by activating N-type calcium channels. *The Journal of Neuroscience*, *21*, 2571–2579.

Buldyrev, I., Tanner, N. M., Hsieh, H. Y., Dodd, E. G., Nguyen, L. T., & Balkowiec, A. (2006). Calcitonin gene-related peptide enhances release of native brain-derived neurotrophic factor from trigeminal ganglion neurons. *Journal of Neurochemistry, 99*, 1338–1350. doi:10.1111/j.1471-4159.2006.04161.x

Canossa, M., Gartner, A., Campana, G., Inagaki, N., & Thoenen, H. (2001). Regulated secretion of neurotrophins by metabotropic glutamate group I (mGluRI) and Trk receptor activation is mediated via phospholipase C signalling pathways. *The EMBO Journal, 20*, 1640–1650. doi:10.1093/emboj/20.7.1640

Davies, A. M. (1988). The trigeminal system: an advantageous experimental model for studying neuronal development. *Development, 103*(Supplement), 175–183.

Davies, A. M. (1997). Studies of neurotrophin biology in the developing trigeminal system. *Journal of Anatomy, 191*, 483–491. doi:10.1046/j.1469-7580.1997.19140483.x

De Koninck, P., Carbonetto, S., & Cooper, E. (1993). NGF induces neonatal rat sensory neurons to extend dendrites in culture after removal of satellite cells. *The Journal of Neuroscience, 13*, 577–585.

Gärtner, A., & Staiger, V. (2002). Neurotrophin secretion from hippocampal neurons evoked by long-term-potentiation-inducing electrical stimulation patterns. *Proceedings of the National Academy of Sciences of the United States of America, 99*, 6386–6391. doi:10.1073/pnas.092129699

Ghosh, A., Carnahan, J., & Greenberg, M. E. (1994). Requirement for BDNF in activity-dependent survival of cortical neurons. *Science, 263*, 1618–1623. doi:10.1126/science.7907431

Griesbeck, O., Canossa, M., Campana, G., Gärtner, A., Hoener, M. C., & Nawa, H. (1999). Are there differences between the secretion characteristics of NGF and BDNF? Implications for the modulatory role of neurotrophins in activity-dependent neuronal plasticity. *Microscopy Research and Technique, 45*, 262–275. doi:10.1002/(SICI)1097-0029(19990515/01)45:4/5<262::AID-JEMT10>3.0.CO;2-K

Hartmann, M., Heumann, R., & Lessmann, V. (2001). Synaptic secretion of BDNF after high-frequency stimulation of glutamatergic synapses. *The EMBO Journal, 20*, 5887–5897. doi:10.1093/emboj/20.21.5887

Heymach, J. V., Krüttgen, A., Suter, U., & Shooter, E. M. (1996). The regulated secretion and vectorial targeting of neurotrophins in neuroendocrine and epithelial cells. *The Journal of Biological Chemistry, 271*, 25430–25437. doi:10.1074/jbc.271.41.25430

Ichikawa, H., Yabuuchi, T., Jin, H. W., Terayama, R., Yamaai, T., & Deguchi, T. (2006). Brain-derived neurotrophic factor-immunoreactive primary sensory neurons in the rat trigeminal ganglion and trigeminal sensory nuclei. *Brain Research, 1081*, 113–118. doi:10.1016/j.brainres.2006.01.027

Krüttgen, A., Möller, J. C., Heymach, J. V., & Shooter, E. M. (1998). Neurotrophins induce release of neurotrophins by the regulated secretory pathway. *Proceedings of the National Academy of Sciences of the United States of America, 95*, 9614–9619. doi:10.1073/pnas.95.16.9614

Kurkowska-Jastrzebska, I., Balkowiec-Iskra, E., Ciesielska, A., Joniec, I., Cudna, A., Zaremba, M. M., et al. (2009). Decreased inflammation and augmented expression of trophic factors correlate with MOG-induced neuroprotection of the injured nigrostriatal system in the murine MPTP model of Parkinson's disease. *International Immunopharmacology*.

Kurkowska-Jastrzebska, I., Balkowiec-Iskra, E., Joniec, I., Litwin, T., Czlonkowski, A., & Czlonkowska, A. (2005). Immunization with myelin oligodendrocyte glycoprotein and complete Freund adjuvant partially protects dopaminergic neurons from 1-methyl-4-phenyl-1,2,3,6-tetrahydropyridine-induced damage in mouse model of Parkinson's disease. *Neuroscience*, *131*, 247–254. doi:10.1016/j.neuroscience.2004.10.027

Lever, I. J., Bradbury, E. J., Cunningham, J. R., Adelson, D. W., Jones, M. G., & McMahon, S. B. (2001). Brain-derived neurotrophic factor is released in the dorsal horn by distinctive patterns of afferent fiber stimulation. *The Journal of Neuroscience*, *21*, 4469–4477.

Lillesaar, C., Eriksson, C., & Fried, K. (2001). Rat tooth pulp cells elicit neurite growth from trigeminal neurones and express mRNAs for neurotrophic factors in vitro. *Neuroscience Letters*, *308*, 161–164. doi:10.1016/S0304-3940(01)01997-8

Lundberg, J. M., Rudehill, A., Sollevi, A., Fried, G., & Wallin, G. (1989). Co-release of neuropeptide Y and noradrenaline from pig spleen *in vivo*: importance of subcellular storage, nerve impulse frequency and pattern, feedback regulation and resupply by axonal transport. *Neuroscience*, *28*, 475–486. doi:10.1016/0306-4522(89)90193-0

Luukko, K., Suvanto, P., Saarma, M., & Thesleff, I. (1997). Expression of GDNF and its receptors in developing tooth is developmentally regulated and suggests multiple roles in innervation and organogenesis. *Developmental Dynamics*, *210*, 463–471. doi:10.1002/(SICI)1097-0177(199712)210:4<463::AID-AJA9>3.0.CO;2-E

MacPhedran, S. E., & Hall, A. K. (2001). Influence of non-neuronal cells on establishment of neuropeptide Y expression by sympathetic neurons in vitro. *Developmental Neuroscience*, *23*, 307–317. doi:10.1159/000048714

Martin, J. L., Jenkins, V. K., Hsieh, H.-Y., & Balkowiec, A. (2009). Brain-derived neurotrophic factor in arterial baroreceptor pathways: Implications for activity-dependent plasticity at baroafferent synapses. *Journal of Neurochemistry*, *108*, 450–464. doi:10.1111/j.1471-4159.2008.05781.x

Nosrat, C. A., Fried, K., Ebendal, T., & Olson, L. (1998). NGF, BDNF, NT3, NT4 and GDNF in tooth development. *European Journal of Oral Sciences*, *106*(Supplement 1), 94–99.

Scanlin, H. L., Carroll, E. A., Jenkins, V. K., & Balkowiec, A. (2008). Endomorphin-2 is released from newborn rat primary sensory neurons in a frequency- and calcium-dependent manner. *The European Journal of Neuroscience*, *27*, 2629–2642. doi:10.1111/j.1460-9568.2008.06238.x

Sun, Y., Rao, M. S., Zigmond, R. E., & Landis, S. C. (1994). Regulation of vasoactive intestinal peptide expression in sympathetic neurons in culture and after axotomy: the role of cholinergic differentiation factor/leukemia inhibitory factor. *Journal of Neurobiology*, *25*, 415–430. doi:10.1002/neu.480250407

Tarsa, L., & Balkowiec, A. (2009). Nerve growth factor regulates synaptophysin expression in developing trigeminal ganglion neurons *in vitro*. *Neuropeptides*, *43*, 47–52. doi:10.1016/j.npep.2008.09.009

Whim, M. D., & Lloyd, P. E. (1994). Differential regulation of the release of the same peptide transmitters from individual identified motor neurons in culture. *The Journal of Neuroscience*, *14*, 4244–4251.

ADDITIONAL READING

Bolay, H., Reuter, U., Dunn, A. K., Huang, Z., Boas, D. A., & Moskowitz, M. A. (2002). Intrinsic brain activity triggers trigeminal meningeal afferents in a migraine model. *Nature Medicine*, *8*, 136–142. doi:10.1038/nm0202-136

Brain, S. D., & Cox, H. M. (2006). Neuropeptides and their receptors: innovative science providing novel therapeutic targets. *British Journal of Pharmacology*, *147*(Supplement 1), S202–S211. doi:10.1038/sj.bjp.0706461

Buonanno, A., & Fields, R. D. (1999). Gene regulation by patterned electrical activity during neural and skeletal muscle development. *Current Opinion in Neurobiology*, *9*, 110–120. doi:10.1016/S0959-4388(99)80014-2

Durham, P. L., & Russo, A. F. (1999). Regulation of calcitonin gene-related peptide secretion by a serotonergic antimigraine drug. *The Journal of Neuroscience*, *19*, 3423–3429.

Eckert, S. P., Taddese, A., & McCleskey, E. W. (1997). Isolation and culture of rat sensory neurons having distinct sensory modalities. *Journal of Neuroscience Methods*, *77*, 183–190. doi:10.1016/S0165-0270(97)00125-8

Goadsby, P. J. (2005). New targets in the acute treatment of headache. *Current Opinion in Neurology*, *18*, 283–288. doi:10.1097/01.wco.0000169746.60029.e5

Kerr, B. J., Bradbury, E. J., Bennett, D. L., Trivedi, P. M., Dassan, P., & French, J. (1999). Brain-derived neurotrophic factor modulates nociceptive sensory inputs and NMDA-evoked responses in the rat spinal cord. *The Journal of Neuroscience*, *19*, 5138–5148.

Lazarov, N. E. (2002). Comparative analysis of the chemical neuroanatomy of the mammalian trigeminal ganglion and mesencephalic trigeminal nucleus. *Progress in Neurobiology*, *66*, 19–59. doi:10.1016/S0301-0082(01)00021-1

Lessmann, V., Gottmann, K., & Malcangio, M. (2003). Neurotrophin secretion: current facts and future prospects. *Progress in Neurobiology*, *69*, 341–374. doi:10.1016/S0301-0082(03)00019-4

Malcangio, M. (2003). GDNF and somatostatin in sensory neurones. *Current Opinion in Pharmacology*, *3*, 41–45. doi:10.1016/S1471-4892(02)00007-3

Malcangio, M., & Lessmann, V. (2003). A common thread for pain and memory synapses? Brain-derived neurotrophic factor and trkB receptors. *Trends in Pharmacological Sciences*, *24*, 116–121. doi:10.1016/S0165-6147(03)00025-7

Mannion, R. J., Costigan, M., Decosterd, I., Amaya, F., Ma, Q. P., & Holstege, J. C. (1999). Neurotrophins: peripherally and centrally acting modulators of tactile stimulus-induced inflammatory pain hypersensitivity. *Proceedings of the National Academy of Sciences of the United States of America*, *96*, 9385–9390. doi:10.1073/pnas.96.16.9385

Mendell, L. M., Albers, K. M., & Davis, B. M. (1999). Neurotrophins, nociceptors, and pain. *Microscopy Research and Technique*, *45*, 252–261. doi:10.1002/(SICI)1097-0029(19990515/01)45:4/5<252::AID-JEMT9>3.0.CO;2-N

Pezet, S., Malcangio, M., & McMahon, S. B. (2002). BDNF: a neuromodulator in nociceptive pathways? *Brain Research. Brain Research Reviews*, *40*, 240–249. doi:10.1016/S0165-0173(02)00206-0

Poo, M. M. (2001). Neurotrophins as synaptic modulators. *Nature Reviews. Neuroscience*, *2*, 24–32. doi:10.1038/35049004

Ren, K., & Dubner, R. (1999). Central nervous system plasticity and persistent pain. *Journal of Orofacial Pain, 13*, 155–163.

Samsam, M., Covenas, R., Ahangari, R., Yajeya, J., Narvaez, J. A., & Tramu, G. (2000). Simultaneous depletion of neurokinin A, substance P and calcitonin gene-related peptide from the caudal trigeminal nucleus of the rat during electrical stimulation of the trigeminal ganglion. *Pain, 84*, 389–395. doi:10.1016/S0304-3959(99)00240-7

Samsam, M., Covenas, R., Csillik, B., Ahangari, R., Yajeya, J., & Riquelme, R. (2001). Depletion of substance P, neurokinin A and calcitonin gene-related peptide from the contralateral and ipsilateral caudal trigeminal nucleus following unilateral electrical stimulation of the trigeminal ganglion; a possible neurophysiological and neuroanatomical link to generalized head pain. *Journal of Chemical Neuroanatomy, 21*, 161–169. doi:10.1016/S0891-0618(01)00088-6

Scholz, J., & Woolf, C. J. (2002). Can we conquer pain? *Nature Neuroscience, 5*(Supplement), 1062–1067. doi:10.1038/nn942

Sessle, B. J. (2000). Acute and chronic craniofacial pain: brainstem mechanisms of nociceptive transmission and neuroplasticity, and their clinical correlates. *Critical Reviews in Oral Biology and Medicine, 11*, 57–91. doi:10.1177/10454411000110010401

Shankland, W. E. (2000). The trigeminal nerve. Part I: An over-view. *Cranio, 18*, 238–248.

Shu, X. Q., & Mendell, L. M. (1999). Neurotrophins and hyperalgesia. *Proceedings of the National Academy of Sciences of the United States of America, 96*, 7693–7696. doi:10.1073/pnas.96.14.7693

Tao, X., West, A. E., Chen, W. G., Corfas, G., & Greenberg, M. E. (2002). A calcium-responsive transcription factor, CaRF, that regulates neuronal activity-dependent expression of BDNF. *Neuron, 33*, 383–395. doi:10.1016/S0896-6273(01)00561-X

Thompson, S. W., Bennett, D. L., Kerr, B. J., Bradbury, E. J., & McMahon, S. B. (1999). Brain-derived neurotrophic factor is an endogenous modulator of nociceptive responses in the spinal cord. *Proceedings of the National Academy of Sciences of the United States of America, 96*, 7714–7718. doi:10.1073/pnas.96.14.7714

Woolf, C. J., & Salter, M. W. (2000). Neuronal plasticity: increasing the gain in pain. *Science, 288*, 1765–1769. doi:10.1126/science.288.5472.1765

KEY TERMS AND DEFINITIONS

Activity-Dependent Plasticity: A feature of neurons and neural networks characterized by the ability to change their properties in response to activation. It comprises of structural (changes in neuronal morphology) and functional (changes in excitability or responsiveness to given transmitters, etc.) components.

Brain-Derived Neurotrophic Factor (BDNF): A small peptide (molecular weight of 13.5 kD) that belongs to the family of neurotrophins and was originally described as a target-derived survival factor for developing neurons. More recent studies indicate prominent roles of BDNF in synaptic transmission and plasticity, including learning and memory, pain modulation, etc.

Electrical Field Stimulation: A method of activating excitable cells, such as neurons and muscle cells, by applying a periodically changing voltage (electrical potential difference) across the space in a vicinity of the excitable cells to allow for a flow of current through that space, which, in turn, leads to transient changes in cell membrane potential.

ELISA: Enzyme-linked immunosorbent assay; an antibody-based technique used for detection of antibodies or proteins (antigens) in liquid samples. For protein detection, samples are added to individual wells of a plate characterized by high-protein binding surfaces, on which the capture antibody has been immobilized. The 'capture antibody-protein of interest' complex is detected by another antibody (sandwich ELISA) which, in turn, is visualized by enzymatic color reaction initiated by an antibody-conjugated enzyme.

Inflammatory Mediator: A factor contributing to the immune reaction. It can either be secreted by cells of the immune system, or come from other sources (such as neurons) and influence the inflammatory response.

Neuroinflammation: An inflammatory process that affects the nervous system. It is a complex biological response of the organism to an infection or injury that involves the immune system. For sensory neurons, neuroinflammation is usually associated with increased sensitivity (i.e. sensitization) to stimuli. Neuroinflammation can also result from an autoimmune response, i.e. without any infection or injury.

Neuropeptides: Peptides that are synthesized by neurons and released at synapses to mediate or modulate synaptic transmission.

Neurotrophins: A family of neuronal growth factors that plays a crucial role in neuronal development. In mammals, it consists of four members: Nerve Growth Factor, Brain-Derived Neurotrophic Factor, Neurotrophin-3, and Neurotrophin-4/5. Neurotrophins exert their biological effects acting through trk tyrosine kinase receptors (TrkA, TrkB, and TrkC) and the low-affinity $p75^{NTR}$ receptor.

Sensory Pathways: A division of neural pathways devoted to transmission of sensory information from peripheral sensory organs (e.g. pain, temperature or touch receptors, retina of the eye, taste buds, etc.) to the brain. Sensory pathways usually consist of a chain of several nerve cells connected through synapses.

Trigeminal Ganglion: A cluster of cell bodies of neurons that transmit sensory information from sensory receptors in the head to second-order neurons in the brainstem. It is located inside the skull, near the apex of the petrous part of the temporal bone. Its name originates from the three branches of the trigeminal nerve: ophthalmic, maxillary, and mandibular, each supplying the respective region of the face.

Section 2
Informatic Tools in Oral Diagnostic Technologies

Chapter 5

Current Molecular Technologies for Assessing the Amount of Microbial Pathogens in Oral Plaque Biofilms

Hans-Peter Horz
RWTH Aachen University Hospital, Germany

Georg Conrads
RWTH Aachen University Hospital, Germany

ABSTRACT

The goal of identifying and quantifying defined oral microbial populations has gained increasing importance in clinical dentistry. Standard laboratory culture-based procedures–despite their importance for the generation of resistance profiles–are unfortunately inadequate to grow the majority of mainly anaerobic species that predominate at pathological sites, such as periodontal pockets or infected root canals. Conversely, the rapidly evolving field of nucleic-acid-based technologies is a promising approach to access the full breadth of the oral microflora. Critical to this development, however, is a proper understanding and application of the methodologies and knowledge of their limitations. In this chapter molecular tools based on real-time quantitative polymerase chain reaction (RTQ-PCR) will be described along with ways showing the computation and analysis of the datasets. RTQ-PCR allows the determination of the amount of almost any given bacterial species or the total bacterial load in oral clinical sample in a sensitive and highly reproducible way. The precise and time-efficient nature of this technique allows to run large numbers of samples and if several bacterial targets are studied in parallel to study the dynamics and potential interactions of microbial populations over space and time. This chapter will be complemented by discussing potential pitfalls that should be taken into consideration for producing proper results along with referring the reader to pertinent literature that will allow an individual deepening into the concept of molecular-based diagnosis in clinical dentistry.

DOI: 10.4018/978-1-60566-733-1.ch005

INTRODUCTION

The human body (primarily the intestinal tract and the oral cavity) harbors approximately 10^{14} microbes which exceed the number of human cells by factor 10 (Bäckhed et al., 2005). In addition, the total gene pool of the human-associated microorganisms (i.e. the human microbiome of approximately 2000 different species) is at least 100 times larger than the human genome (Turnbaugh et al., 2007). Co-evolution of humans and microbes has led to mutual interdependencies with the human body benefiting from the unique metabolic capacities of the adapted microbes. Besides providing us with nutrition and vitamins and "shaping" our immune system our microflora protects us from invasion by pathogenic species through complex competitive interactions. Conversely, the microbes are provided with a rich buffet of glycans and a protected anoxic environment. The symbiotic relationship, however, depends on the stability of the protecting microflora. Shifts in the microbial community composition can occur quite frequently leading possibly to the development of disease or at least to the predisposition for a disease. Classical examples are oral diseases, such as periodontitis and caries but also extra-oral diseases such as inflammatory bowel disease (Crohn's disease). These chronical infectious diseases can be viewed as the result of an "ecological disaster" within the microbial community (Marsh, 2003). Knowledge about the amount and kind or microbial consortia responsible for the development of disease is becoming increasingly important with the recognition that most chronical infectious diseases are polymicrobial (Brogden et al., 2004).

In recent years, recovery of sequence-based signatures of life (using the 16S rRNA gene as target) direct from natural environments and the human body have revealed an extremely high diversity of microorganisms of which at least 90% are resistant to cultivation in the laboratory and thus with as-yet unknown functions (Amann et al., 1995). Conversely, clinical microbiology continues to rely heavily upon cultivation-based methods. The strong bias toward bacteria that are amenable to cultivation is illustrated by the fact that in a 6-year period 65% of all published microbiological research focused on just 8 bacterial genera (Hugenholtz, 2002). While there is certainly no dearth of known microbial pathogens it is even so plausible to assume that the existence of pathogens is not restricted to those being best adaptive to laboratory culture conditions. In this regard it should be noted that traditional diagnostic methods applied to syndromes of suspected infectious etiology, such as pneumonia, encephalitis, lymphocyte-predominant meningitis, pericarditis, acute diarrhea, and sepsis quite frequently fail to give a microbiological explanation. Furthermore the etiology of a large list of chronic inflammatory diseases with features of infection remains poorly understood.

Hence, nucleic acid based technologies may not only help improve daily routine diagnosis in microbiology but also to screen for novel, previously unrecognized microbial pathogens. In addition - combined with principles and concepts of microbial ecology – cultivation-independent approaches will enable to better understand the beneficial effects of the endogenous microflora as well as the consequences coming along with changes from the physiological to a pathological community. In this regard oral microbiology is a multidisciplinary research field which is equally relevant to general microbiologists as well as for dentistry. Since most oral diseases are associated with pathogenic microflora (e.g. caries, periodontitis and infected root canals with necrotic pulp tissue) knowledge of the amount and types of microorganisms involved is important for the dentist in order to choose the optimal treatment therapy. For the microbiologist the oral microflora is of interest because it can be considered as a model microbial system, with which fundamental ecological principles also valid for more complex microbial ecosystems in nature can be studied.

In either case knowledge of population size and diversity of the microflora are important. In the next section the basic concept of quantifying oral microbes based on real-time quantitative PCR (RTQ-PCR) will be discussed. The following section will focus on general parameters that have to be considered when RTQ-PCR experiments are planned. The section thereafter is dedicated to a representative application along with the discussion of problems as well as possibilities to obtain reasonably interpretable results. References to pertinent literature which provides overviews of the major existing platforms, chemistries and software will be given in the text, where it is appropriate.

THE GENERAL CONCEPT OF RTQ-PCR

Background

Numerous nucleic-acid based approaches have been developed to characterize microbial communities, most of which employ the polymerase chain reaction (PCR) which has, since its development by Kary Mullis more than 20 years ago (Mullis and Faloona, 1987) become one of the most important tools in molecular diagnostics. This technique, based on in vitro replication of DNA through repetitive cycles of denaturation, primer annealing and extension steps, provides a high sensitivity and specificity for detection of gene fragments even if present in low copy numbers in clinical samples. Clinical laboratory diagnosis was one of the first fields to embrace PCR methodology, initially in form of endpoint-PCR in which product verification was performed by detection of DNA-bands of expected size by electrophoresis on agarose gels. Although this technique is still being used a major cornerstone has been the development of RTQ-PCR, which uses the kinetics of product formation for quantification of initial target amount, and - supported by sophisticated software tools - enables product verification in real-time without the need for electrophoresis. RTQ-PCR exists in a variety of modifications and underlying technology is fairly complex when dealing with every parameter in detail. For getting in depth insights into the techniques including the biochemical and genetic background the reader will be referred to specialized review articles that address distinct forms of applications. It should further be noted that for the understanding of the current chapter a minimum background in molecular biology (e.g. DNA structure, basic PCR principle and microbiology) is required since a presentation of all molecular details would go beyond the scope of this book. It should further be noted that the term RTQ-PCR should not be mixed up with RT-PCR, the latter of which is reserved for "reverse transcriptase-PCR".

Detection Strategies of Amplified Products in RTQ-PCR

In contrast to endpoint-PCR (also referred to in literature as conventional PCR) RTQ-PCR is a closed-tube methodology with continuous detection of the amplification products. Quantification is possible because kinetic information about product accumulation is collected after or during each cycling step. There exist two major RTQ-PCR approaches for measuring the increase in PCR product based on different chemistries, namely SYBR Green, and fluorescently labeled oligonucleotides, (Wittwer et al., 1997, Holland et al., 1991, Heid et al., 1996) of which so-called hydrolysis probes and hybridization probes will be described below. The RTQ-PCR technology (that is equipment including software and corresponding reagents) is commercially available by the following companies: Roche Applied Science (http://www.roche-applied-science.com/lightcycler-online/), ABI (http://www3.appliedbiosystems.com/AB_Home/index.htm), Cepheid (http://www.cepheid.com/systems-and-software/systems-overview/), Corbett Research (http://

www.corbettresearch.com/home.htm), BioRad (http://www.bio-rad.com/), Stratagene (http://www.stratagene.com/homepage/), MJ Research (http://www.mjr.com/), and Genetic Discovery Technology (http://www.biogene.com/index.cfm). Specifications for these available real-time PCR instruments, including the nucleic acid probe formats supported, excitation and detection wavelengths, maximum number of samples per run, reaction volumes, and relative thermocycling times are provided in Espy et al., 2006. The easiest and most cost-efficient way is use of the fluorescence dye SYBR Green which intercalates into double-stranded amplification products, and thus increases fluorescence emission. This method has a limited specificity, as the dye binds to all double-stranded DNA, so that false amplification products or primer-dimers which also increase fluorescence cannot be distinguished in the amplification curve. Therefore, after completion of RTQ-PCR melting curve analysis is performed for verification of the correct PCR product. By gradually increasing the temperature, the double-stranded PCR product gradually separates into single strands thus allowing measurement of the decline in fluorescence. Since denaturation is a function of PCR product size and sequence, the correct PCR Product can be identified by its characteristic melting point, generally referred to as T_m. The T_m indicates the temperature at which a given DNA fragment exists as 50% each double- and single-stranded DNA. Melting curve analysis alone may in some cases not be accurate enough to predict that the correct target has been amplified, since the T_m-value of different DNA fragments can be identical or highly similar. In case of doubt electrophoresis on an agarose-gel can give additional evidence. It should be noted here, that the problem of unspecific PCR products is a general problem attributable to any form of PCR. Primer sequence, target gene, type of clinical samples as well as the selected temperature profile for PCR are amongst the most important factors influencing the quality of the PCR reaction. A higher specificity in detecting (not generating) the correct PCR product can be achieved by use of a target specific and fluorescently labeled oligonucleotide probes. For instance, the so-called hydrolysis probe (also referred to as TaqMan-probe), usually 20- to 30 bp in size, is labeled with a 5'-terminal reporter dye and a 3'-terminal fluorescence quencher and is specific to the target in a region between the two primer-binding sites. As long as this probe does not hybridize to its target it remains intact and the quencher prevents fluorescence emission. During the extension step of the RTQ-PCR, the Taq DNA polymerase cleaves the hybridized probe by its 5'-exonuclease activity, both fluorescence dyes are physically separated, so that fluorescence emission from the reporter dye occurs and can be measured. The increased specificity of this approach is based on the rationale that the likelihood of TaqMan-probe hybridization to unspecific PCR-products is very low. Increase in fluorescence during RTQ-PCR is therefore generally directly linked to successful amplification of the correct target gene. Critical for this technique is the careful design of the TaqMan-probe. The T_m needs to be substantially high, so that the probe still binds during the extension step, which is usually performed at a temperature of 60 °C. Since separation of reporter dye from quencher is irreversible the TaqMan probe cannot be used for melting curve analysis.

Another strategy is based on use of Fluorescence resonance energy transfer (FRET) in which fluorescent labels of two (instead of one) different hybridization probes "communicate". Detection of the amplified target sequence is achieved by hybridization of these two probes in close proximity. Once having hybridized to the target the fluorescence dye at the 3'-end of the so-called donor probe (mostly labelled with fluorescein) transfers its activation energy to the acceptor dye, which then emits long-wave fluorescent light, that is measured. Hence, with increase of the amplification product the amount of hybridized probes during the PCR annealing step increases leading to an increase of measurable fluorescent light. The overall specificity of this system is even higher than with the TaqMan probe, since two probes are necessary here, decreasing the likelihood of reporting the presence of false PCR product. Again, the likelihood that two primers mis-anneal and generate a false PCR product and that this wrong product shares two specific inner hybridization sites identical to those of the correct target is highly unlikely. In contrast to hydrolysis probes, where cleavage of the probe is required, in order to obtain a signal, hybridization probes are not degraded and fluorescence is reversible. This allows melting curve analysis after the PCR run, providing additional confidence for the correctly amplified target.

A variety of further signal detection formats exist such as molecular beacons, light-up probes, sunrise primers and scorpion primers (e.g. described in Kaltenboeck and Wang, 2005). In the following we will focus on SYBR Green as the most straight-forward and cost efficient strategy. Although SYBR Green is less specific than oligonucleotide probes, the reader should bear in mind that the quality of any PCR performance depends on its primer/probe-design and the appropriate temperature profile. Even the best technique for specifically reporting the correct amplicon cannot compensate for a badly designed PCR assay. If primer dimer or other unspecific products dominate over generation of the correct PCR product accurate identification and quantification of the target microbes is hardly possible.

The Quantification of Target DNA

Although frequently misunderstood, the term "real-time PCR" does not itself imply any quantification but merely the fact that product accumulation can be monitored at the moment when the PCR reaction occurs. In order to quantify the amount of microbial DNA in patient samples control reactions with a template of known amounts (standards) have to be performed and thought must be given to the type and number of controls required. For the quantification of microorganisms most commonly an exogenous control is used, either based on a purified and/or cloned fraction of the amplicon itself. This amplicon has to be quantified by means of nucleic-acid quantification methods using for instance PicoGreen (Molecular Probes, Leiden, Netherlands). By amplifying different amounts of the quantified amplicon (for instance 10-fold dilutions) an external standard curve can be generated and the concentration of an unknown sample, which is amplified in the same PCR run but in a separate reaction tube, can be deduced from the standard curve. For quantitative analysis, the kinetic of product accumulation is the base for evaluation. As mentioned above, the amplification process is monitored either through the fluorescence of dsDNA-specific dyes (like SYBR Green) or of sequence-specific probes. Principally, each amplification curve consists of at least three distinct phases: 1) an initial lag phase in which no product accumulation can be measured, 2) an exponential phase, and 3) a plateau phase. For exact quantifications, the efficiency of the amplification reaction must be known and it is crucial that the amplification efficiencies of standards and unknowns are identical. The PCR efficiency is usually referred to as "E", with values ranging between 1 and 2, the latter of which indicating that the amount of product is exactly doubled in each PCR cycle. While this would be the ideal case, the experimental value of E usually varies between 1.5 and 1.9. Regardless of detection format (SYBR Green or probes) the amount of initial target is determined based on the number of cycles required for the fluorescence signal to exceed a certain threshold value. This threshold value (also referred to as threshold cycle = Ct or as crossing point = Cp) can be arbitrary chosen within a certain range as long as it is kept constant for all samples. One frequently used definition for the Cp is the PCR cycle in which the fluorescence signal exceeds 10 standard deviations of the mean baseline fluorescence, using data taken from cycles

3-15. Although the equipment and software provided by the manufacturer automatically calculates the efficiency based on the standard curves the user should know the underlying mathematics, which does not require an ingenious mind. The basic assumption is that at the threshold cycle the number of molecules (N_{Cp}) of the target DNA has been increased as described in the following equation:

Equation 1: $N_{Cp} = N_0 \times E^{Cp}$, with N_0 being the number of initial target molecules.

This formula can be linearized to:

Equation 2: $\log N_{Cp} = \log N_0 + Cp \times \log E$

Solving for Cp leads to *Equation 3*, which describes the linear relationship between the Cp-values determined and the log of the initial template concentration N_0.

Equation 3:
$Cp = -(\log E)^{-1} \times \log N_0 + (\log E)^{-1} \times \log N_{Cp}$

With $m = -(\log E)^{-1}$ and $b = (\log E)^{-1} \times \log N_{Cp}$, *Equation 3* can be simplified to *Equation 4*:

Equation 4: $Cp = m \log N_0 + b$

The parameters m and b of this classical linear equation can be determined by a regression analysis of the Cp-values of the standards. When solved for N_0 the equation serves as calibration curve for the calculation of the unknown samples according to *Equation 5*:

Equation 5: $N_0 = 10^{(Cp-b)/m}$

The calculation of unknowns based on external standards assumes equal and constant efficiency of all samples. This may be not the case considering that each DNA preparation may contain individual amounts of PCR inhibiting substances. Use of internal controls in every reaction tube can solve this problem. However, for clinical routing diagnostics this approach seems impractical, unless such internal controls are readily available within the reagents of the commercial RTQ-PCR kits used. In this case defined amounts of control-DNA would go into the master mix and would then be evenly distributed into the individual reacting tubes. However, technical challenges remain, since fluorescence detection of the resulting control-amplicons must not interfere with the detection of the target DNA and appropriate methods to correct for unequal PCR efficiencies across samples must be applied. Fortunately, in cases, in which relatively large levels of target DNA are present (and this is usually the case with microbial DNA from oral samples) PCR inhibition may not severely affect the accuracy of quantification. Hence, being aware of this limitation along with careful interpretation of the results should allow reasonable and useful conclusions from the data, even in the absence of internal controls.

PERFORMING RTQ-PCR

In the following paragraphs all individual steps from sample collection to preparation of genomic DNA, quantification of oral microbes will be discussed. Limitations and possible pitfalls will be addressed as they occur.

The Target Gene

Although a variety of different genes can be used for the identification of microorganisms, the most commonly target for broad-range or species-specific microbial identification is the 16S rDNA encoding for small subunit ribosomal RNA (generally referred to as 16S rRNA gene). Ribosomal RNAs are integral parts of the protein synthesis apparatus and thus present in all cellular life forms. On the one hand these molecules and their encoding genes are highly conserved among all prokaryotes (i.e. bacteria and archaea). On the other hand they contain sufficient sequence variability so that evolutionary relationships between different bacteria can be assessed. In addition, with the development of the PCR- and sequence technology and recognition of the 16S rRNA gene as outstanding phylogenetic marker gene, specific probes and primers at almost every taxonomic level have been designed and used for detection and phylogenetic characterization of known and novel human pathogens. Since then 16S rRNA gene databases (i.e. the Ribosomal Database Project [http://rdp.cme.msu.edu/] or Genbank [http://www.ncbi.nlm.nih.gov/]), have been constantly growing and becoming increasingly robust, leading in turn to an increased usefulness and attractiveness of the 16S rRNA gene. Meanwhile, numerous oligonucleotides-based test systems for different periodontal pathogens have been developed and prior to the relatively laborious attempt to design and experimentally validate own primers one should first screen the literature for the existence of primers specific to the target microorganism of interest (see paragraph: The selection of primers). As mentioned above the 16S rRNA gene is a phylogenetic marker, which means that it can be used as a chronometer to determine the evolutionary relationship of any two microbial species including those that are uncultivable. This means that 16S rRNA gene analysis enables the identification of uncultivated microbial species. As important as such cultivation-independent detection of microbes is, conclusions about the function of the species merely on the 16S rRNA gene sequence are only partially possible, because even closely related bacterial species may have dramatic physiological differences. As a promising alternative, functional genes which encode for key enzymes involved in a particular metabolic step, such as sulphate-reduction or others which lead to the production of compounds (e.g. proteases) contributing to halitosis may be used as a target. In this case broad-range primers would enable to detect a whole functional guild of different microbes that are otherwise only distantly related to each other (Vianna et al., 2008). This approach has very practical implications however, for the sake of simplicity the focus in this chapter will be on the 16S rRNA gene, which is still the "gold standard" for detecting and quantifying clinically relevant bacteria.

The Target Organisms

Depending on the clinical question that has to be answered different microbial species may be the diagnostic target, for instance *Streptococcus mutans* in caries, or *Porphyromonas gingivalis* in periodontitis or *Enterococcus faecalis* in persistent root canal infections. In these cases the higher specificity of RTQ-PCR in combination with probes would enable to better distinguish target pathogens from the numerous closely related species in the oral cavity as opposed to the SYBR Green detection formate, in which one has to rely on the mere specificity of the primers.

In some cases we might even not be interested in the amount of individual species but rather in the amount of the entire microflora at a pathological site (preferably in form of cell numbers). For instance, it is known that bacteria that have invaded in a tooth's root canal both initiate and perpetuate periapical inflammatory lesions. Thus, the principal goal of root canal treatment is to reduce the number of bacteria. Conversely, the principal cause of treatment failure is considered to be the residual bacteria in the apical part of the root canal. To evaluate the efficacy of any antimicrobial therapy it can therefore be important to determine the total number of bacteria in the root canal before and after treatment. In this case it is evident that knowledge about individual bacterial species is not very informative for the endodontic clinician. The total amount of bacteria (or the entire bacterial load) can be determined by RTQ-PCR using broad-range primers that bind at highly conserved regions of the 16S rRNA gene. The term "universal primers" frequently found in literature should be avoided, because no primer system exists that can really encompass the complete spectrum of bacteria. If we wish to know the abundance of individual bacterial species, species specific primers can be applied. But even then knowledge of the entire bacterial load is useful in order to determine the relative proportions of individual species compared to the entire community size. Such proportion may help assessing the ecological role of the species analyzed and may allow a better comparison among samples. This is, because the variability in biomass of each individual patient, in the sampling procedure, in DNA extraction and PCR efficiency, which is hardly identical between runs, may lead to biases in absolute cell numbers. However, the proportion of a single species relative to the total microbial community may be less skewed. Clearly, the choice of target organisms depends on the type of infectious disease and thus the type of clinical samples to be analyzed. Whether species, genera, divisions or the entire bacterial domain is to be quantified, numerous primer-systems have been developed and are readily available from the literature (see following paragraph)

Thc Selection of Primers

For any PCR, whether quantitative or conventional, the primer selection is not trivial. In this chapter, we discuss this problem based on broad-range primers that bind at highly conserved regions of the 16S rRNA gene. For more phylogenetically focused primers, (i.e. with intended target specificity of defined pathogenic species associated with periodontitis, oral malodor, advanced caries, and pulp inflammation or of anaerobic pathogens in general the reader is referred to the review-articles of Conrads (2002), Song (2005) and Suzuki et al., (2005), which provide a wealth of information about primer sequences, target gene and detection platforms. When studying the primary literature the reader will find quite a high number of broad-range PCR assays. A critical analysis of any article of interest (with respect to the design of the primers, their validation, and the scientific question that the article aims to address) is important. This is, because so-called universal (or broad-range) primers –also referred to as "eubacterial" primers by clinical microbiologists – do not have the potential to encompass the entire spectrum of bacteria. This is simply due to the fact that absolute conserved regions with the 16S rRNA gene although existing, are generally too short to function as primer-binding regions (Baker et al., 2003). While several PCR-based pitfalls due to cell lysis techniques or PCR conditions have well been recognized (Suzuki and Giovannoni, 1996; von Wintzingerode et al., 1997), the lack of universality of "universal" PCR primers and its consequences for routine diagnosis are generally not considered. Numerous broad-range 16S-directed primers and probes have been developed with the intention of targeting all bacteria present in clinical or environmental samples. To this end, the quality of primer assays is usually confirmed by testing representative species of a wide range of bacterial taxa. However, since it is impossible to empirically test all bacterial strains, it cannot be proven whether those PCR assays considered to be "universal" actually encompass the entire bacterial spectrum. For example, some evidence exists, that even the prominent primer pair, "27F" and "1492R" (Weisburg et al., 1991), targeting highly conserved regions of the 16S rRNA gene, is not completely universal (Frank et al., 2008). For every PCR-based bacterial diagnosis of clinical samples it is therefore crucial to know the taxa coverage of the primer systems used, since dramatic qualitative differences exist (Horz et al., 2005). It is also important to note that for RTQ-PCR the size of the amplicon must not exceed a certain value. As an optimal amplicon-size usually 150 to 300 bp are recommended, however according do our experience good results can also be obtained with amplicons with a size of up to 600 bp. Reason for this restriction in size is, that the PCR efficiency decreases with increasing amplicon size and thus reduces the accuracy of quantification. We found in our laboratory the primer system described by Nadkarni et al., (2002) which amplifies a 16S rRNA gene fragment of 466 bp valuable for quantifying oral microbes in association with periodontitis and endodontic infections. However, with ever increasing public 16S rRNA gene-databases a re-evaluation and possibly re-design of primers is possible and advisable to improve the intended target-specificity.

The Sample Collection and DNA Extraction

Specimens are taken from the regions associated with infectious disease: supragingival dental plaque with dental caries, subgingival plaque with periodontitis, carious dentine with infected pulp or chronic caries and tongue surface debris with oral malodor.

Quantification of oral bacteria is usually performed for comparative analysis. For instance, we wish to compare the entire bacterial load in infected root canals or in periodontal pockets before and after treatment. Or we wish to compare the entire bacterial load in subgingival plaque samples with analogous healthy control sites. The comparability of different samples depends on the standardized and well defined collection of the samples. Sterile paper tips are usually applied and here, knowledge about the collected liquid volume and the recovery of liquid volume from the filter tips into reaction tube is important in order to assess the amount of target-bacteria per volume (Hartroth et al., 1999).

Special care has to be taken in order to avoid contamination during sampling. In the case of endodontic specimens the surrounding area has to be properly isolated and cleaned prior to sampling. A detailed description of the sampling technique is described in Ng et al. (2003). Due to the anaerobic life style of most oral bacteria, rapid transportation into the molecular laboratory is necessary to avoid or limit cell death and subsequent degradation of free DNA.

DNA extraction strongly influences the outcome of any PCR reaction. Basic issues are efficient release of bacterial DNA (consider different cell wall properties of gramnegative and grampositive bacteria), co-extraction of PCR-inhibiting substances, accurate storage of DNA extracts (for long-term storage freezing at -70 °C is recommended, for short durations storage at 4 °C is possible). Frequent freeze-thawing procedures lead to degradation of genomic DNA and should be avoided. If samples have to be used repeatedly aliquots should be made prior to freezing.

PCR inhibiting substances co-extracted from human samples can be bile salts, complex polysaccharides in feces, heme, immunoglobulin G, and lactoferrin in blood (Kaltenboeck and Wang, 2005). The latter three substances may also be of importance when DNA-samples obtained from bleeding oral sites are analyzed. Besides these substances human DNA itself which is usually co-extracted may interfere with the detection and diagnosis of pathogens (Cadieux et al., 1993; Chen et al., 1989). Detection of pathogens might in particularly be hampered in samples in which human DNA is present in dominating concentration, such as blood, cerebrospinal fluid, or in other primary sterile sites. Problems associated with human DNA are not restricted to sterile sites but also occur when oral samples are analyzed. We have encountered this problem frequently in our lab especially in cases of low-copy targets (i.e. use of primers specific to single bacterial species which are present in low numbers). To address this problem two different extraction strategies have been developed that aim at the selective isolation of bacterial DNA from clinical specimen. These strategies are based on use of two commercially available kits MolYsis® (Molzym GmbH & Co. KG, Bremen, Germany) and Pureprove® (SIRS-Lab GmbH, Jena, Germany), both of which were originally developed to enrich bacterial DNA from blood samples. These kits can also be used for oral samples, however, according to our experiments undesired loss of bacterial DNA is currently still too high (Horz et al., 2008). Further improvement of these kits may make them more suitable for oral diagnostics in future.

Commercial DNA extraction kits are available for a variety of samples including clinical samples, such as tissue or blood. Some of the most frequently used manual kits as reported in peer reviewed publications are presented in Espy et al., 2006. Note that some kits have been developed in order to extract human DNA rather than bacterial DNA from clinical samples. In addition, those kits that were developed for extracting DNA from bacterial cells are usually based on the evaluation of selected grampositive and gramnegative pure cultures. However, diagnosis of bacteria directly from clinical specimen (i.e. culture-independent) is much more demanding and the best DNA extraction procedure and extraction kit has sometimes to be tested experimentally. In our lab we compared different extraction procedures based on chemical and mechanical lysis steps and found the following protocol as useful: Microbial DNA from subgingival plaque was extracted and purified with a Qiamp DNA Mini kit ("tissue protocol"; QIAGEN, Hilden, Germany) according to the manufacturer's instructions, with the following modification: 0.8 g of zirconia-silica beads (0.1 mm in diameter; Biospec, Bartlesville, OK) was added prior to the addition of proteinase K. Samples were then agitated in a FastPrep FP 120 instrument (Qbiogene, Carlsbad, CA) at 6.5 m/s for 45 s. All further steps followed the original protocol. In preliminary tests this protocol proved to be superior over a chemical lysis or physical lysis alone.

Pre-Conditions for Proper Application of RTQ-PCR

For reliable quantitative results the design of robust real-time PCR assays is important. This is achieved through a finely tuned mixture of reagents and thermal reaction parameters. Even minor changes in any component may change the overall efficiency of the PCR reaction. The basic chemical components are similar to conventional PCR. This includes a thermostable DNA polymerase, oligonucleotide primers, nucleotides, $MgCl_2$, KCl and Tris-HCl. Specific to RTQ-PCR assays are dsDNA-binding fluorophores (e.g. SYBR Green) or fluorescently labeled oligonucleotide probes (e.g. TaqMan probes or hybridization probes). By changing both the chemical composition as well as thermal cycling parameters real-time PCR assays can be optimized. However, we recommend the use of commercially available RTQ-PCR reaction kits, which enable PCR performance under standardized chemical conditions. Hence, chemical components cannot be altered, except for the concentration of primers and the template which are added separately into the reaction tubes. The major control tool for the user is the thermal profile in order to optimize PCR reactions. As in any scientific experiment, it is critically important to change only one parameter at a time, and to keep the overall reaction chemistry and protocol constant throughout the measurements, once established in order to guarantee comparability of different runs. Samples should be run in replicates (for instance in triplicate) in order to compensate for pipette errors and biases caused by PCR drift. If the Cp-values of the replicates are within an acceptable range (i.e. not more than half a cycle within the same run, or not more than one cycle deviation between runs) the mean value can be used for analysis. Cross-contamination of different samples has to be avoided and special care has to be taken to avoid contamination from previously generated PCR products. The risk of specimen-to-specimen contamination can only be minimized by consequent physical separation of processes, equipment and reagents. Ideally, four different work areas are suggested, one for nucleic acid extraction, one for preparation of the PCR master mix, one for adding the target DNA (template) obtained from the specimen to the PCR master mix in the reaction tubes, and lastly the amplification area where thermocycling and probe detection occurs.

DETAILED PROTOCOL

Clinical Procedures of Root-Canal Treatment

Based on RTQ-PCR we have performed an in vivo evaluation of the microbial reduction after chemo-mechanical preparation of human root canals containing necrotic pulp tissue. This assessment is useful since remaining microorganisms in the root canal are one major cause of recurring root-canal infections. The experiment described here represents only an example of how quantitative microbial data can be obtained but of course modifications of the described protocols are possible. A detailed description of the clinical background of the patients, root-canal treatment and microbiological sampling is described in Vianna et al., 2006. Briefly, selected teeth were uniradicular, asymptomatic, did not respond to sensitivity testing, had not received previous endodontic treatment and showed radiographic evidence of periapical bone loss. After comprehensive isolation and disinfection of the surrounding area an access cavity was prepared with sterile high-speed diamond burs. The samples (pre and post clinical procedures) were collected with four sterile paper points, which were consecutively placed into each canal to the total length calculated from the preoperative radiograph and then pooled in a sterile tube containing 1 ml reduced transport fluid. The samples were transported to the laboratory within 15 min for DNA extraction and subsequent RTQ-PCR analysis. Post-treated samples were generated and processed accordingly. Irrigation of the filed root canal was performed with 5 ml of 2.5% NaOCl solution. Inactivation of NaOCl was accomplished with a rinse of 5 ml of sterile 0.5% sodium thiosulphate, for 1 minute, before the post-treatment sample was taken. Finally, the teeth were filled and the access cavities were restored with 2 mm of Cavit® and resin (Z-250, 3M Dental Products, St. Paul, USA).

DNA Extraction and General Conditions for RTQ-PCR

The DNA was extracted and purified with a Qiamp DNA Mini Kit (Qiagen, Hilden, Germany) according to the manufacturer's instructions except for the modification outlined above. Using this extraction method, DNA from both grampositive and gramnegative bacteria was retrieved with no apparent discrimination against either bacterial group (Vianna et al. 2005). The DNA concentration (A_{260}) and the purity (A_{260}/A_{280}) were calculated using Gene Quant II photometer (Pharmacia Biotech, Cambridge, England).

For broad-range bacterial RTQ-PCR we chose the afore mentioned primers that were designed from highly conserved regions of the 16S rDNA by Nadkarni et al. (2002); forward primer EuF: 5'-TCCTACGGGAGGCAGCAGT-3', reverse primer EuR: 5'-GCACTACCAGGTATCTAATC-CTGTT-3', amplifying 466 bp from the 16S-region 331 to 797 (according to *E. coli* position). Amplification and detection of DNA by RTQ-PCR was performed on a Light Cycler 2.0 (Roche Applied Science, Penzberg, Germany) using LightCycler FastStart DNA Master^{plus} SYBR Green I in a total volume of 20 µl. Data acquisition and subsequent analysis was performed using LightCycler Software 4.05 (Roche Applied Science). The temperature profile for RTQ-PCR was 95°C (10 min); 40 cycles of 95°C (10 s), 60°C (10 s), and 72°C (25 s); fluorescence read was performed during each of the 40 cycles at a defined temperature of 78°C.

The amount of initial target DNA was calculated by determining the crossing point (Cp), the cycle at which the fluorescence exceeds a threshold value significantly higher than the background fluorescence. Quantification was performed using the automated (default) algorithm, a strategy that calculates the crossing point as the first maximum of the second derivative of the amplification curve. The conversion of crossing points to initial gene target molecule numbers was based on dilution series of target DNA with defined target molecules amounts as described below.

Establishment of the Standards

Genomic DNA of *F. nucleatum was* used for establishing the standard curve. Using the broad range bacterial primers PF1 5'-AGAGTTTGATC-CTGGCTCAG-3' and PR1 5'-GGCTACCTTGT-TACGACTT-3' (Edwards et al., 1989) a PCR amplicon with the size of approximately 1500 bp was generated using the temperature profile: 94°C (2 min); 33 cycles of 94°C (30 s), 55°C (30 s), and 72°C (90 s) based on conventional PCR. The resulting amplicons was purified using the QIAGEN purification kit (QIAGEN, Hilden, Germany) according to the manufacturer's instruction.

Purified PCR products were subsequently quantified with the PicoGreen dsDNA quantification kit (Molecular Probes, Leiden, Netherlands) according to the manufacturer's instruction. Nucleic acid quantification was performed with the LightCycler using the following program: Increase of temperature at a constant value of 40°C, followed by 20 cycles of a single fluorescence read for 1 s. Knowing the exact size of the amplicons and using the average molecular weight of a single DNA base pair, the measured DNA amount could then be converted to target molecule numbers per µl ($=C_S$) with the following formula: $C_S = C_W \times N_A / N \times M_N$, with C_W being the measured concentration of the amplicon in ng/µl, N the size of the amplicon in base-pairs, M_N the average molecular weight of G/C or A/T base-pair (i.e. 650 ng/nmol), and N_A the Avogadro constant (i.e. $6.022 \times 10^{23} \times 10^{-9}$/nmol). A ten-fold dilution series of this PCR product was then used as calibration standard for measuring samples with unknown content of bacteria using the universal bacterial assay primers of Nadkarni et al. (2002) for RTQ PCR.

Preparing the Master Mix

Once good quality DNA for the standards and from the unknown oral samples was obtained the RTQ-PCR reaction assay was set up. A master mix of reagents for a pre-determined number of 20 µl reactions was prepared in a PCR-workstation equipped with a UV-lamp for sterilization to reduce the risk of contamination. The number of reactions set up in the master mix should be n +1 (for n reactions), in order to guarantee that the final mixture will enable to load n capillaries with equal volume. The master mix was calculated based on the composition of a single reaction as given in Table 1. After careful mixture of the master mix a volume of 19 µl was distributed into n capillaries after which the template DNA was added individually. Detailed information of the PCR-set up is provided with the RTQ-PCR kit.

RESULTS

Figure 1 shows the result of six dilutions of the standard along with one representative endodontic sample before and after root canal treatment and one negative control (NTC), in which sterile water was added instead of a DNA template.

When fluorescence intensity is plotted against cycle number the ideal amplification curve has a sigmoidal shape. Early amplification cannot be seen because of a basic level of background fluorescence which masks the emission. Once the emission has exceeded a given signal inten-

Table 1. Chemicals used for RTQ-PCR

Reagents	Volume Σ 20µl
LightCycler FastStart DNA Master^plus SYBR Green I	4µl
Sterile water (provided by the kit	14,8µl
Forward primer	0,1µl (0.5 µM)
Reverse primer	0,1µl (0.5 µM)
Template	1µl

Figure 1. (A) Amplification curves of a dilution series containing 600 to 60,000,000 16S rRNA gene target molecules (curves with dots, 1 to 6) and of two endodontic samples before and after chemo-mechanical preparation of one root canal with necrotic pulp tissue (solid curves, S1 and S2). Note that each single amplification curve has its individual number of cycles that characterize the three PCR phases, which are for simplicity collectively shown on the right side. The reaction was monitored with SYBR Green. NTC = non-target control. (B) Standard curve constructed from the data in Figure 1 A through linear regression analysis based on the Cp-values of the standards. The slope of the line is the negative reciprocal of the log of the efficiency, which was in this case 1.838. The error of 0.0136 (which is actually 1 - r^2), indicates the goodness-of-fit of linear regression and is a measure of the extent of scattering of the points. In this example the points almost exactly lie on the regression line, which is the result of accurate dilution and pipetting of the samples.

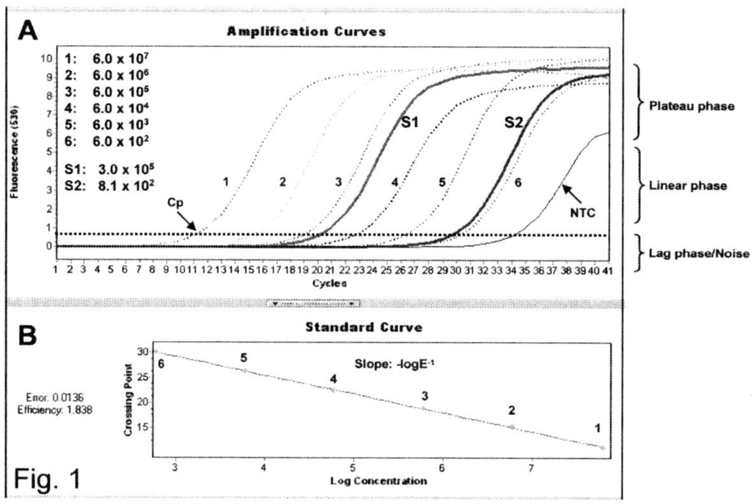

sity an exponential (or log-linear) increase in fluorescence can be measured each cycle (linear phase, Figure 1 A). During this "log"-phase the relationship between initial target amount and the amount of amplification product at any cycle can be expressed with *Equation 1* mentioned before. Eventually, primers or enzyme become limiting or end products become inhibitory to the PCR reaction, leading to the plateau phase, in which no further PCR product is formed.

After completion of the RTQ-PCR, the reactions were heated to 95°C for 0 s, and then cooled down to 65°C (15 s), a value below the expected T_m of the double stranded PCR product. During subsequent gradual reheating by 0.1°C-steps fluorescence was continuously measured until 95°C were reached. Because of denaturation of the double-stranded amplicon SYBR Green is released from the DNA resulting in a decrease in fluorescence signal (Figure 2A). The negative first derivative of the fluorescence over temperature produces a peak at the point of highest change in signal, which indicates the transition of 50% of the DNA into single strands (Figure 2 B). The congruence of the T_m of the standards and the unknowns confirms that the correct target sequence has been amplified in the clinical samples. Verification of the identity of the correct amplicon can be done by agarose-gel electrophoresis (cave: risk of contamination!) and in case of species-specific RTQ-PCR by sequencing of the amplicon. These additional control steps are usually only necessary at the beginning when a novel primer system has been tested for the first time.

In the case of a first RTQ-PCR run, the target specific T_m has to be determined before the routine RTQ-PCR runs for the actual quantification can be

Figure 2. Melting curve analysis for T_m determination and assessment of reaction specificity. For more information see body text.

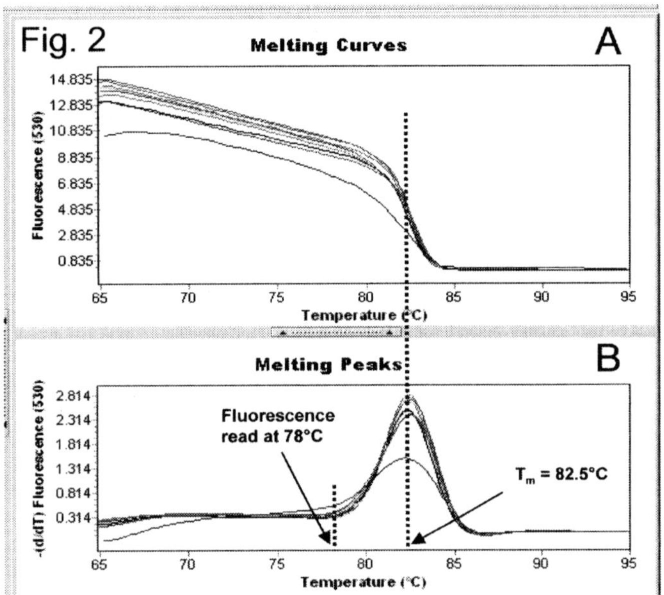

performed. This is because the ideal temperature for the fluorescence read during amplification has to be assessed which should be adjusted to a degree just below the melting point of the amplification product (i.e. in our case 78°C, Figure 2 B). With this temperature it is guaranteed that any possible primer dimers or false amplification products with a lower T_m would interfere with the quantification of the correct target.

Based on the exact amounts and Cp-values of the standards compared to the Cp-values of the clinical samples (S1=Cp: 19.93; S2=Cp: 29.54), the software automatically deduces the target-concentrations of the two unknown samples. The total amount of bacteria in the initial endodontic sample was 2.92×10^5, while after root-canal treatment this amount was reduced to 8.18×10^2 target molecules. This experiment shows that the endodontic bacterial load has been substantially reduced, namely by 99.72%. Several issues can be discussed based on this result:

Relative Versus Absolute Quantification

Since the number of 16S rRNA operons varies among bacterial taxa and can range from 1 to 15 copies depending on the species (Farelly et al., 1995) absolute values of cell numbers are difficult to assess. However, in the case of oral infections, anaerobic microorganisms dominate, which usually contain only few 16S rRNA gene copies (approximately one to four) due to the nature of their metabolism which yields relatively few energy (Klappenbach et al., 2000). Hence, 16S rRNA gene target molecules may be a reasonable approximation of the actual cell numbers of oral bacteria. However, even if we do not know the absolute values of our standards, the relative information (i.e. the ten-fold dilution steps) is sufficient information to calculate the PCR efficiency E. With knowledge of E, the percent reduction of the bacterial load can be calculated based on the subtraction of the Cp-values (ΔCp) as follows: Percent reduction = $100 - 100 \times E^{-\Delta Cp}$

$\Delta Cp = 29.54 - 19.93 = 9.61$; $100 - 100 \times 1.838^{-9.61} = 99.72\%$.

This shows that relative quantification of the bacterial load before and after clinical treatment may already allow the assessment of the efficacy of endodontic procedures.

Viability of Bacteria

One drawback of RTQ-PCR in clinical microbiology is its potential to detect not only DNA from intact bacterial cells but also from dead bacteria. While this aspect may be discussed with controversial opinion depending on the question to be answered, it should be noted that for proper root canal treatment it is not only important to kill bacteria, but also to remove cell debris (Martin 1991). Any organic remaining in the root canal can be a risk factor because it serves as substrate for viable microbes present in dentine tubules and might induce an inflammatory host response in the surrounding tissues. Some substances, such as released endotoxin (i.e. LPS) of gramnegative bacteria can even cause inflammatory reactions themselves. Thus, DNA from lysed or nonviable cells measured by RTQ-PCR could serve as a marker for remaining cell debris in the root canal.

Background Contamination

As can be seen in Figure 1 A, the negative control (NTC) is not entirely free of bacterial DNA. This is a general problem of broad-range 16S rRNA gene targeting PCR assays, because of the ubiquity of traces of bacterial DNA in chemical reagents and aerosols. This poses in particular a problem for diagnosis of pathogens in clinical samples such as blood, in which the target concentration is usually low. In contrast, oral infections such as periodontitis and root canal infections are characterized by a high bacterial load. The above experiment shows, that even after treatment, remaining DNA-levels are ways beyond background contamination, the latter of which therefore can be considered as negligible for interpretation of the results. In addition, the closed system for amplification and detection used with RTQ-PCR reduces the risk of amplicon contamination caused by the opening and closing of reaction vessels which is problematic with conventional PCR and detection methods. Amplicon contamination is usually much stronger pronounced than mere background contamination, reducing the Cp of the NTC significantly, so that the entire RTQ-PCR run is impossible to be analyzed. Even with the closed system of RTQ-PCR, the laboratory is therefore advised to add uracil-*N*-glycosylase to the PCR mix in conjunction with the nucleotide uracil instead of thymidin (readily available with many commercial RTQ-PCR kits) which allows degradation of carry-over PCR products from previous runs, while the natural DNA template remains intact for subsequent PCR.

Interpreting RTQ-PCR Results

The experiment shown here is representative for a larger number of endodontic samples that we have monitored by RTQ-PCR in our laboratory. In no case have we observed an entire removal of bacterial cells. Parallel determination of bacterial load by cultivation and plate counting confirmed the presence of viable cells after treatment although on average recovery of bacterial cells was lower by culture analysis compared to RTQ-PCR. This underscores the higher sensitivity of RTQ-PCR (e.g. detection of uncultivable bacteria and free DNA). Apparently, for a successful endodontic treatment complete removal of bacteria may not be necessary. The question of how much trace levels are acceptable cannot be easily answered and may vary with the overall clinical situation and with several host factors, including the immune system. However, the collection of quantitative data about the amount of endodontic pathogens before and after treatment for a large number of patients will certainly help understand in future the role that the persistent endodontic microflora may play for recurring root canal infections/inflammations.

FINAL REMARKS

The assessment of the total bacterial load in clinical samples (including oral infections) by broad-range PCR will have an increasing impact on future microbiology, and one important format will be RTQ-PCR. The meaningfulness of this technology depends on the question that has to be answered, on the careful design of the experiment, and on the thorough knowledge of the limitations or the drawbacks of the methods. Since its first application, a number of early shortcomings have been corrected. However, one major remaining problem associated with RTQ-PCR whether relative or absolute is the underlying assumption that the PCR efficiency of the clinical samples is identical to standard samples. This problem can be solved by using internal standards in every reaction. This approach involves the use of internal amplification controls of known amounts in all samples. These controls are amplified simultaneously with the target DNA and are used to detect the presence of inhibitors and can be used to correct for such inhibition leading to more accurate quantification. Alternately, a dilutions series can be run on the unknown samples, which for routine applications would be impractical. In more recent attempts the quantification in RTQ-PCR has become the subject of in-depth mathematical modeling. By modeling individual samples, such approaches will allow in future an objective, highly accurate quantification due to their insensitivity to differences in PCR efficiency (Ramakers et al., 2003). Finally, the largest present limitation of RTQ-PCR may not be inherent in the technology itself but rather stem from human error: improper assay development, incorrect data analysis, or unwarranted conclusions. Therefore, as with any other technology careful experimental design, execution and analysis along with a reasonable portion of healthy skepticism will be the key for successful application of RTQ-PCR.

REFERENCES

Amann, R. I., Ludwig, W., & Schleifer, K. H. (1995). Phylogenetic identification and in situ detection of individual microbial cells without cultivation. *Microbiological Reviews*, *59*, 143–169.

Bäckhed, F., Ley, R. E., Sonnenburg, J. L., Peterson, D. A., & Gordon, J. I. (2005). Host-bacterial mutualism in the human intestine. *Science*, *307*, 1915–1920. doi:10.1126/science.1104816

Baker, G. C., Smith, J. J., & Cowan, D. A. (2003). Review and re-analysis of domain-specific 16S primers. *Journal of Microbiological Methods*, *55*, 541–555. doi:10.1016/j.mimet.2003.08.009

Brogden, K. A., Guthmiller, J. M., & Taylor, C. E. (2004). Human polymicrobial infections. *Lancet*, *365*, 253–255.

Cadieux, N., Lebel, P., & Brousseau, R. (1993). Use of a triplex polymerase chain reaction for the detection and differentiation of *Mycoplasma pneumoniae* and Mycoplasma genitalium in the presence of human DNA. *Journal of General Microbiology*, *139*, 2431–2437.

Chen, K., Neimark, H., Rumore, P., & Steinman, C. R. (1989). Broad range DNA probes for detecting and amplifying eubacterial nucleic acids. *FEMS Microbiology Letters*, *48*, 19–24. doi:10.1111/j.1574-6968.1989.tb03213.x

Conrads, G. (2002). DNA probes and primers in dental practice. *Clinical Infectious Diseases*, *35*, 72–77. doi:10.1086/341924

Edwards, U., Rogall, T., Blocker, H., Emde, M., & Bottger, E. C. (1989). Isolation and direct complete nucleotide determination of entire genes. Characterization of a gene coding for 16S ribosomal RNA. *Nucleic Acids Research*, *17*, 7843–7853. doi:10.1093/nar/17.19.7843

Espy, M. J., Uhl, J. R., Sloan, L. M., Buckwalter, S. P., Jones, M. F., & Vetter, E. A. (2006). Real-time PCR in clinical microbiology: applications for routine laboratory testing. *Clinical Microbiology Reviews*, *19*, 165–256. doi:10.1128/CMR.19.1.165-256.2006

Farrelly, V., Rainey, F. A., & Stackebrandt, E. (1995). Effect of genome size and rrn gene copy number on PCR amplification of 16S rRNA genes from a mixture of bacterial species. *Applied and Environmental Microbiology*, *61*, 2798–2801.

Frank, J. A., Reich, C. I., Sharma, S., Weisbaum, J. S., Wilson, B. A., & Olsen, G. J. (2008). Critical evaluation of two primers commonly used for amplification of bacterial 16S rRNA genes. *Applied and Environmental Microbiology*, *74*, 2461–2470. doi:10.1128/AEM.02272-07

Hartroth, B., Seyfarth, I., & Conrads, G. (1999). Sampling of periodontal pathogens by paper points: evaluation of basic parameters. *Oral Microbiology and Immunology*, *14*, 326–330. doi:10.1034/j.1399-302X.1999.140510.x

Heid, C. A., Stevens, J., Livak, K. J., & Williams, P. M. (1996). Real time quantitative PCR. *Genome Research*, *6*, 986–994. doi:10.1101/gr.6.10.986

Holland, P. M., Abramson, R. D., Watson, R., & Gelfand, D. H. (1991). Detection of specific polymerase chain reaction product by utilizing the 5'-3' exonuclease activity of Thermus aquaticus DNA polymerase. *Proceedings of the National Academy of Sciences of the United States of America*, *88*, 7276–7280. doi:10.1073/pnas.88.16.7276

Horz, H.-P., Scheer, S., Huenger, F., Vianna, M. E., & Conrads, G. (2008). Selective isolation of bacterial DNA from human clinical specimens. *Journal of Microbiological Methods*, *72*, 98–102. doi:10.1016/j.mimet.2007.10.007

Horz, H.-P., Vianna, M. E., Gomes, B. P., & Conrads, G. (2005). Evaluation of universal probes and primer sets for assessing total bacterial load in clinical samples: general implications and practical use in endodontic antimicrobial therapy. *Journal of Clinical Microbiology*, *43*, 5332–5337. doi:10.1128/JCM.43.10.5332-5337.2005

Hugenholtz, P. (2002). Exploring prokaryotic diversity in the genomic era. *Genome Biology*, *3*, 1–8. doi:10.1186/gb-2002-3-2-reviews0003

Kaltenboeck, B., & Wang, C. (2005). Advances in real-time PCR: Application to clinical laboratory diagnostics. *Advances in Clinical Chemistry*, *40*, 219–259. doi:10.1016/S0065-2423(05)40006-2

Klappenbach, J. A., Dunbar, J. M., & Schmidt, T. M. (2000). rRNA operon copy number reflects ecological strategies of bacteria. *Applied and Environmental Microbiology*, *66*, 1328–1333. doi:10.1128/AEM.66.4.1328-1333.2000

Marsh, P. D. (2003). Are dental diseases examples of ecological catastrophes? *Microbiology*, *149*, 279–294. doi:10.1099/mic.0.26082-0

Martin, H. (1991). Cleanliness, disinfection, and sterilization of the root canal. *Current Opinion in Dentistry*, *1*, 734–736.

Mullis, K. B., & Faloona, F. A. (1987). Specific synthesis of DNA in vitro via a polymerase-catalyzed chain reaction. *Methods in Enzymology*, *155*, 335–350. doi:10.1016/0076-6879(87)55023-6

Nadkarni, M. A., Martin, F. E., Jacques, N. A., & Hunter, N. (2002). Determination of bacterial load by real-time PCR using a broad-range (universal) probe and primers set. *Microbiology*, *148*, 257–266.

Ng, Y. L., Spratt, D., Sriskantharajah, S., & Gulabivala, K. (2003). Evaluation of protocols for field decontamination before bacterial sampling of root canals for contemporary microbiology techniques. *Journal of Endodontics*, *29*, 317–320. doi:10.1097/00004770-200305000-00001

Ramakers, C., Ruijter, J. M., Lekanne-Deprez, R. H., & Moorman, A. F. M. (2003). Assumption-free analysis of quantitative real-time polymerase chain reaction (PCR) data. *Neuroscience Letters*, *339*, 62–66. doi:10.1016/S0304-3940(02)01423-4

Song, Y. (2005). PCR-based diagnostics for anaerobic infections. *Anaerobe*, *11*, 79–91. doi:10.1016/j.anaerobe.2004.10.006

Suzuki, M. T., & Giovannoni, S. J. (1996). Bias caused by template annealing in the amplification of mixtures of 16S rRNA genes by PCR. *Applied and Environmental Microbiology*, *62*, 625–630.

Suzuki, N., Yoshida, A., & Nakano, Y. (2005). Quantitative analysis of multi-species oral biofilms by TaqMan real-time PCR. *Clinical Medicine & Research*, *3*, 176–185. doi:10.3121/cmr.3.3.176

Turnbaugh, P. J., Ley, R. E., Hamady, M., Fraser-Ligett, C. M., Knight, R., & Gordon, J. I. (2007). The human microbiome project. *Nature*, *449*, 804–809. doi:10.1038/nature06244

Vianna, M. E., Holtgraeve, S., Seyfarth, I., Conrads, G., & Horz, H.-P. (2008). Quantitative analysis of three hydrogenotrophic microbial groups - methanogenic archaea, sulfate-reducing bacteria, and acetogenic bacteria - within plaque biofilms associated with human periodontal disease. *Journal of Bacteriology*, *190*, 3779–3785. doi:10.1128/JB.01861-07

Vianna, M. E., Horz, H.-P., Gomes, B. P., & Conrads, G. (2006). *In vivo* evaluation of microbial reduction after chemo-mechanical preparation of human root canals containing necrotic pulp tissue. *International Endodontic Journal*, *39*, 484–492. doi:10.1111/j.1365-2591.2006.01121.x

von Wintzingerode, F., Goebel, U. B., & Stackebrandt, E. (1997). Determination of microbial diversity in environmental samples: pitfalls of PCR-based rRNA analysis. *FEMS Microbiology Reviews*, *21*, 213–229. doi:10.1111/j.1574-6976.1997.tb00351.x

Weisburg, W. G., Barns, S. M., Pelletier, D. A., & Lane, D. J. (1991). 16S ribosomal DNA amplification for phylogenetic study. *Journal of Bacteriology*, *173*, 697–703.

Wittwer, C. T., Herrmann, M. G., Moss, A. A., & Rasmussen, R. P. (1997). Continuous fluorescence monitoring for rapid cycle DNA amplification. *BioTechniques*, *22*, 130–138.

KEY TERMS AND DEFINITIONS

Crossing Point: This term, also abbreviated as Cp, indicates the number of PCR cycles at which the fluorescence exceeds a threshold value significantly higher than the background fluorescence. This value is individual to any PCR sample and is used for calculating the amount of initial target DNA. Depending on the RTQ-PCR platforms this term is also referred to as "threshold cycle" (or "Ct").

Hybridization Probes: DNA detection strategy during RTQ-PCR based on use of Fluorescence resonance energy transfer (FRET) in which fluorescent labels of two different hybridization probes "communicate". Detection of the amplified target sequence is achieved by hybridization of these two probes in close proximity. Once having hybridized to the target the fluorescence dye at the 3'-end of the so-called donor probe transfers its activation energy to the acceptor dye, which then emits long-wave fluorescent light, that is measured.

Hydrolysis Probes: DNA detection strategy during RTQ-PCR based on use of one oligonucleotide (also referred to as TaqMan-probe), labeled with a 5'-terminal reporter dye and a 3'-terminal fluorescence quencher. This probe specifically binds to the target DNA in a region between the two primer-binding sites. During the extension step of the RTQ-PCR, the Taq DNA polymerase cleaves the hybridized probe by its 5'-exonuclease activity, both fluorescence dyes are physically separated, so that fluorescence emission from the reporter dye occurs and can be measured.

Melting Curve Analysis: After completion of RTQ-PCR melting curve analysis is performed for verification of the correct PCR product. By gradually increasing the temperature, the double-stranded PCR product separates into single strands thus allowing measurement of the decline in fluorescence. The characteristic melting point of the target DNA (also referred to as T_m) indicates the temperature at which the DNA exists as 50% each double- and single-stranded.

PCR Efficiency: This term usually referred to as "E" indicates the overall performance of a PCR reaction, with values ranging between 1 and 2. A value of 2 means, that the amount of PCR product is exactly doubled in each PCR cycle. The experimental value of E usually varies between 1.5 and 1.9, and is usually determined by testing a series dilution of standard templates with known DNA amount.

RTQ-PCR: Abbreviation for real-time quantitative polymerase chain reaction. This is a general term for the in vitro replication of DNA through repetitive cycles of denaturation, primer annealing and extension steps and simultaneous measurement of increase in fluorescence due to product accumulation.

SYBR Green: Name of the most frequently used fluorophore in RTQ-PCR that intercalates into double-stranded DNA thereby exhibiting fluorescence. Due to its binding potential to any double stranded DNA, SYBR Green is less specific than oligonucleotide probes.

Chapter 6
HPV Detection and Genotyping Using the Luminex xMAP Technology

Marios Kambouris
Yale University School of Medicine, USA

Vasiliki Chini
Shafallah Medical Genetics Center, Qatar

Andriani Daskalaki
Max-Planck-Institute for Molecular Genetics, Germany

ABSTRACT

The Human Papillomavirus (HPV) is playing an important role in oral cancer. The molecular detection of HPV is based on the fact that the viral DNA is present in all the epithelial layers of the affected tissue and it can be detected easily with PCR or Real-Time PCR. The major disadvantage of PCR is that it cannot provide genotype information and the Real-Time PCR can only detect very few types in a multiplex assay. Although the HPV typing assays are capable of typing a relatively large spectrum of HPV genotypes, they cannot be automated or deployed in a high-throughput platform. The bead-based technology (Luminex suspension array technology) provides a rapid and cost-effective method to simultaneously detect different HPV genotypes.

BACKGROUND

Over the past 20 years, high-risk human papilloma-virus (HPV) infection has been evolving as a risk factor for the development of head and neck squamous cell carcinoma (Hennessey et al. 2009). In particular, HPV is strongly associated with the development of oropharyngeal cancer and a small minority of oral cavity cancers. In 2008, 47,500 people were diagnosed with head and neck cancer in the United States, representing approximately 3% of new cancer diagnoses, and 11,260 people died (Jemal et al., 2008).

Cervical cancer is the leading cause of cancer mortality among women in developing countries.

DOI: 10.4018/978-1-60566-733-1.ch006

There are estimated to be approximately 500,000 new cases of cancer, leading to about 239,000 deaths each year (World Health Report, 2004). Over 99% of cervical cancer cases are linked to genital infection with human papillomavirus, which is the most common viral infection of the reproductive tract worldwide and infects an estimated 660 million people. While HPV infection resolves spontaneously in the majority of people, it can develop into chronic infection and in some women, cervical cancer (WHO, 2005).

The data from combined research studies have revealed the causative role of certain HPV types in cancer. There is sufficient evidence for carcinogenicity of the anogenital tract for types 16, 18, 31, 33, 35, 39, 45, 51, 52, 56, 58, 59 and 66 (the "high-risk" types of HPV). Jo S et al. (2009) studied the presence of high-risk HPV-16 in patients with HNSCC, assess the impact of HPV status on treatment response and survival in patients treated with combined therapy and the differences in HIF-1alpha and VEGF expression in HPV-positive and -negative tumors. Some case-control studies also also point to a role of HPVs 26, 68, 73 and 82 in cervical cancer, but they are found relatively rarely. There is possible carcinogenicity for HPV 6 and 11, which although not been associated with cervical cancer, are consistently detected in the rare Buschke-Löwenstein tumours converting into verrucous carcinomas of the vulva. In the skin, some types of HPV Genus are possibly carcinogenic to humans. HPV 5 and 8 are considered as carcinogenic for patients with epidermodysplasia verruciformis (WHO, 2005).

There is a strong need not only to detect the virus, but mostly to identify individual HPV types, in order to investigate the epidemiology and the clinical behaviour of particular types and, also to decide the appropriate therapy. Strategies assessed have included vaccination (initiated at age 12 years or at a later age), cytological screening (varying numbers of screening visits using different screening methods, e.g. direct visual inspection, Pap smear, or HPV testing, at different ages), and combined vaccination and screening strategies. The identification of high-risk HPV types prompted the development of new methods for early cancer screening. Furthermore, HPV genotyping is also valuable for investigation of the clinical behavior and epidemiology of particular types, for the characterization of study populations in HPV vaccination trials and for monitoring the efficacy of HPV vaccines.

The molecular detection of HPV is based on the fact that the viral DNA is present in all the epithelial layers of the affected tissue and it can be detected easily with PCR or Real-Time PCR. The major disadvantage of PCR is that it cannot provide genotype information and the Real-Time PCR can only detect very few types in a multiplex assay. In addition, a number of HPV typing assays have recently been reported, such as solid–phase microarrays (Klaassen *et al*, 2004; Oh *et al*, 2004), GP5+/6+ - linked enzyme immunoassay (EIA) (van den Brule *et al*, 2002), the Roche AMPLICOR HPV test, and the INNO-LiPA HPV assay (Labo Biomedical Products; van Ham *et al*; 2005). Although these assays are capable of typing a relatively large spectrum of HPV genotypes, they cannot be automated or deployed in a high-throughput platform. On the contrary, the bead-based technology (Luminex suspension array technology) provides a rapid and cost-effective method to simultaneously detect different HPV genotypes.

The Luminex xMAP technology uses 5.6 μ polystyrene microspheres which are internally dyed with two spectrally distinct fluorophores, red and infrared. Using different ratios of these flurorochromes, different microspheres sets – up to 100 - can be created, each with a unique spectral signature determined by its red/infrared mixture. Different microspheres sets may be combined within an assay. Since each microsphere carries a unique signature, the xMAP detection system can identify to which set it belongs. Therefore multiplexing up to 100 tests in a single reaction volume is possible. The surface chemistry of the

Figure 1. Schematic overview of HPV genotyping of GP5+ /6+ PCR products by bead-based multiplex assay (Adapted from Schmitt et al, 2006)

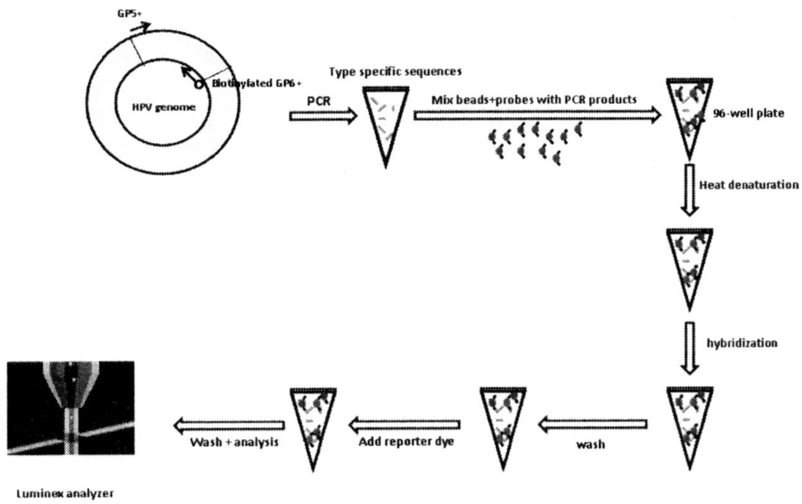

xMAP microspheres allows simple chemical coupling of capture reagents such as antibodies, oligonucleotides, peptides or receptors.

Detection of the multiplexed results is carried out using the Luminex system and is based on a combination of flow cytometry and spectal photometry. Assays are carried out in a 96-well plate, with up to 100 tests per well. Special fluidics causes the stream of suspended microspheres to line up in a single file prior to passing through the detection chamber. As the microsphere passes through the detection chamber a red laser excites both the internal red and infrared dyes allowing the proper classification of each microsphere to one of the 100 sets (classification channel reading). A third fluorochrome coupled to a reporter molecule detects the hybridization occurring at the microsphere surface. A green laser excites any orange fluorescence associated with the binding of the analyte (reporter channel reading). Since both the classification and the reporter readings are made on each individual particle, the Luminex system is able to precisely determine multiplex assay results.

The HPV bead array detection method is based on the amplification of the HPV DNA by a general primer set and the subsequent detection of the products with type-specific oligonucleotide probes coupled to fluorescent-labeled beads. General primers GP5+ /6+ (the reverse GP6+ primer is biotynlated) are used for the amplification of a 150 bp fragment of the viral L1 open reading frame. Following amplification, PCR products are hybridized with type-specific probes coupled to beads. The hybridized products are labeled with streptavidin-R-phycoerythrin witch binds to the already existing biotyne of the PCR products. Beads are analyzed for internal bead color and R-phycoeryhtrin reporter fluorescence on the Luminex 100 analyzer [Figure 1] (Schmitt et al, 2006).

This simple bead-based high-throughput hybridization method allows the simultaneously detection and genotyping of up to 100 HPV types. The technology described here is been applied for the genotyping of 33 HPV types, including 16 high-risk HPV types (16, 18, 31, 33, 34, 35, 39, 45, 51, 52, 56, 58, 59, 68, 73, 82), two putative high-risk types (53, 66) and the 15 most prevalent low-risk types (6, 11, 13, 30, 40, 42, 43, 44, 54, 57, 55, 61, 62, 70, 74) [Table 1] (Munoz et al, 2003). Among them, 29 microspheres sets possess an HPV type-specific probe on its surface, while

Table 1. Bead targets used for multiplexed HPV genotyping

High-risk HPV types	16, 18, 31, 33, 34, 35, 39, 45, 51, 52, 56, 58, 59, 68, 73, 82
Putative high-risk HPV types	53, 66
Low-risk HPV types	6, 11, 13, 30, 40, 42, 43, 44, 54, 57, 55, 61, 62, 70, 74
Human DNA internal control	Amel X, Amel Y
Viral DNA internal control	univeral

two sets are able to detect two HPV-types each of them, 54/57 and 66/68. Each of those beads only contains one probe, but the probe is cross-reactive to another type. The probe on bead 54 is designed to be specific for type 54. However, there is a high degree of homology to type 57, and therefore, type 57 is detected as well. The same is true for bead specific for types 66 and 68.

So they can be combined, allowing up to 33 different HPV targets to be measured simultaneously in a single reaction vessel. In addition, there are two microspheres sets harboring two sex-specific probes permitting the sex determination and the control of the DNA quality. Finally, there is one bead set tagged with a universal probe that serves as an internal control, since it binds to viral DNA and ensures the presence of viral DNA and the PCR's success. The probes are specific for the L1 region and the universal probe is also designed to hybridized to the L1 region.

The method described here is a high-throughput multiplex assay that allows fast and simple genotyping of all clinically relevant genital HPV types in a single reaction. It seems to have higher sensitivity, comparing to other methods, because of the improved detection of variants by novel probes, the improved detection limits of novel probes and the overall higher sensitivity of the beads technology (Schmitt et al, 2006). In addition, suspension arrays have some advantages over solid-phase microarrays. Hybridization kinetics with suspension arrays closely approximate the kinetics of solution-phase hybridization (Wallace *et al*, 2005). This results in short hybridization times and faster turn-around times, than those possible with solid-phase microarrays. Another advantage is the fast instrument readout (30 s for each specimen) and the rapid and automated analysis.

REFERENCES

Hennessey, P. T., Westra, W. H., & Califano, J. A. (2009). Human papillomavirus and head and neck squamous cell. *Journal of Dental Research, 88*(4), 300–306. doi:10.1177/0022034509333371

Jemal, A., Siegel, R., Ward, E., Hao, Y., Xu, J., & Murray, T. (2008). Cancer statistics, 2008. *CA: a Cancer Journal for Clinicians, 58*, 71–96. doi:10.3322/CA.2007.0010

Jo, S., Juhasz, A., Zhang, K., Ruel, C., Loera, S., & Wilczynski, S. P. (2009). Human Papillomavirus Infection as a Prognostic Factor in Oropharyngeal Squamous Cell Carcinomas Treated in a Prospective Phase II Clinical Trial. *Anticancer Research, 29*, 1467–1474.

Klaassen, C. H., Prinsen, C. F., de Vals, H. A., Horrevorts, A. M., Jeunink, M. A., & Thunnissen, F. B. (2004). DNA microarray format for detection and subtyping of human papillomavirus. *Journal of Clinical Microbiology, 42*, 2152–2160. doi:10.1128/JCM.42.5.2152-2160.2004

Melchers, W. J. (2005). Comparison of two commercial assays for detection of human papillomavirus (HPV) in cervical scrape specimens: validation of the Roche AMPLICOR HPV test as a means to screen for HPV genotypes associated with a higher risk of cervical disorders. *Journal of Clinical Microbiology, 43*, 2662–2667. doi:10.1128/JCM.43.6.2662-2667.2005

Munoz, N., Bosch, F. X., de Sanjose, S., Herrero, R., Castellsague, X., & Shah, K. V. (2003). Epidemiologic classification of human papillomavirus types associated with cervical cancer. *The New England Journal of Medicine, 348*, 518–527. doi:10.1056/NEJMoa021641

Oh, T. J., Kim, C. J., Woo, S. K., Kim, T. S., Jeong, D. J., & Kim, M. S. (2004). Development and clinical evaluation of a highly sensitive DNA microarray for detection and genotyping of human papillomaviruses. *Journal of Clinical Microbiology, 42*, 3272–3280. doi:10.1128/JCM.42.7.3272-3280.2004

Schmitt, M., Bravo, I. G., Snijders, P. J. F., Gissmann, L., Pawlita, M., & Waterboer, T. (2006). Bead-based multiplex genotyping of human papillomaviruses. *Journal of Clinical Microbiology, 44*, 504–512. doi:10.1128/JCM.44.2.504-512.2006

Van de Brule, A. J., Pol, R., Fransen-Daalmeijer, N., Schouls, L. M., Meijer, C. J., & Snijders, P. J. (2002). GP5+/ 6+ PCR followed by reverse line blot analysis enables rapid and high-throughput identification of human papillomavirus genotypes. *Journal of Clinical Microbiology, 40*, 779–787. doi:10.1128/JCM.40.3.779-787.2002

Van Ham, M. A., Bakkers, J. M., Harbers, G. K., Quint, W. G., Massuger, L. F., & Melchers, W. J. (2005). Comparison of two commercial assays for detection of human papillomavirus (HPV) in cervical scrape specimens: validation of the Roche AMPLICOR HPV test as a means to screen for HPV genotypes associated with a higher risk of cervical disorders. *Journal of Clinical Microbiology, 43*, 2662–2667. doi:10.1128/JCM.43.6.2662-2667.2005

Wallace, J., Woda, B. A., & Pihan, G. (2005). Facile, comprehensive, high-throughput genotyping of human genital papillomaviruses using spectrally addressable liquid bead microarrays. *The Journal of Molecular Diagnostics, 7*, 72–80.

World Health Organization (WHO). (2005). *Report of the Consultation on human papillomavirus vaccines*. Geneva, April.

KEY TERMS AND DEFINITIONS

Amplification: A process leading to multiple copies of a chromosomal region.

Cervical Cancer: Malignant transformation of cells in the area of cervix uteri

Fluorophore: A component of a molecule which causes a molecule to be fluorescent.

Genotype: Set of genes characterizing the hereditary information in the organism.

High-Risk: HPV types that lead to cancer.

Hybridization: Process of joining two complementary strands of DNA.

HPV: A human papillomavirus (HPV) is a non-enveloped DNA virus that infects the epidermis and mucous membranes of humans.

PCR: Polymerase chain reaction (PCR) is a DNA amplification technique, a laboratory technique for creating multiple copies of small segments of DNA.

Chapter 7
Time-Sequencing and Force-Mapping with Integrated Electromyography to Measure Occlusal Parameters

Robert B. Kerstein[1]
Tufts University School of Dental Medicine, USA

ABSTRACT

Computerized Occlusal Analysis technology records, and quickly displays for clinical interpretation, tooth contact timing sequences of .003 second increments, and each tooth contacts' fluctuating force levels which occur during functional jaw movements. These measurements are recorded intraorally with an ultra-thin, mylar-encased sensor that is connected to a computer via a USB interface. This sensor is placed between a patients' teeth during functional jaw movements to record changing tooth-tooth interactions. The displayed occlusal data aids in the examination and treatment of occlusal abnormalities on natural teeth, dental prostheses, and dental implant prostheses. The software can be linked to an Electromyography software program that simultaneously records the electromyographic potential of 8 head and neck muscles. This combination of dynamic tooth contact force and time data, and functional muscular data, affords a dentist detailed, precise, and unparalleled diagnostic and treatment information, with which to address many differing clinical occlusal pathologies.

INTRODUCTION

Computerized Occlusal Analysis technology (T-Scan III for Windows®, Tekscan Inc., S. Boston, MA, USA) records, and quickly displays for clinical interpretation, tooth contact Time-Sequences while simultaneously Force-Mapping each tooth contacts' fluctuating *relative occlusal force* levels which occur during functional jaw movements (*known as* Occlusal Events) (Maness 1993, Montgomery and Kerstein 2000, Kerstein 2001, Kerstein and Wilkerson 2001). These *occlusal event* measurements are recorded intraorally, with an ultra-thin, electronically charged, mylar-encased sensor that is connected to a computer via a USB interface.

By measuring *Relative Force*, the T-Scan III system can detect whether an occlusal force on one set of contacting opposing teeth is greater, equal

DOI: 10.4018/978-1-60566-733-1.ch007

to, or less than, the occlusal forces occurring on other contacting teeth all throughout the dental arches. Determining relative force is important to the user-Dentist, as relative force illustrates measured differences of varying applied loads within all contacting tooth locations. The T-Scan III software displays the relative occlusal force, at any instant within a recorded occlusal event on all contacting teeth, as a percentage of the maximum occlusal force obtained within the recording.

Detected relative force variances can be employed clinically to:

- Precisely balance an unbalanced occlusal force distribution with targeted time-based and force-based occlusal adjustments
- Diagnose excessively high occlusal load present in one area of the occlusion, while simultaneously diagnosing where there is little, moderate, or no occlusal load in other areas of the same occlusion

After various occlusal events are recorded, the retrieved occlusal contact time-sequence data and relative force data are mapped for analysis in 4 different quantifiable ways:

- By real-time increments that measure the sequential order of each individual tooth contacts' loading occurrence. The real-time sequence can be separated into increments as short as .003 seconds duration
- By *force location* on the contacting surfaces of many teeth individually and collectively within the 2 dental arches
- By relative changing *force percentage values* on all individual contacting teeth
- By a changing, moveable *occlusal force summation icon* and trajectory, that describes the changing concentrated force position within the 2 dental arches of all the collective tooth contacts' relative occlusal forces

The mapped contact time-sequence and relative occlusal force data, when analyzed by a user-Dentist, aids in the clinical determination of, and occlusal treatment of, many time premature contacts, and occlusal force abnormalities, which occur during occlusal events on natural teeth, dental prostheses, and dental implant prostheses (Kerstein Chapman and Klein 1997, Kerstein 1997, Kerstein and Wilkerson 2001, Kerstein and Grundset 2001,).

This technology's ability to isolate time-premature tooth contacts, and excessive occlusal contact forces, is vastly superior to the commonly utilized, non-technology based occlusal indicators which dentists routinely employ (articulating paper, wax imprints, silicone imprints, and articulated stone dental casts). None of these dental materials have any scientifically proven capability to time-sequence tooth contacts, or force-map occlusal forces. Additionally, they all necessitate the user-Dentist to "subjectively interpret" their occlusal representations.

The most commonly employed occlusal indicator is dental Articulating Paper. It is comprised of ink-impregnated strips of either Mylar, or various thicknesses and forms of papers. To date, no study has shown Articulating Paper to be reliably accurate when it is used to describe occlusal forces (Reiber Fuhr and Hartmann 1991, Millstein and Maya 2001, Carossa Lojacono Schierano and Pera 2001, Saraçoğlu and Ozpinar 2001, Carey Craig Kerstein and Radke 2007, Saad Weiner and Ehrenberg 2008). Therefore, user-Dentist's subjective interpretation of the size and shape, and color intensity of various Articulating Paper markings, can lead to incorrect clinical determinations of where in the dental arches occlusal problems exist, and where occlusal treatment should be performed or not performed. These incorrect clinical determinations occur because the user-Dentist is taught (incorrectly), to perceive widespread and uniform shaped markings' appearance on the teeth as representative of "time simultaneous" tooth contact sequences with "normal and balanced" occlusal forces present within the dental arches.

Figure 1. T-Scan III Evolution Handle with sensor

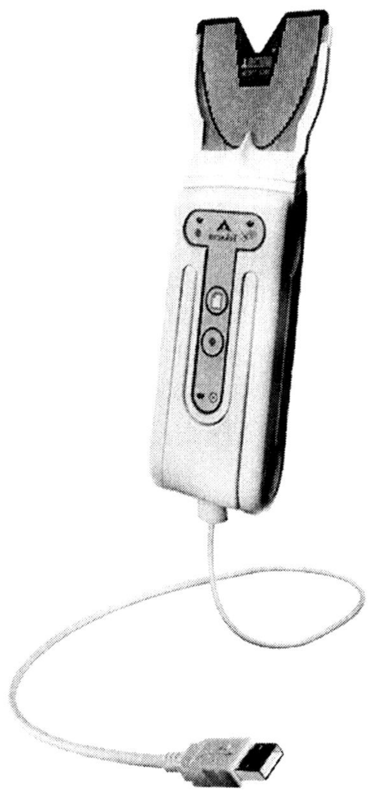

EVOLUTION OF TIME SEQUENCING AND RELATIVE OCCLUSAL FORCE-MAPPING BY COMPUTERIZED TECHNOLOGY

The evolution of pressure sensitive ink-Mylar encased sensor technology that could time-sequence and force-map relative occlusal forces, was introduced as the T-Scan® I computerized occlusal analysis system (Maness Benjamin Podoloff and Bobick and Golden 1987). Occlusal data was obtained by instructing patients to occlude through an intraoral recording sensor that was connected to a stand-alone computer. The computer screen displayed a Force Movie *(Maness 1988)*, which illustrated a dynamic columnar time and force display of the recorded occlusal contacts for playback and analysis.

The original T-Scan I Recording Sensor was comprised of a flexible laminated epoxy matrix surrounding a pressure sensitive ink grid, which was formed in the shape of a dental arch. When inserted intraorally, and occluded into and through by a patients teeth, the sensor relayed occlusal contact *real-time* and relative force-mapping information to compatible software that was capable of interpreting 16 levels of intraoral relative force in approximately .01 second time increments. The resultant occlusal analysis was displayed in two or three dimensions, as a Snapshot *(Maness 1988)*, or as a continuous Movie *(Maness 1988)* of the entire occlusal contact event the patient made. The data could be played forwards, backwards, or in individual .01 second time increments.

In 1998, the entire T-Scan I system was redeveloped as the T-Scan II Occlusal Analysis System for Windows®. The changes included hardware, software, and further sensor advances. T-Scan II was a Microsoft Windows® (Microsoft Corp, Seattle WA, USA) compliant system that was integrated into a clinical diagnostic computer workstation. An IBM compatible PC with a Pentium processor, and a minimum of 4-8 megabytes of RAM, were required to properly operate the system (Figure 1 and Figure 2). The graphical interface used familiar Windows® toolbar icons, to display the software features that analyzed recorded occlusal contact information.

In 2006, the T-Scan II hardware was altered to interface with the PC via a USB plug that replaced a serial parallel port interface. Then, in 2008, the T-Scan III USB with *Turbo Mode Recording* was introduced. A recording handle hardware improvement resultant from increased speeds with which computer chips process commands, made it possible to significantly increase the recording speed of a given occlusal event. The *Evolution Handle* of the T-Scan III USB System, when operated in Turbo Mode, can record time-sequences and map relative occlusal force data in increments of .003 seconds, thereby capturing 3 times more occlusal data for analysis than was possible with the T-Scan

Figure 2. T-Scan III Evolution Handle connected to a personal computer

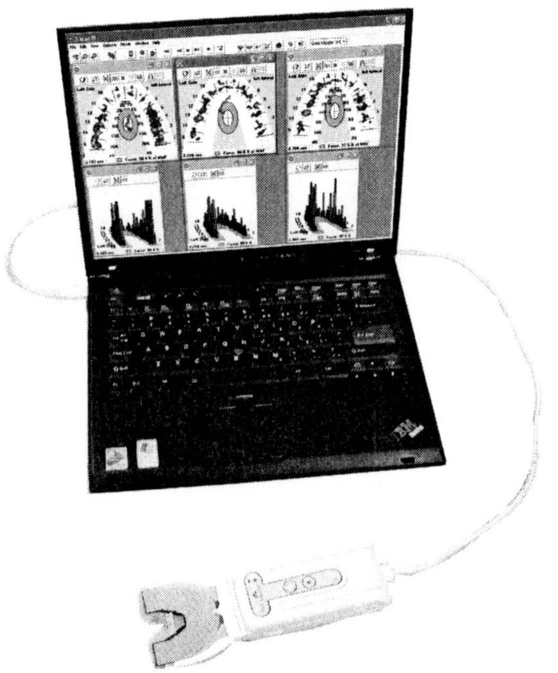

III USB. Turbo Mode data acquisition provides a user-Dentist with an increased ability over the conventional non-Turbo Mode recording, to locate more non-simultaneous tooth contact sequences and aberrant occlusal force concentrations within a patient's occlusion.

T-SCAN III SENSOR DESIGN

The most current available recording sensor for the T-Scan III system represents the 4th generation of T-Scan system sensors. It is known as the *High Definition sensor (HD)*. The HD sensor is dental arch-shaped such that it fits between a patient's maxillary and mandibular teeth during the recording of occlusal events. When correctly positioned between a patients 2 maxillary Central Incisor teeth, and held stable by a hard plastic *Sensor Support (Figure 1),* the sensor is then clenched upon, and chewed over by a patient, so as to record and precisely map changing tooth-to-tooth occlusal force interactions in *real-time*.

A number of different occlusal events can be captured by the recording sensor:

- Single or multiple patient-self closures into complete tooth intercuspation
- Dentist-assisted patient closure into the Centric Relation mandibular position
- Patient self-closure into complete tooth intercuspation followed by a mandibular excursion to the left, right, or forward, out of the complete intercuspated position
- Patient clenching and grinding motions in and around complete tooth intercuspation
- Habitual Occlusal Force Patterns

The HD sensor's structural design consists of two layers of Mylar encasing a grid of resistive ink rows and columns printed between them (Figure 3 and Figure 4). The high definition design has both larger *Sensels* (the Tekscan proprietary force recording element within each sensor; a sensel is 1.61 mm^2) and less space between the sensels than all of the previous T-Scan I and II sensor designs. Within the HD sensor, the sensels are packed closer together within the recording grid, resulting in increased recording surface area available for teeth to occlude upon. When compared to all pervious sensor designs, the HD configuration specifically limits the amount of inactive, non-recording grid areas between the sensels.

Figure 3. Sensor schematic

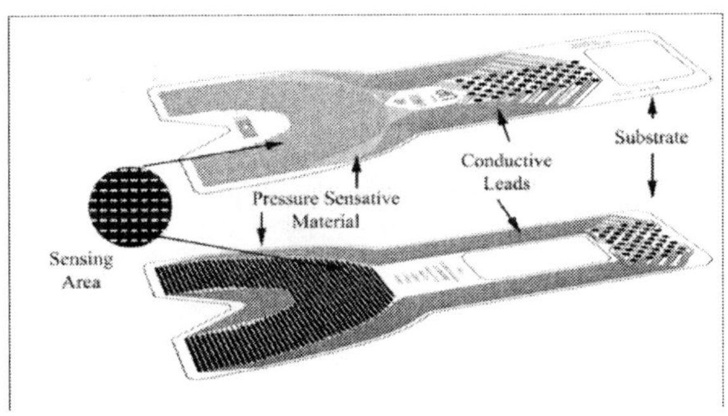

Figure 4. HD sensor

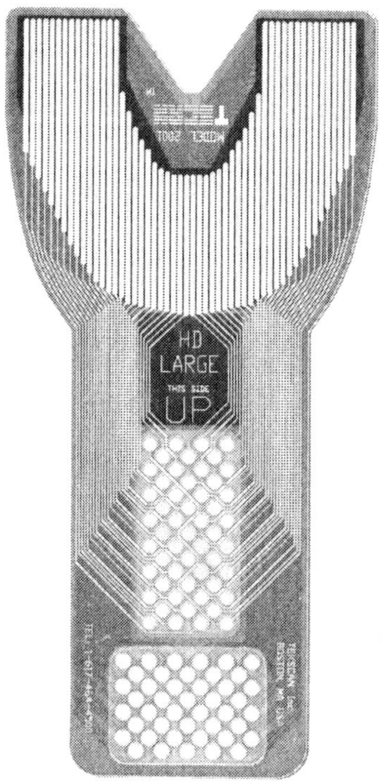

A published performance study (Kerstein Lowe Harty and Radke 2006) comparing Generation-3 (G3) sensors against HD sensors revealed that the HD sensor reproduced more consistent force levels than the older G-3 sensor. The G-3 sensor mean force variances were significantly larger than for the same 6 occlusal contact locations measured with the HD sensor. Additionally, the HD sensor exhibited consistent force reproduction in at least 20 in-laboratory crushing cycles (Kerstein Lowe Harty and Radke 2006).

SENSOR RECORDING DYNAMICS

When tooth contact is made with a T-Scan III sensor, the applied force on individual sensels changes their resistance. Larger applied forces produce larger resistance changes and lower occlusal forces produce lesser resistance changes.

The electronics in the Recording Handle of the T-Scan III system excites the sensor by applying voltage to each column of recording sensels in succession, Then, as a T-Scan III sensor is occluded upon, a change in the applied force at various tooth contacts results in a change in the resistance of the resistive ink at each of the contacted sensels. This resistance change is measured by the system's hardware electronics as a change in *Digital* Output Voltage (DO). Higher forces on contacting teeth result in larger decreases in the resistance of the loaded sensels, and therefore, a higher measured output voltage from the loaded sensels. The greater the applied force to the contacting teeth then the higher the output voltage that is measured.

The electronics in the recording handle reads the output voltage of each row of sensels in a process called Scanning. The output signal is conditioned and converted to an 8-bit digital value so that the measured resistance change is proportional to force applied to each sensel with a range between 0 and 255 raw counts. The raw count for an individual sensel can be conceptualized as the minimum pressure that is on that sensel. And, because each sensel has an area of 1.61 mm^2, the raw count can also be conceptualized as a force. A map in the software receives from the recording handle, the stream of changing sensel digital voltage output values, and organizes them for display to the user-Dentist into the same orientation pattern that the sensels have on the sensor.

Within the software, the user-Dentist can raise or lower the *Recording Sensitivity* across 16 differing levels to compensate for varying occlusal strengths of individual patients. This allows the user-Dentist to modify the sensor recording behavior to select a pressure range which will record optimum individual patient occlusal data for analyses, regardless of a patients' absolute occlusal strength.

RELATIVE FORCE MEASUREMENT VS. ABSOLUTE FORCE MEASURED IN ENGINEERING UNITS

As stated in the Introduction, the T-Scan III system records relative force. It therefore, does not provide absolute occlusal force in engineering units (calibrated force numbers) such as in Newtons (*n*) or pounds per square inch (*lb/in²*).

To obtain accurate numeric force values in engineering units, a T-Scan sensor would need to undergo pre-use *Equilibration, some surface preparationand thenCalibration:*

- Sensor *Equilibration* is accomplished by applying a uniform load all over a sensor at three levels (low, near the load of interest, and at a high load) to determine that each sensel has a uniform digital output from a uniform applied load. This can be accomplished by using an air bladder with the sensor being compressed on a flat surface.
- Next, the recording sensor would need to be covered with a *shim material* – The shim would prevent sensor crinkling when loaded, while at the same time, distribute the load amongst a greater sensor surface area than the surface areas of individual tooth contact points. The shim helps avoid individual sensor saturation. This shim material increases the sensor thickness from approximately 0.1 mm (no shim) to about 3 mm (with shim). This is a "clinical use problem" for the user-Dentist because a modified sensor thickness increase does not allow a patient's teeth to completely and fully intercuspate against each other.
- Lastly, the sensor must undergo sensor with shim *Calibration* - This would be performed on a set of articulated dental casts made from a patient's dental arches, by applying 1 or 2 representative occlusal loads to a modified sensor that are within the patient's occlusal force range. Calibration is performed to correlate the digital output of the sensels to engineering units (force or pressure) and confirms and improves the uniformity of output from sensel to sensel throughout the entire recording grid.

Because individual patients have variable occlusal strengths, and the dental community continually resists the use of a thickened sensor which interferes with complete tooth contact intercuspation, and there are no commercially available dental calibration devices with which to apply known test loads to a modified T-Scan sensor, it is not possible to use the T-Scan III system to obtain force values in engineering units. Therefore, throughout the remainder of this chapter, all references made forward from here regarding occlusal force *are to be describing* relative occlusal force.

For any measurement of force in engineering units, the I-Scan system is commercially available (I-Scan for Windows®, Tekscan Inc. S Boston, MA. USA). I-Scan is a general purpose research product designed for industrial applications that lacks many software features which aid in the understanding of dental occlusion (such as those related to time-sequencing analyses). Alternatively, the I-Scan's software features include equilibration, calibration, general purpose analysis graphs, and the ability to export arrays of X–Y sensel pressure data into ASCII format into other applications. These features make the I-Scan a more versatile absolute force analysis system than is the T-Scan III system.

RECORDED T-SCAN III MOVIE ANALYSES

A T-Scan III recording of an occlusal event is captured in a dynamic Movie (Maness 1988) which reveals all the varying occlusal contact forces, as time evolves within a given occlusal event. Once recorded, the Movie is retrieved for review in a 2-Dimensional View window, a 3-Dimensional View window, and two Force vs. Time Graph windows (Figure 5). The mapped occlusal force data is converted into colors so each frame of the Movie is an image of the pressure at varying tooth contact locations at that instant of time. This pressure results from the tooth contact forces that dissipate between opposing teeth as they interact during a recorded occlusal event. By advancing the Movie or going back in time, all force changes that occur between sets of interacting teeth are observed in the exact order with which they occurred throughout the entire recorded occlusal event.

A Legend with Color Spectrum (Figure 5) depicts a scale of relative occlusal forces. Darker, cooler colors, such as dark blue through light blue, represent lower forces. Brighter, warmer colors such as yellow, orange and red, indicate higher occlusal contact forces. Pink indicates that the sensel has saturated, or reached its maximum digital output. Pink sensels may have an unknown amount of greater force than red sensels.

In 2 or 3 dimensions, the occlusal contact timing sequence can be played forwards or backwards continuously, or in either .01-second increments when recorded non-Turbo Mode, or in .003 second increments when recorded in Turbo Mode. In the 3 dimensional (3-Dimensional) playback window the force columns change both their height and color designation. In the 2 dimensional (2-D) contour view, the color-coded force concentration zones change size, shape, and color, as occlusal forces change.

Below the 2-Dimensional view and 3-Dimensional view windows are 2 *Force vs. Time Graph* windows (Figure 6). It is here where Time-Sequencing is mapped incrementally, through changing Red and Green colored lines that represent the changing force percentages found in both dental arch halves over the entire recorded occlusal event. 4 additional moveable, vertical, hyphenated lines denote *key* Time-Regions within a recorded occlusal event. Lastly, a Data Window to the far right describes the occlusal *Time Parameters* that can be calculated from the recorded occlusal event.

Figure 5. Legend with color spectrum

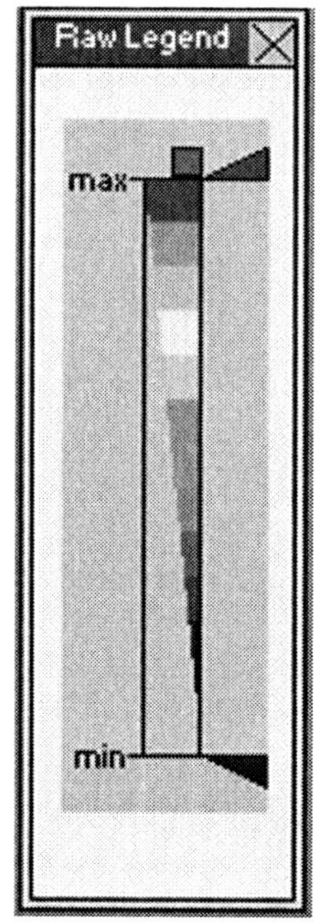

The Occlusal Time Parameters that can be displayed for analyses within the graph Data Window are:

- Occlusion Time **(OT):** The elapsed time from 1st tooth contact to the complete intercuspation of all occluding teeth. <.2 seconds duration is considered optimal bilateral tooth contact simultaneity (Kerstein and Grundset 2001)
- Disclusion Time **(DT):** The elapsed time required for a patient to exit their complete intercuspated position, and move their mandible either right, left, or forward, so as to disclude (completely separate) all posterior teeth, including and behind the 1st premolar tooth, so that only Canines and/or Incisors are making tooth contact. <.4 seconds duration is considered optimal so as to reduce long periods of tooth interaction

Figure 6. T Scan III playback windows

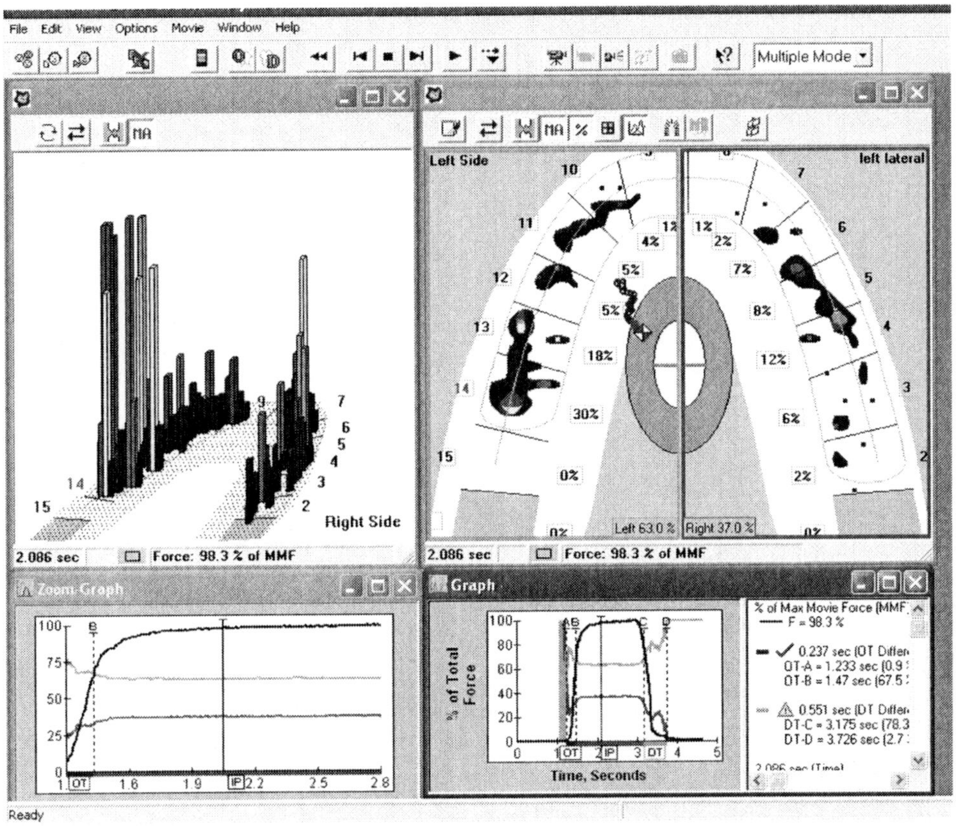

friction, and lessen masticatory muscle hyperactivity (Kerstein and Wright 1991)

Warning Icons located next to the Time Parameters inform a user-Dentist whether the recorded occlusal Time Parameters are clinically physiologic (green check mark), borderline physiologic (yellow triangle) or non-physiologic (pink triangle) occlusal function. The tolerance settings for these warning thresholds can be altered by the user-Dentist within the software's User Preference settings.

The lower left graph is a *Zoom Graph,* which shows .75 seconds of occlusal function from before and after the Movie frame that is being displayed in the 2-Dimensional and 3-Dimensional windows above. The Zoom Graph affords a user-Dentist greater visual clarity in comparison to the regular Force vs. Time Graph (Figure 7), of the subtleties present within all the changing colored force lines.

All 4 playback windows can be kept together to move as a unit around the desktop as a connected group. Or, they can be separated into individual windows for comparison to other similar type playback windows that come from other Movies recorded on the same patient when treatment is rendered to improve their occlusion (Figure 8).

OCCLUSAL PARAMETER TIME CALCULATION USING THE FORCE VS. TIME GRAPH

Occlusal Parameter time calculations can be precisely accomplished by using the Force vs.

Figure 7. Force vs. time graph

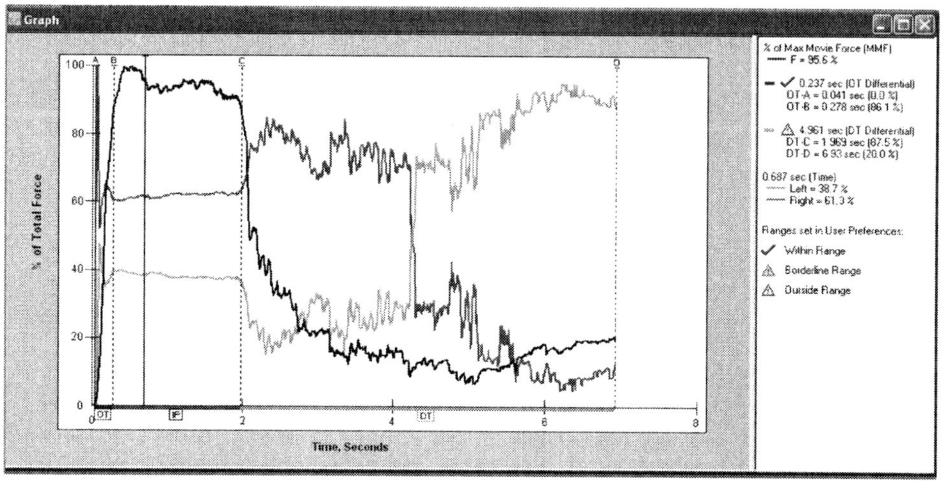

Time Graph. There are 3 distinct graph types that illustrate 3 different diagnostic occlusal event types that can be recorded from a patient's occlusal scheme. They are:

- Closure Graphs: A patient occludes into complete tooth intercuspation, holds their teeth together firmly and fully intercuspated for 1-3 seconds, then opens to disarticulate their teeth completely.

Figure 8. 2D playback window and 4 quadrant force vs. time graph

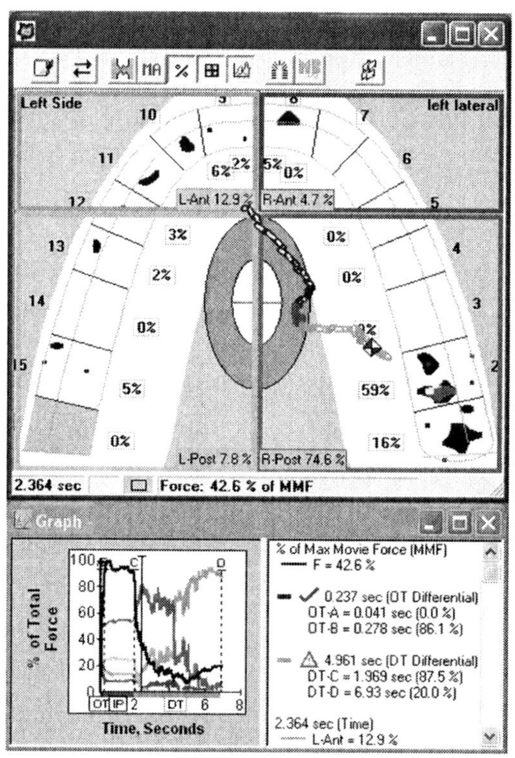

- Excursive Graphs: A patient occludes into complete tooth intercuspation, holds their teeth firmly and fully intercuspated for 1-3 seconds, and then slides their lower teeth across and over their maxillary teeth to either the left, right, or forward by leaving their complete intercuspated position.
- Multi-Bite Graphs: A patient occludes into complete tooth intercuspation, holds their teeth together firmly and fully intercuspated for 1-3 seconds, then opens to disarticulate their teeth, then re-closes their teeth back together into complete intercuspation, holds their teeth firmly together again for 1-3 seconds, and then reopens to disarticulate all occluding teeth. This can be repeated again and again in 1 continuous recording.

A recorded occlusal event contains certain key Time-Regions, which are graphically depicted with colored portions on the x-axis of a Force vs. Time Graph. The different time regions displayed directly relate to specific mandibular movements within a recorded occlusal event. Time Regions are mapped within each graph by 3 non-vertical force lines, and 5 vertical moveable time position *l*ines (Figure 9). The distances between all these lines both vertically and horizontally, describes the time-sequencing and force-mapping of specific parts of a recorded occlusal event.

The 3 non-vertical Force Lines are:

- **A non-vertical Black line:** This line denotes the *Total Force* changes that are mapped throughout the entire recorded event
- **A non-vertical Red line:** This line denotes the *Right arch-half* force changes that are mapped throughout the entire recorded event

Figure 9. Pre operative and post operative COF trajectory

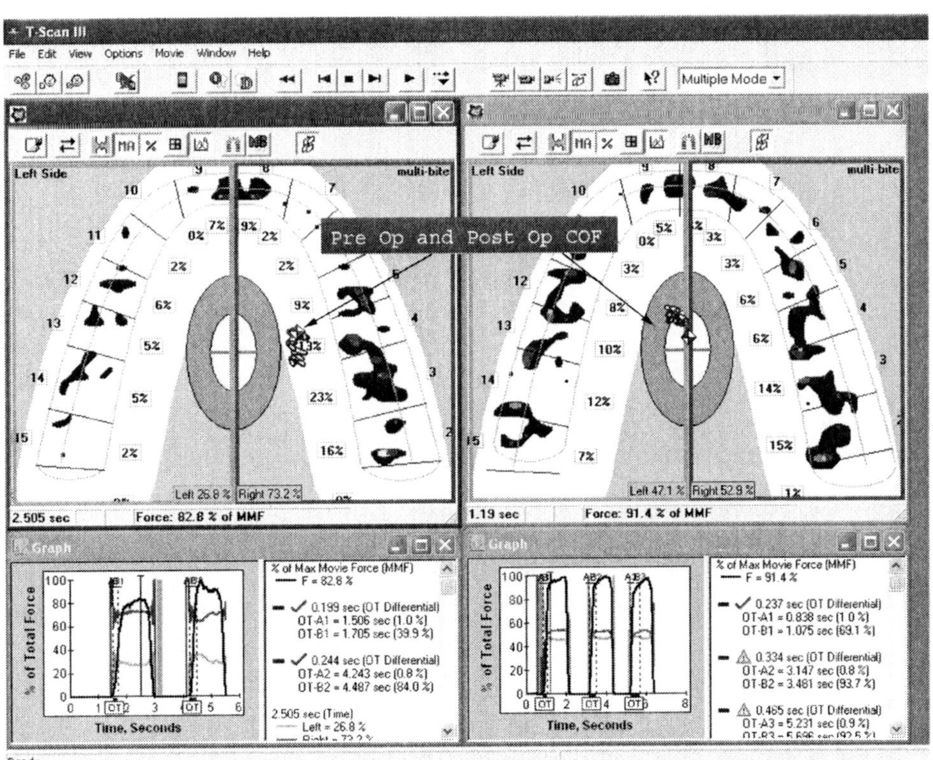

- **A non-vertical Green line:** This line denotes the Left arch-half force changes that are mapped throughout the entire recorded event

The 5 Time Position Lines are:

- **A Black vertical Time Line:** This line denotes how much time has elapsed within the recorded occlusal event and marks the time location of the Movie frame being displayed in the 2-D and 3-Dimensional windows
- **4 Black vertical hyphenated A, B, C, & D Lines:** The A-B line separation, and the C-D line separation, can be used to calculate the Occlusion Time *(A-B)* and the Disclusion Time (*C-D*) of the recorded event. The separation between these line-pairs is color coded along the x-axis of the graph; OT (Occlusion Time) is denoted in blue; Intercuspation (IP) when teeth are held firmly together is denoted in green; and DT (Disclusion Time) is denoted in orange.

Figure 7 depicts an Excursive Graph. During the A-B increment (*OT; x-axis blue area*), teeth in the right and left arch halves are occluding sequentially so the Red and Green lines change from 0% left (*no occlusal contact*) and 100% right (*1st and only contact*) to 40% left and 60% right. The Total Force line (*non-linear black line*) rapidly rises to the top of the graph, peaks near 100%, and then slightly lessens in the IP period (*x-axis green area*) as the patient firmly holds their teeth together at 95% total force for 1.69 seconds duration. The calculated OT is .237 seconds duration, which is marked in the graph data box as "physiologic" by a green *check mark.*

The green IP period denotes the distance from the B line to the C line, while the patient firmly holds their teeth together fully intercuspated. The Total Force line and the Red and Green lines stay horizontal and unchanging during the IP period, as there are no occlusal force changes during this time period of the recorded event.

At C, the Total Force line sharply declines when the mandibular excursion to the left begins because there is a major force drop when the patient disarticulates their teeth to commence moving to their left. After C, the Red line rises indicating forces on the right arch-half are increasing while the left side forces drop (Green line declines). Then later in the excursion, the Green and Red lines cross each other because the forces reverse between the arch-halves. During the excursion, low total occlusal force is generated when the teeth are no longer intercuspated and move over each other. Therefore, the Total Force line stays near the x-axis. Throughout the entire C-D increment, the x axis is orange. The DT is extremely prolonged at 4.961 seconds duration, hence a pink *Warning Triangle* in the graph data box denotes this time duration as "non-physiologic" for the user-Dentist. This DT warrants correction to reduce tooth frictional engagement of the posterior teeth, and decrease applied muscular hyperactivity to the teeth and Temporomandibular Joints during left excursive function.

4-QUADRANT FORCE VS. TIME GRAPH

The same Force vs Time Graph can display 4 quadrants (instead of only 2 quadrants) for even more detailed time-sequencing and occlusal force-mapping. A button on the 2-Dimensional view window tool bar divides the force plot into 4 quadrants instead of 2. As a result, within a 4-quadrant graph, 2 new lines are created by the software;

- **Purple line:** This *right posterior quadrant line* denotes the force changes that are mapped in the posterior right region of the dental arch (from right 3rd molar up to the right 1st premolar) throughout the entire recorded event.

- **Aqua line:** This *left posterior quadrant denotes* the left arch-half force changes that are mapped in the posterior left region (from left 3rd molar up to the left 1st premolar) throughout the entire recorded event.

The Red and Green lines now denote force changes in the anterior right and anterior left arch-halves, respectively (from canine to central incisor).

Figure 8 depicts a 4-quadrant graph that describes the left excursion seen in figure 7. As this patient attempts to move their mandible to her left, the posterior right teeth engage thereby limiting the patient's ability to easily move left. This occlusal phenomenon is denoted in the *4-quadrant graph* after the C line, where the posterior right Purple line rises highest from horizontal while the left anterior Green line struggles to rise. Only much later in the movement to the left does the Purple line decline and the Green line rise. This indicates a transfer of movement control from the earlier controlling right posterior teeth to the later controlling left anterior teeth near to D.

FORCE-MAPPING SOFTWARE FEATURES

In addition to the playback windows, there are several force-mapping software features that enhance the user-Dentists' ability to locate problem occlusal force concentrations:

- **The Center of Force Trajectory (COF):** The history of changing total occlusal force summation can be mapped positionally throughout the dental arches by a software feature known as the Center Force Trajectory. As forces evolve on individual teeth in sequence, the force summation will move towards higher force concentrations and away from lesser concentrations throughout the occlusal event. These force summation changes are graphically displayed during playback within the 2-Dimensional view window, by a red and white diamond-shaped icon followed by its' colored-line trailer (Figure 6). Each *leg* of the trailer represents .01 seconds (in *non-Turbo Mode recording*) or .003 seconds (in *Turbo Mode recording*). The incremental positions of the movement of the COF icon creates its' trailer.

The COF icon pinpoints the location of the sum of the total force of the occlusal contacts by the software's calculation of the sum of the medio-lateral and antero-posterior force moments of the recorded occlusal contacts. This data is presented to the user-Dentist by superimposing the COF marker within the tooth contact data. The shorter in length, and the less number of individual legs in total that constitute the COF trajectory, the more simultaneous is the time-sequence of a closure occlusal event. The more centered along the midline of the 2-Dimensional view window the COF trajectory travels, the more balanced are the occlusal forces between the right and left halves of the dental arch.

An off-center COF trajectory, which indicates poor occlusal force balance, can be rerouted and centered within the occlusal contacts by the user-Dentist performing both time-sequence and force-based correction occlusal adjustments. In figure 9, the left-positioned 2-Dimensional view window details a right-sided COF that begins posteriorly and moves anteriorly (physiologic abnormal). The overall force summation is skewed to the right side of the dental arch. This represents a right side early-left side late time-sequence of non-simultaneous occlusal contacts which demonstrate very poor occlusal balance.

After T-Scan III guided occlusal adjustments are accomplished on both the pre-operative locations of time-sequence early contacts, and the areas of occlusal force excess, the mapped direction and position of the new COF has been improved in the right-positioned 2-Dimensional view window. The total occlusal force summation is shared equally between the right and left arch halves, and the COF moves from anterior to posterior (physiologic normal). This clinical rerouting of the COF indicates improved contact time simultaneity, and equally shared occlusal force evolution between the right and left arch halves.

Another unique T-Scan III force analysis software feature is:

- **Force Percentage per Tooth:** During both recording and playback, the percentage of changing force per individual tooth is mapped in the 2-Dimensional view window in either .01 or .003 seconds,. *Force % per Tooth* describes unequal, or equal, individual tooth loading between each arch half as time elapses. Corrective occlusal adjustments can be accomplished to equalize force % per tooth discrepancies, which are based upon the right % per tooth comparison to its left % per tooth counterpart (i.e. % 1st molar right - % 1st molar left).

Figure 10, Figure 11 and Figure 12 illustrate the differing force percentages per tooth being displayed as a Movie of a patient self closure into intercuspation evolves. These 3 sequential individual 2-Dimensional Movie frames map the changing percentage per tooth of the occlusal forces on all 14 individual teeth involved within the occlusion. Note that the COF trajectory moves towards the teeth with the most force percentage at different stages of the patient self closure.

3-DIMENSIONAL SIMULTANEOUS TIME-SEQUENCING AND FORCE-MAPPING

To observe changing occlusal forces across passing time, a user-Dentist can employ the 3-Dimensional view window with its' changing heights of force

Figure 10. Early closure contact force % per tooth

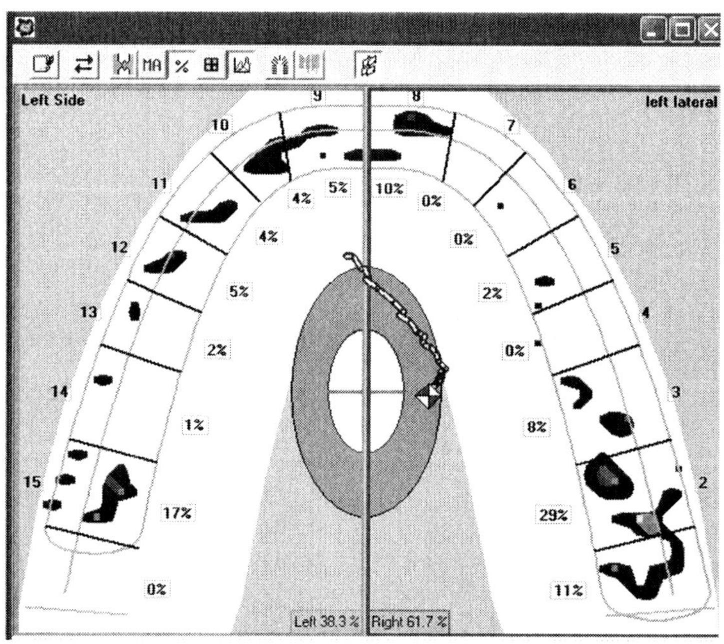

Figure 11. Mid closure contact force % per tooth

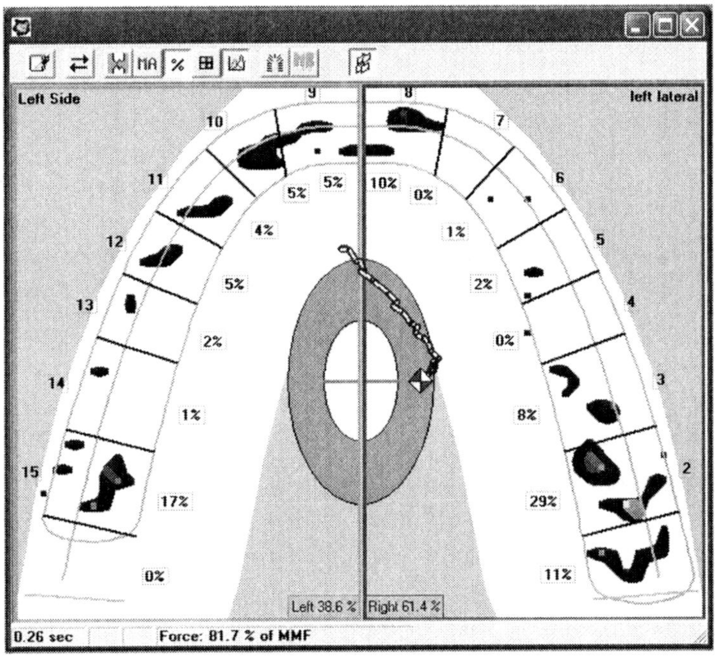

columns. This columnar view displays the same data as the 2 dimensional window, but in a force-wise, more visually descriptive fashion.

Figure 13, Figure 14 and Figure 15 are the same 3 time moments depicted in Figure 10, Figure 11 and Figure 12. Here they are represented in the

Figure 12. Late closure contact force % per tooth

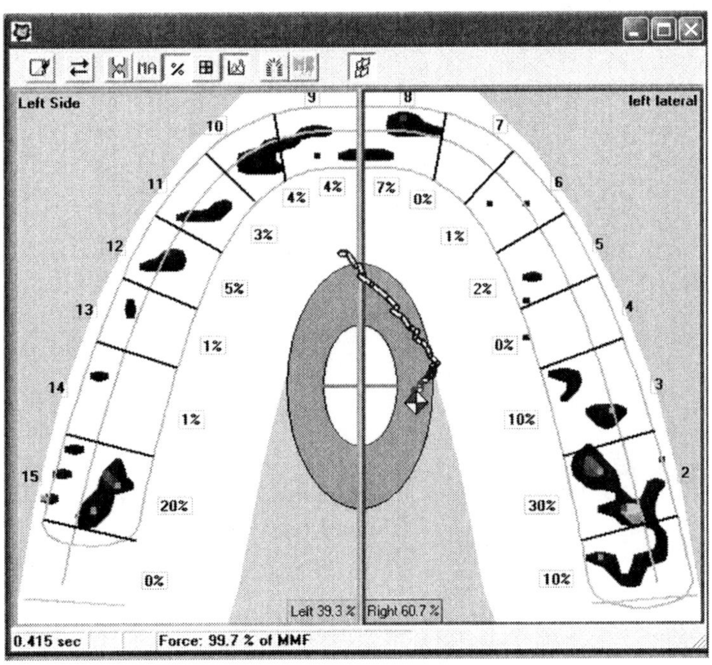

3-Dimensional columnar view. The progression of rising forces on the closure occlusal contacts is displayed as differing column heights in different regions of the dental arch beginning in Figure 13 (early contact forces), thru Figure 14 (mid–closure contacts), to Figure 15 (complete intercuspated contacts). Note how the posterior right teeth demonstrate consistently taller column heights, indicating they are absorbing more occlusal force, than their left side counterparts during each stage of the patient's closure.

INTEGRATED ELECTROMYOGRAPHY SYNCHRONIZED WITH COMPUTERIZED OCCLUSAL ANALYSIS

Computerized Occlusal Analysis and Electromyography technologies have been synchronized together so that a user-Dentist can record, and playback, their separate diagnostic data simultaneously (Kerstein 2004). The T-Scan III system can be linked together thru software integration with the BioPAK Electromyography System (*Bioresearch, Assoc., Milwaukee, Wisconsin. USA.*). The T-Scan III/BioEMG Integration uniquely combines the simultaneous mapping of time-sequencing, force-mapping, and muscle activity.

The integration of these two technologies allows the user-Dentist to analyze and correlate specific time-sequences and occlusal event contact force moments to specific electromyographic changes that result from these occlusal moments. Their combined desktops can be seen in Figure 16, which places the recorded occlusal event data beside the recorded electromyographic data of up to 8 head and neck muscles. The Time Line in the T-Scan III is synchronized with a Time Line in the EMG playback window (vertical grey line) such that the displayed occlusal data and displayed electromyographic data are mapped simultaneously.

Figure 13. 3D columnar view early closure contacts

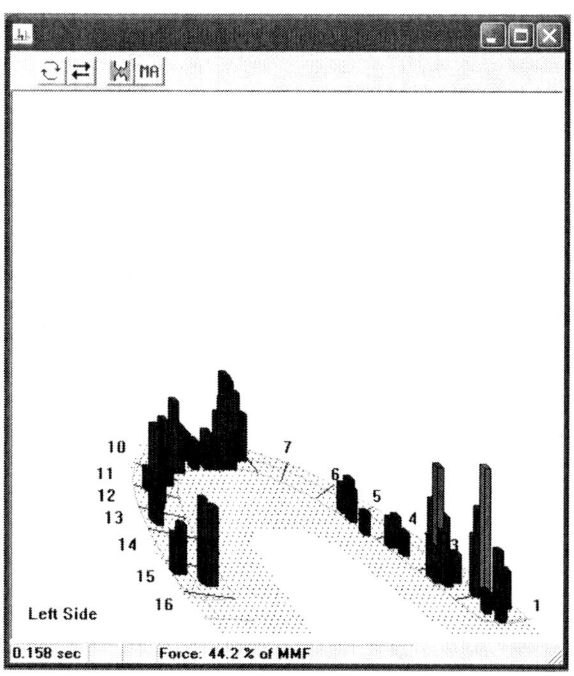

Figure 14. 3D columnar view mid closure contacts

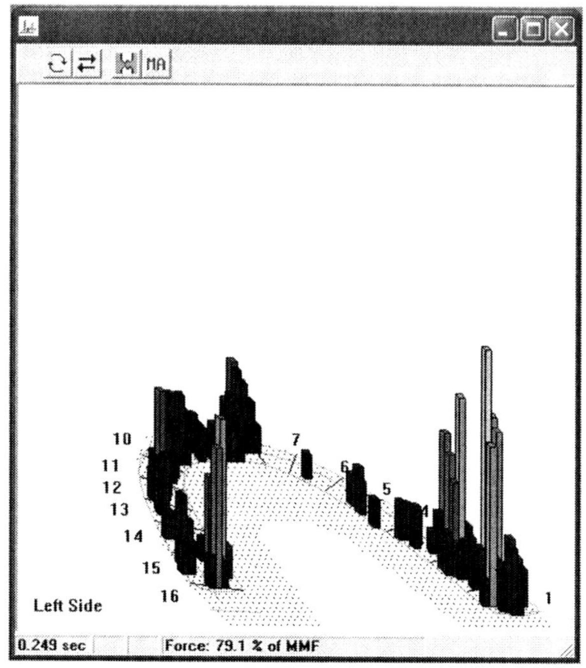

Figure 15. 3D columnar view late closure contacts

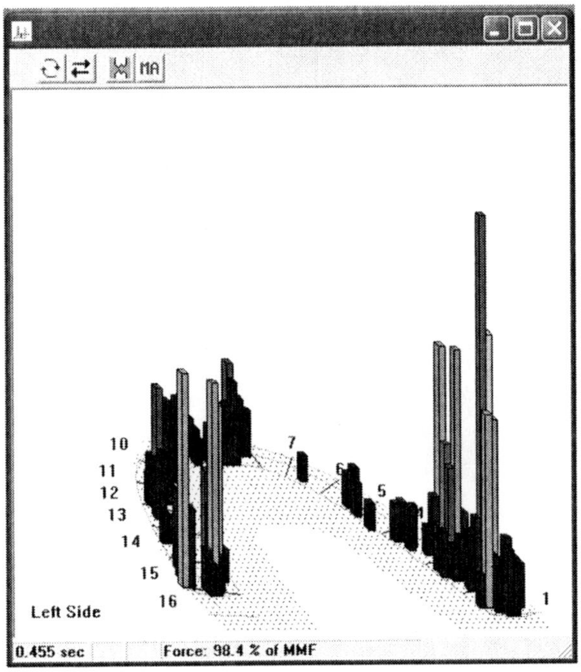

This T-Scan III/BioEMG synchronization affords the user-Dentist a unique method to ascertain the relationship of the muscle activity levels resultant from any occlusal contact time-sequence, and/or contact force map

BIOPAK ELECTROMYOGRAPHY SYSTEM

The BioPAK electromyography system records electrical (bio-potential) activity from eight muscles simultaneously. Bilaterally, the anterior temporalis, massetter, digastric, and sternocleidomastoid muscles, can be measured. The user-Dentist can choose which muscle combinations are to be analyzed.

Surface EMG measurements are obtained by means of conductive adhesive gel-based bipolar electrodes. The electrodes are attached to the skin, over the palpated main bulk of the contracted muscle, and oriented parallel to the general direction of the muscle fibers (Figure 17). An IBM/PC-compatible computer (*or Macintosh with Intel Processor*) samples the individual muscular activity level signals sequentially through a USB interface at the rate of 1000-6000 samples per second (*with a resolution of 12 or 16 bits*).

Before analysis, the filtered raw myoelectric signals are amplified to 5000 times their original levels. The signals are displayed on a computer as *real-time time-domain waveforms* and off-line as *frequency-domain waveforms,* as average levels that disclose contraction patterns and relative muscle contraction intensities. After the data are recorded, they are digitally filtered to remove virtually all (*99%*) of any 50/60-cycle noise content from the electromyographic signals. NOTE: A reduction of 40 dB (on a logarithmic scale) is equivalent to a 99% reduction in noise amplitude. Subsequently, specific occlusal event muscle contraction actions (*clench, swallow, excursion, etc.*) can be quantified in microvolts. An optional, special module, is available that is specifically designed for the analysis of masticatory function.

SYSTEM INTEGRATION DYNAMICS

The integration and synchronization of these 2 separate systems affords the user-Dentist real-time recording of occlusal contacts and the electrical potential of selected masticatory muscles in a dynamic "Movie Form". The T-Scan III system initiates the acquisition of both types of data when its recording function is activated. At that exact moment, the electromyographic recording initiates, as well. As tooth contact time-sequence and force data is recorded, so is the muscle activity recorded (Kerstein 2004).

In the Biopak EMG playback windows, the recorded electromyography data is displayed as a real-time EMG Movie that is time-stamped to match the occlusal contact data time-stamps recorded by the T-Scan III system. 2 EMG play-

Figure 16. T-Scan III/BioEMG desktop with long disclusion time and hyperactive EMG data

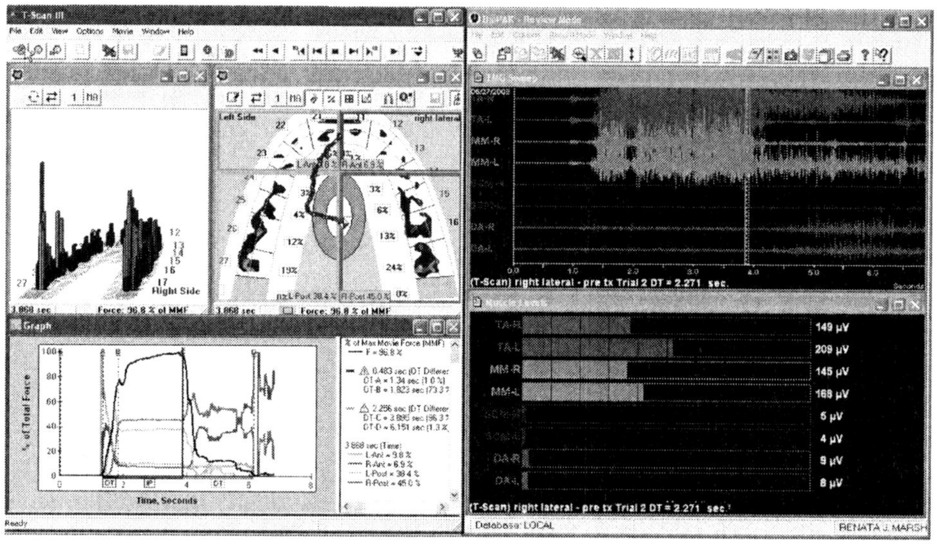

back windows are present; one that shows the recorded muscle activity in wave-form (above) with a vertical time curser that moves through the wave forwards or backwards (time-synchronized with the T Scan). The other window *below* is a horizontal bar graph which contains changing bar lengths that illustrate the changing quantitative muscle activity levels in micro-volts. Both the wave-form and bar graphs can be played forwards and backwards continuously, or as .01 second frames (*non-Turbo Mode)* or in .003 second frames (*Turbo Mode*) in stop-action, at the same time, and in the same manner as the T-Scan III Movie playback.

The time synchronization of the 2 systems insures that transitory occlusal contact variances

Figure 17. T-Scan III Handle and Bio/EMG leads placed on 8 head and neck muscles

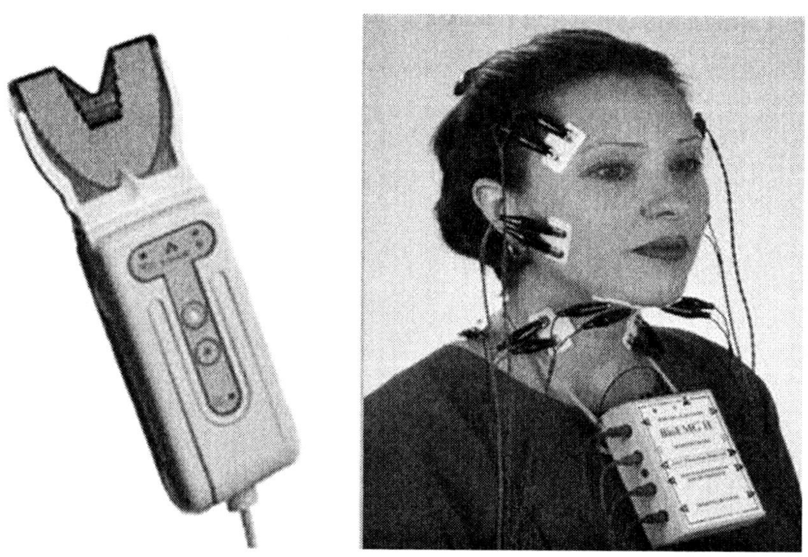

in time-sequencing and force-mapping, which occur throughout a recorded Movie, can be time-correlated to specific changes in muscle activity levels that are the result of these variances. This is an occlusal "first" as at no prior time has it been possible to record simultaneously dynamic occlusal contact information and its corresponding muscle activity information.

EXAMPLE OF CLINICAL OCCLUSAL PARAMETER OPTIMIZATION

Because of the precision simultaneous data capture of the T-Scan III and the Bio EMG integration module, crucial occlusal optimization procedures and their impact on muscle function can all be quantified, understood, and manipulated through computer-guided occlusal adjustments. Computer-guidance insures the treated occlusion is measurably optimized. For example, when a user-Dentist performs an occlusal adjustment procedure known as a Disclusion Time Reduction *(Kerstein and Wright 1991, Kerstein 1992, Kerstein 1993, Kerstein 1994, Kerstein 1995, Kerstein Chapman and Klein 1997, Kerstein and Radke 2006)* the recipient patient will undergo Clinical Occlusal Parameter Optimization, which is designed to shorten the elapsed time that all posterior teeth engage during functional jaw movements. Disclusion Time Reduction reduces the frictional forces that are shared between teeth as they mill together during chewing, and clenching and Bruxism. Less frictional force applied to the engaging teeth, reduces their potential for long-term tooth wear, while simultaneously lessening masticatory muscle hyperactivity (Kerstein and Wright 1991, Kerstein 2004, Kerstein 1995, Kerstein Chapman and Klein 1997) that is often a factor in muscular overload of the Temporomandibular Joints.

Within the pre operative EMG data (Figure 12), note that to the direct right of the vertical Time Line, there is excursive muscle hyperactivity in the right temporalis and left massetter muscles, while the left temporalis and right massetter muscles demonstrate almost no elevated muscle activity. The observed elevated muscle activity is the result of prolonged tooth socket compressions that occur when the patient's Disclusion Time is prolonged (2.256 seconds). The longer is the Disclusion Time, the longer the opposing occluding posterior teeth compress each other into their respective tooth sockets (Kerstein 1993). Because of the unique neuroanatomy of the molar periodontal mechanoreceptors, which synapse directly with muscles of mastication within the Central Nervous System (Haines 2000) prolonged tooth socket compressions can trigger an equally prolonged time-duration of masticatory muscle contraction. In Figure 12, when the patient is moving their mandible to their right, the prolonged Disclusion Time present within this patient's occlusion, contracts the right temporalis and left massetter muscles for a equal time duration of 2.256 seconds. This observed hyperactivity can be minimized therapeutically by shortening the Disclusion Time, which directly shortens the tooth socket compression time.

Figure 18 illustrates the optimized right excursive Disclusion Time after the pre-operative prolonged Disclusion Time is shortened to .279 seconds duration. Within the EMG data (*Figure 18*), note that just to the right of the vertical Time Line post-treatment, there is almost no hyperactivity remaining in the right temporalis and left massetter muscles. This muscular effect is observed because of the dramatically shortened compression time of the contacting opposing teeth within their respective tooth sockets. This therapeutic action is resultant from shortening the pretreatment prolonged Disclusion Time to <.4 seconds (Kerstein and Wright 1991) on the occlusal surfaces of the involved teeth. A comparison of Figure 19 and Figure 20 shows that the pre-operative excessive muscle activity visible to the right of the vertical Time Line (Figure 19), is absent in the post-treatment corrected occlusion (Figure 20).

Figure 18. Short disclusion time post treatment of the long disclusion time depicted in Figure 16

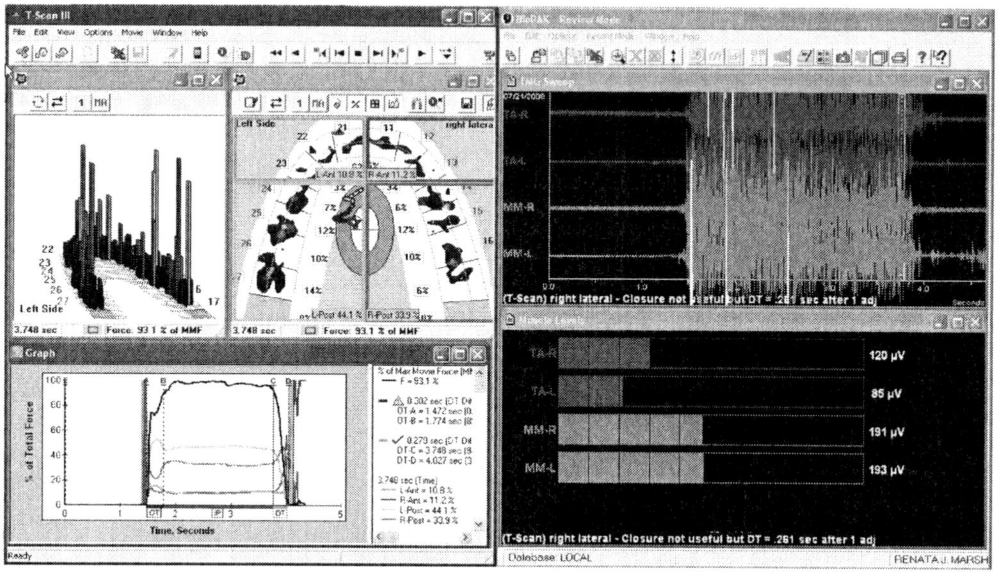

Figure 19. EMG data of pre operative long disclusion time depicted in Figure 16

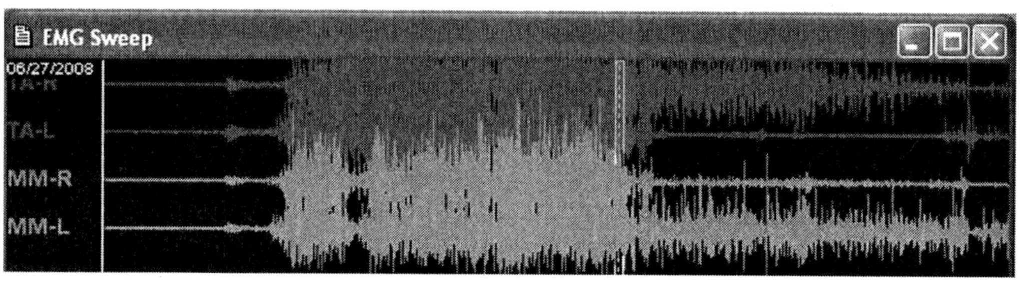

Figure 20. EMG data of post operative short disclusion time depicted in Figure 18

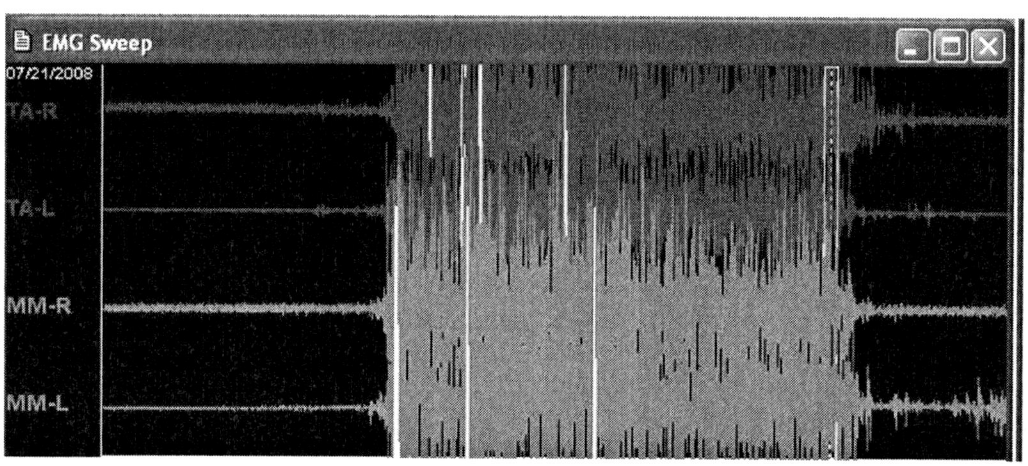

CHAPTER SUMMARY

Time-sequencing and relative occlusal force-mapping with Computerized Occlusal Analysis technology displays for clinical interpretation, tooth contact timing sequences of .003 second increments, with each tooth contacts' fluctuating relative occlusal force levels that occur during functional jaw movements. The displayed occlusal time-sequence and force data aids in the examination and treatment of occlusal abnormalities on natural teeth, dental prostheses, and dental implant prostheses. The software can also be linked to an Electromyography software program that simultaneously records the electromyographic potential of 8 head and neck muscles. This combination of dynamic tooth contact time-sequencing and force-mapping, with functional muscular electromyographic data affords a user-Dentist detailed, precise, and unparalleled diagnostic and treatment information, with which to diagnose and treat many differing clinical occlusal pathologies.

REFERENCES

Carey, J.P., Craig, M., Kerstein, R.B., Radke, J. (2007). Determining a relationship between applied occlusal load and articulating paper mark area. *The Open Dentistry Journal,* (1), 1-7

Carossa, S., Lojacono, A., Schierano, G., & Pera, P. (2000). Evaluation of occlusal contacts in the dental laboratory: influence of strip thickness and operator experience. *The International Journal of Prosthodontics, 13*(3), 201–204.

Haines, D. E. (2000). *Neuroanatomy: An Atlas of Structures, Sections, and Systems*, (5th Ed.) (pp. 175, 193). Baltimore, MD: Lippincott, William and Wilkins.

Kerstein, R. (2001). Current Applications of Computerized Occlusal Analysis in Dental Medicine. *General Dentistry, 49*(5), 521–530.

Kerstein, R. B. (1992). Disocclusion time-reduction therapy with immediate complete anterior guidance development to treat chronic myofascial pain-dysfunction syndrome. *Quintessence International, 23*(11), 735–747.

Kerstein, R. B. (1993). A Comparison of Traditional Occlusal Equilibration and Immediate Complete Anterior Guidance Development. *Cranio, 11*(2), 126–140.

Kerstein, R. B. (1994). Disclusion Time Measurement Studies: Stability of disclusion time. a 1 year follow - up study. *The Journal of Prosthetic Dentistry, 72*(2), 164–168. doi:10.1016/0022-3913(94)90075-2

Kerstein, R. B. (1994). Disclusion time measurement studies, Part 2: A comparison of disclusion time length of 49 chronic myofascial pain dysfunction syndrome patients to 40 non - patients. A population analysis. *The Journal of Prosthetic Dentistry, 72*(5), 473–480. doi:10.1016/0022-3913(94)90117-1

Kerstein, R. B. (1995). Treatment of myofascial pain dysfunction syndrome with occlusal therapy to reduce lengthy disclusion time - a recall study. *Cranio, 13*(2), 105–115.

Kerstein, R. B. (1999). Computerized Occlusal Management of a Fixed/ Detachable Implant Prosthesis. *Pract Periodontol Aesthet Dent, 11*(9 November/December), 1093-1102.

Kerstein, RB Grundset, K. (2001). Obtaining Measurable Bilateral Simultaneous Occlusal Contacts with Computer-Analyzed and Guided Occlusal Adjustments. *Quintessence International, January, 32*(1), 7-18.

Kerstein, R. B. (2004). Combining Technologies: A Computerized Occlusal Analysis System Synchronized with a Computerized Electromyography System. *Cranio, 22*(2), 96–109.

Kerstein, R. B., Chapman, R., & Klein, M. (1997). A Comparison of ICAGD (Immediate Complete Anterior Guidance Development) to Mock ICAGD for Symptom Reductions in Chronic Myofascial Pain Dysfunction Syndrome Patient. *Cranio*, *5*(1), 21–37.

Kerstein, R.B., & Lowe, M., Harty, Radke, J. (2006). A Force reproduction analysis of two recording sensors of a computerized occlusal analysis system. *Cranio*, *24*(1), 15–24.

Kerstein, R. B., & Radke, J. (2006). The effect of Disclusion Time Reduction on maximal clench muscle activity level. *Cranio*, *24*(3), 156–165.

Kerstein, R. B., & Wilkerson, D. (2001). Locating the Centric Relation Prematurity with a Computerized Occlusal Analysis System. *Compend Contin Educ Dent*, *22*(6), 525–532.

Kerstein, R. B., & Wright, N. (1991). An electromyographic and computer analysis of patients suffering from chronic myofascial pain dysfunction syndrome; pre and post - treatment with immediate complete anterior guidance development. *The Journal of Prosthetic Dentistry*, *66*(5), 677–686. doi:10.1016/0022-3913(91)90453-4

Maness, W. L. (1988). Force Movie: A Time and Force View of Occlusal Contacts. *Compend Contin Educ Dent*, *10*(7), 404–408.

Maness, W. L. (1993). Computerized Occlusal Analysis, Hi-Tech, Hi-Care. *Dental Journal*, *59*(8).

Maness, W. L., Benjamin, M., Podoloff, R., Bobick, A., & Golden, R. F. (1987). Computerized occlusal analysis: a new technology. *Quintessence International*, *18*(4), 287–292.

Millstein, P., & Maya, A. (2001). An evaluation of occlusal contact marking indicators descriptive quantitative method. *The Journal of the American Dental Association*, *132*(9), 1280–1286.

Montgomery, M., & Kerstein, R. B. (2000). Mapping Occlusal Forces on Rebuilt Anterior Guidance. *Contemporary Esthetics*, *4*(4), 68–72.

Reiber, T., Fuhr, K., & Hartmann, H. (1989). Recording pattern of occlusal indicators, influence of indicator thickness, pressure, and surface morphology. *Deutsche Zahnarztliche Zeitschrift*, *44*(2), 90–93.

Saad, M.N., Weiner, Ehrenberg D., et al. (2008). Effects of load and indicator type upon occlusal contact markings. *Journal of Biomedical Materials Research. Part B, Applied Biomaterials*, *85*(1), 18–22. doi:10.1002/jbm.b.30910

Saraçoğlu, A., & Ozpinar, B. J. (2002). In vivo and in vitro evaluation of occlusal indicator sensitivity. *The Journal of Prosthetic Dentistry*, *88*(5), 522–526. doi:10.1067/mpr.2002.129064

KEY TERMS AND DEFINITIONS

Absolute Force: Force measured in Engineering Units.

Articulating Paper: Colored ink-impregnated strips of Mylar or paper that is employed by Dentists to mark occlusal contact locations between occluding teeth. Scientific studies have repeatedly determined that Articulating Paper cannot measure or map occlusal forces, or describe occlusal contact time-sequences.

Disclusion Time Reduction: A computer-guided occlusal adjustment procedure that shortens prolonged durations of frictional occlusal surface engagement shared between opposing molars and premolars during a mandibular excursive movement (right working, left working or protrusive). Prolonged occlusal surface engagement creates an equal time duration of prolonged molar and premolar compressions into their respective tooth sockets and Periodontal Ligaments. The objective of the "Disclusion Time Reduction" procedure is to shorten the pre-treatment prolonged frictional interaction of the involved posterior teeth such that, there is an equal time reduction of the time duration that these molar and premolar compress their respective Periodontal Ligaments. By reducing the compression time of the Periodontal Ligaments, excess masticatory muscle hyperactivity created in the masticatory muscles from the prolonged compressions of the periodontal Ligament, is physiologically lessened. Muscular symptoms of Myofascial Pain Dysfunction Syndrome (MPDS) can be effectively and rapidly treated with Disclusion Time Reduction (average published treatment times are 3 -5 treatment visits spread over 1-2 months of total treatment time).

Electromyography: The recording of the electrical activity in muscles using conductive adhesive gel-based bipolar surface electrodes. The BioPAK Electromyography system can be synchronized with the T-Scan III System so that the 2 data sets (muscle activity levels, and tooth contact force-mapping and time-sequencing) can be recorded simultaneously.

Force-Based Occlusal Adjustments: The technique of correcting relative occlusal force abnormalities by utilizing the location of measured and excessive relative occlusal force levels as a guide for the dentist to where to reshape specific affected occlusal surface regions of the dental arches.

Force-Mapping: The spatial locating and displaying of relative occlusal force levels that result from the frictional interaction of the occlusal surfaces of sets of upper and lower contacting teeth as a patient makes functional mandibular movements when recorded over elapsed time.

Force Movie (or Movie): The playback of a digital recording of numerous simultaneous and non-simultaneous changing occlusal forces that evolve over elapsed time during Occlusal Events. It can be displayed in 2 or 3 dimensions and played forwards or backwards continuously, or in individual time increments of .01-.003 seconds in duration.

HD Sensor: 4th generation T-Scan III sensor design with the most active recording surface area and the least inactive non-recording surface area.

I-Scan System: An alternative Tekscan computer program that measures absolute force in engineering units.

Occlusal Force: Force that is generated between the occlusal (bite) surfaces of contacting teeth.

Occlusal Event: A functional movement of the mandible, like chewing, opening and closing, or sliding the mandible across the maxilla, during which opposing teeth from the mandible and maxilla frictionally generate occlusal forces over fractions of seconds of elapsed time

Occlusal Parameter Optimization: The improvement of prolonged pre treatment non-ideal Occlusion Times and/or Disclusion Times to more physiologic durations through corrective computer-guided occlusal adjustments.

Occlusal Time Parameters: The measured elapsed time of opposing tooth contact interactions that occur during recorded Occlusal Events. Occlusion Time (OT) and Disclusion Time (DT) are 2 occlusal time parameters.

Recording Sensitivity: Variable levels of sensor "activeness" that can be selected by the user-Dentist, to optimize the quality of the occlusal force recording so as to compensate for varying individual patient occlusal force strength capacity.

Recording Sensor: The dental arch-shaped recording element of the T-Scan system. It is comprised of rows and columns of "sensels" surrounded by rows conductive ink. When compressed by occluding teeth, the individual sensels register a voltage output that is proportional to the applied load.

Relative Occlusal Force: Describes different occlusal force levels as greater to, equal to, or less than each other.

Timed-Based Occlusal Adjustments: The technique of correcting prolonged occlusal contact time engagement abnormalities by utilizing the measured and elongated occlusal contact time durations to guide the dentist as to where to reshape affected occlusal surface regions of the dental arches.

Time Regions: Colored portions on the time axis (x-axis) of a Force vs. Time Graph that quantify tooth contact durations that occur between interacting teeth within a recorded occlusal event. These regions are defined within the Graph between 2 sets of hyphenated vertical lines (A-B and C-D lines).

Time-Sequence: The order of individual tooth contacts that occur between sets of upper and lower interacting occlusal surfaces when recorded over elapsed time and measured in .001-003 second real-time increments as a patient makes functional mandibular movements.

T-Scan III System: This is a Microsoft Windows® compliant clinical occlusal diagnostic computer workstation. An IBM compatible PC with a Pentium processor and a minimum of 4-8 megabytes of RAM are required to properly operate the system. The graphical interface uses Windows® toolbar icons, to display the software features that analyze recorded occlusal contact information.

User-Dentist: A dental clinician who employs the T-Scan System to map occlusal forces and time-sequence occlusal contacts.

ENDNOTE

1. Practice limited to prosthodontics and computerized occlusal analysis

Chapter 8
Selective Laser Melting in Dentistry

Roland Strietzel
BEGO Bremer Goldschlaegerei, Germany

ABSTRACT

Although casting is currently the first choice to produce metallic frame work selective laser melting (SLM) has established. Based on a CAD/CAM system the digital data of the frame work are transferred to the production machine. The three dimensional data set of the transferred in to numerous quasi 2-dimensional data. Each of these data sets represents a single slice, which is then produced. Due to the production process complex geometries and outstanding mechanical and chemical properites can be realized. Advantageously is also the large number of simultaneously fabricated parts, which makes this method very economic.

INTRODUCTION AND PRESENT STATUS

In dentistry destroyed enamel and/or dentine has to be replaced by artificial materials. If the defects are too big also complete teeth have to be replaced. Therefore materials for fillings (e. g. composites, amalgams, alloys or ceramics) and for crown and bridges (acrylics, ceramics, metals) have to be distinguished. The present article will focus on metallic materials for the production of frameworks.

DOI: 10.4018/978-1-60566-733-1.ch008

The most common way to fabricate metallic frameworks is casting. In this process the dental technician transfers the impression made by the dentist into a model (most made of gypsum). Then the framework is molded with wax. After this he invests the wax modelations and sprueings in special investment materials. In special furnaces the wax is burned out. In those hollow spaces the alloy is than cast. After embedding the framework is polished or veneered with ceramics or composites.

Several different hundred metals are available for frameworks. They may be classified due to their usage (e. g. inlays/onlays, crown and bridges or for

Table 1. Overview of dental alloys classified according to their main component

Precious alloys	Non precious alloys
Gold-based	**Cobalt-based**
Pure gold (galvano technique)	For partial dentures
High gold content	With ceramics venerable
Gold reduced	**Nickel-based**
Palladium-based	Nickel-chromium alloys
Palladium-copper	High chromium content
Palladium-silver	Low chromium content
Silver-based	Nickel-titanium alloys
Silver-Palladium	**Iron-based**
Silver-gold	**Titanium**
	Pure Titanium
	Titanium alloys

partial dentures), their fabrication (e. g. casting, sintering) or their composition (Table 1).

In the present the price of the restorations is getting more and more important. The US and the European markets have great difficulties to compete with the Asian laboratories because of the low labor costs there. One possible way to over come this is to automate the production process. This is one of the reasons CAD/CAM systems are entering the market in Europe successfully.

In general on have to divide the automated production process in to two parts. The first part is the CAD step (CAD: computer aided design). In this step the geometry of the parts which should be produced is defined. Than the second step, the CAM (CAM: computer aided manufacturing), follows. Here the information for the production is merged. Mostly the control of the production machines is made here.

CAD/CAM in dentistry is discussed since over 20 years (Strietzel & Lahl, 2007). One of the pioneers is the French Duret who published basic ideas for 20 years (Duret, 1992, 1993; Duret, Blouin, & Duret, 1988; Duret & Preston, 1991). Another important (among others) is the working group of Rekow (D. Rekow, 1987; E. D. Rekow, 1991; E. D. Rekow & Erdmann, 1985; E. D. Rekow, Erdmann, & Speidel, 1985).

For decades CAD/CAM systems were not successful. As the zirconium dioxide entered the market the number of installed systems increased strongly in a short time because this material could only be produced with CAD/CAM systems. A production with conventional methods was not possible.

Figure 1. Production machine for SLM technique

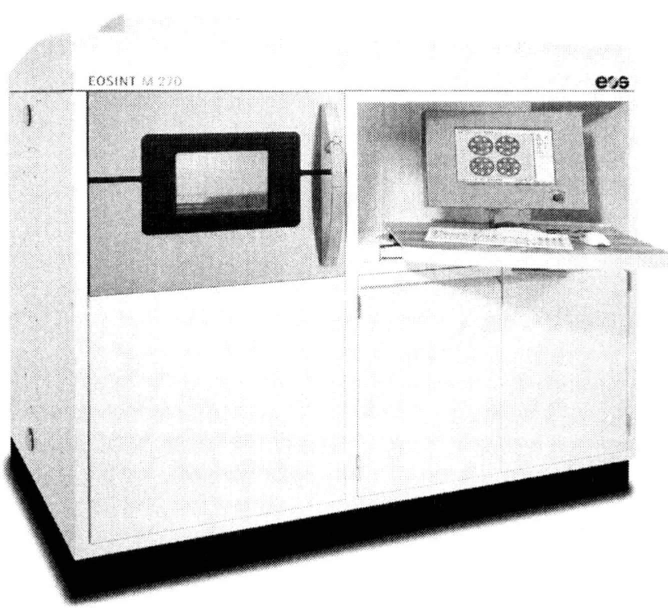

Looking at the CAD/CAM production one can distinguish between several major steps:

Scanning (digitalizing the oral situation)

- Optically
  - Light
  - Laser
- Mechanically

Virtual construction (CAD step)

Production (CAM step)

- Material for the production
  - Metals
  - Ceramics
  - Resin based material
- Location of the production
  - Centralized
    - Chair side by the dentist
    - In the dental laboratory
  - Decentralized (production center)
    - Subtractive production
      - Milling (ceramics, metals, resin based metals)
      - Sparc erosion (metals)
    - Additive production
      - Stereolitography (for resin based materials)
      - SLM (metals)

Independent from the production process the oral situation has to be converted into the virtual world for a CAD/CAM based production. In the conventional process the dentist takes an impression as pointed out already. From this impression (mostly made of silicones) a gypsum model is made by the dental technician. With help of this model he builds up the framework in wax. In case of the CAD/CAM systems the gypsum model is scanned optically (by light or laser) or mechanically (seldom). The virtual situation is than transferred in a CAD program where the construction of the framework is made by the dental technician.

After construction the data is transferred into a CAM program for the production. The production facilities may be located in the dental surgery (so called "chair side systems"), in the dental laboratory or in a production center. Therefore it may be distinguished by a central or decentralized production. In case of the SLM process only a central production (production center) makes sense due to the high investment costs. The question if the production should be central or decentralized is discussed (Pfeifer & Riquier, 2006).

Zirconia (= zirconium dioxide, ZrO_2) may be milled or grind in two different states (Luthard, Rudolph, Sandkuhl, & Walter, 2001; Luthardt, Rudolph, Sandkuhl, & Walter, 2001). Meanwhile the most systems are milling zirconia in a white state. After milling the material has to be sintered. If presintered zirconia is used this material is most often "hipped" (hip: high isostatic pressure). This is done to reduce amount and size of porosities. The hipped material is more dense than the "white zirconia" which has to be sintered after the grinding process. The disadvantage is the high hardness. Therefore the grinding process is very long lasting and demanding.

Because of the brittleness of ceramics porosities or cracks will lead to failure of the restoration. Looking closer to this material it have to be stated that no pure zirconia is used (Cramer von Clausbruch, 2003; Kappert & Krah, 2001). One has to give certain percentages of other oxides to the basic material to be able to use it. The most important component is the Yttrium oxide. This compound is responsible for the "self healing" property of zirconia. Due to phase transformation cracks are hindered in growth. Aluminum oxide is another important compound.

The milling of metals is possible but not in every case economic due to the large amount of unused material. The milling of titanium (Andersson, Carlsson, Persson, & Bergman, 1996) and cobalt chromium alloys is state of the art. Precious alloys may also be produced this way but this is very uneconomic.

CAD/CAM systems are using most often milling systems for the production. For titanium spark erosion is used for the fabrication (Berg,

Davik, Hegdahl, & Gjerdet, 1996). All subtractive processes have the disadvantage of the waste of material. This is maybe acceptable for ceramics, resin based materials or titanium but not for precious metal alloys. Even nickel or cobalt alloys are too expensive to throw away up to 90% of the alloy. Therefore additive processes seem to be more economic. Besides this aspect the milling of cobalt alloys is very demanding for the machines.

Another way to fabricate frameworks, especially for partial dentures, is to plot the virtual data in to wax or resin based material, embed and cast those (Negrel, 2006). This technology, discussed under the name of "CAD cast", is a possible link between CAD/CAM and conventional (Witkowski, 2001) but industrial casting of crown and bridge frameworks.

Another way for the production of frameworks made out of zirconia has established (Cramer von Clausbruch, 2006, 2008; Steger, 2005) in the past few years. The pantograph is somehow a "hybrid technology", settled somewhere between the conventional and CAD/CAM process. This technology is known since several years in dentistry (Eidenbenz & Schärer, 1994; Rinke, Hüls, & Chafizadeh, 1995; Rinke, Markgraf, Jahn, & Hüls, 1994) but undergoes nowadays a renaissance. Those systems need a modellation made out of wax or resin based material. The modellation is than copied mechanically (Steger, 2005) or with a laser scanner (Völkl, 2001). As material presintered ("white") zirconia is used by those systems. After milling the restoration have to be sintered.

In 2008 one may consider that CAD/CAM systems are standard procedures in the dental laboratory. Even though the production of ceramic frameworks is the most used method (Suttor, 2004), also metallic materials are in the focus. But due to the success of the zirconia one links dental CAD/CAM mostly to milling or grinding ceramics.

SELECTIVE LASER MELTING

In industrial research it is necessary to have models of certain objects at a very early state of the research. Therefore several so called rapid prototyping methods were developed (Gebhardt, 2000). For example stereo lithographic processes are used to test new chassis for mobile phones. Similar to that is the laser sintering/melting (SLM) process. In this method the objects are build up by layer by layer. In the industrial SLM process several metals were used. Often two different metals were needed. One of those was a low melting alloy. Those alloys functioned as a binding agent. For dental application this was no option. The available metals (except titanium) were not biocompatible because they were not corrosion resistant and stable in the oral environment. Especially the two phased systems seemed not to meet the requirements of dental alloys regarding mechanical, chemical and biological properties. Last but not least the dental technician couldn't handle those industrial metals. The milling and polishing properties were not appropriate. Also the coefficients of thermal expansion were not suitable to commercial available veneering ceramics. Therefore it was necessary to develop also metal powders that could be fabricated by SLM and meet the dental requirements. The handling of the powder is one key to the success of the SLM process and therefore kept as a secret by the producers. One point of interest is the grain size and contribution.

In 2001 BEGO Medical entered the German market as first dental company with a SLM process (Strietzel, 2004). Two alloys were introduced, a venerable cobalt chromium alloys (Wirobond® C+) and a venerable high gold content alloy (Bio PontoStar® ++). Those two alloys are chemically identical to the alloys used in the conventional casting process (Kirches, Pack, & Schoofs, 2000; Oppacher, 2000). Pure titanium was possible to process, but the market share was too small. Therefore the titanium was not introduced into the market with the SLM technology.

Figure 2. SLM produced lot of dental restorations (BEGO Medical/Bremen, Germany)

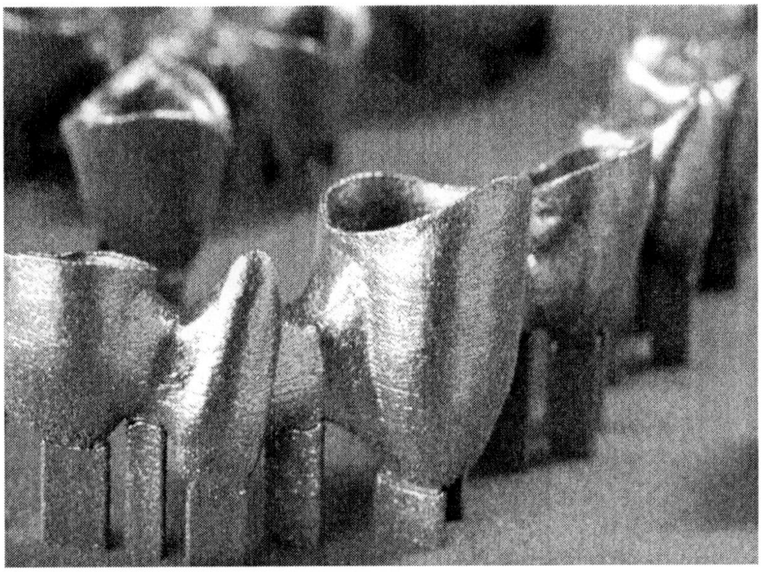

What is noticeable that it was the first industrial usage of SLM for a regular (mass) production. Since than this production method has established in dental technology (Bressem, 2006, 2007).

The Principle of Selective Laser Melting

SLM (selective laser melting) is an additive production process (Strietzel & Lahl, 2007). In contrast to the subtractive processes like milling or spark erosion the objects are building up. They seem to rise out of dust (Niemann, 2003).

For the milling process a virtual model is used to calculate the course of the milling cutter for the milling machine. Then a block of the material is placed into the machine and the milling process is started. In case of SLM also a virtual model is used. But in contrast to the milling process the virtual framework is cut in virtual slices (slicing). The three dimensional model is converted to numerous "two dimensional" files. The third dimension, the constant height of each slice, is responsible for the speed of the process and the accuracy of the final object.

In the next step all objects to be fabricated are placed on a virtual production tablet. One advantage of the SLM process is that a big number of objects may be fabricated parallel (Figure 2). This means a very low production time per unit, which reduces costs.

Afterwards the powder is given on a production platform. This platform can be heated and is moveable in the vertical direction. The whole production room is filled with an inert gas to prevent unwanted oxidation reactions due to high temperatures during the sintering and melting processes.

The laser used for the production is a Nd-YAG laser system. This type of a laser is suitable for metals because they couple into this wave length.

When the first powder layer is applied a laser beam surrounds the border of every slice of each object (Figure 3). When the borders are solidified, the inner material is molten by the laser beam (so called hatch process, hatching). For this process specific strategies have been developed. Those influence the speed and the quality of the process.

After the first layer is solidified the production platform is lowered by the amount of the virtual

Figure 3. Scheme of SLM, shown is the production platform with the applied powder layer

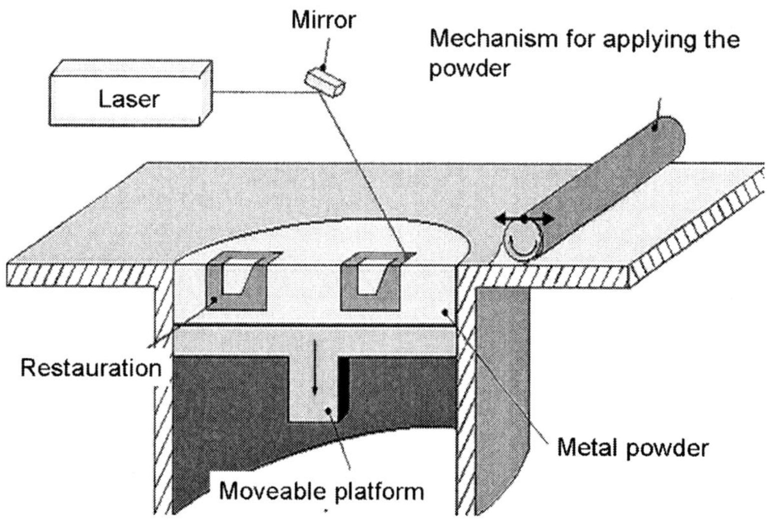

thickness of the next slice to be produced and a new layer of powder is applied. Than the solidification process starts over. The whole procedure is than carried out until all slices are produced.

Because the powder is applied mechanically the danger is big that produced slices are moved horizontally. This unwanted movement would cause a distortion of the framework and has to be avoided. Therefore supporting structures are needed. They are constructed with the CAM software when the virtual models are given into the production machine. After the production the supporting structures have to be removed from the restorations. This is the only material wasted. Together with the short production time per part this is the reason for the economic benefit of the SLM process, even it is discussed contradictory (Riquier, 2006).

The results of the SLM process are objects with a high density and outrageous mechanical properties. Due to the high resolution of the process and the slice by slice technique very complex objects may be produced. For example an under cut is no problem for the production. This means for the dental technician that he must avoid those. An appropriate method is to block out the model before scanning.

One of the parameter which may be influenced is the density of the framework. To speed up the process a low density would be favorable. But this would lower the mechanical integrity of the framework. Therefore it is wanted to achieve a high density. But looking at frameworks for bridges it is thinkable that one can save time and cost when the pontics are not manufactured completely dense. Due to the ductility of metals and when a sufficient thickness of the surrounding walls may be assured it thinkable to produce porous structures in the interior space of the pontics. Problematic is when the dental technician opens those structures. Then problems will appear during firing the ceramics. Due to the hollow structures big volumes of air will expand. The results will be bubbles in the veneering ceramic. This will lead to cracks and therefore to the failure of the veneering.

In general all metals may be fabricated with the SLM process. In dentistry cobalt chromium and high gold content alloys are available (Strietzel, 2004). Titanium was processed also with SLM process by the BEGO Medical Company, but due to the low market share withdrawn from the market quickly.

The Advantages of SLM

As pointed out there are several advantages of the SLM process, which are also discussed by dental technicians (Becker, 2008; Riquier, 2006). Due to the large amounts of units (many dozen) that may be produced in one process parallel the production time per unit is very short, which makes it very economical.

Another big advantage of SLM in contrast to milling is the possibility to control the quality of the fabrication. For each production lot several test specimens are produced simultaneously to the dental parts by BEGO Medical. Those can be tested than (e. g. in a tensile test) and archived. This is not possible with subtractive processes like milling.

Except of the material of the supporting structures there is almost no loss of material. The not used powder can be given in the production process again. Also therefore the SLM process is very economic. The economic production of frameworks consisting out of precious metal alloys is possible this way by a CAD/CAM process.

Also cobalt chromium alloys may be fabricated by SLM very good. Milling this type of alloy is possible but the wearing of the machine is very high and therefore problematic.

Due to the slice by slice technique very complex structures may be produced as stated already. Besides some thinkable problems (s. above) the advantages of the SLM process over weigh clearly. There is nearly no restriction concerning the geometries of the produced objects.

Because the dental technician receives frameworks of the same material as he is used, he can continue in the usual way in his work. He doesn't need to change his work flow or use new/other materials (e. g. veneering ceramics). For example the cobalt chromium bonding alloy Wirobond® C+ (BEGO Medical, for SLM production) has the same composition as the Wirobond® SG (BEGO, cast version).

Besides the numerous advantages of the SLM process there are also disadvantages. For example the powder management is quite difficult. Also one has high investment cost. Last but not least there are also difficulties occurred during production. Due to the production in layers one can observe distortions of the frameworks. There are several possibilities discussed (Eisen & Hinterseher, 2008) to over come those negative effects.

Properties of Dental Alloys Produced by SLM

As mentioned above the chemical composition of the alloys used in the SLM process is identical with the cast version also the mechanical properties should be same. But this is not true. Because of the other structure of the alloys due the SLM process the mechanical and chemical properties are other.

Looking at the etched framework of Wirobond® C+ (Figure 4) one can observe crystallites with a diameter of probably 1 – 3 µm. In case of cast material the crystallites are roundabout ten times larger. The smaller grain size is responsible for the changed mechanical values (Figure 5). The deviations of the modulus of elasticity are not so big. But the 0,2% yield strength and the tensile strength are clearly higher (SLM), which is positive. In contrast the elongation limit is lower and the hardness is higher, which is less favourable. But in any case the international standards for dental alloys are fulfilled (DIN_EN_ISO_9693, 2001). In an investigation of the University of Halle/Germany it was shown that veneered copings showed the same high mechanical stabilities (Rudolph, Beoeckler, & Setz, 2007) regardless if they were cast or fabricated with the SLM process.

Even though it is not as decisive for metals as for ceramics one has to look at porosities. They influence the mechanical stability of the framework. When they are too big and near the surface

Figure 4. Microstructure of Wirobond® C+ (CoCr alloy), etched

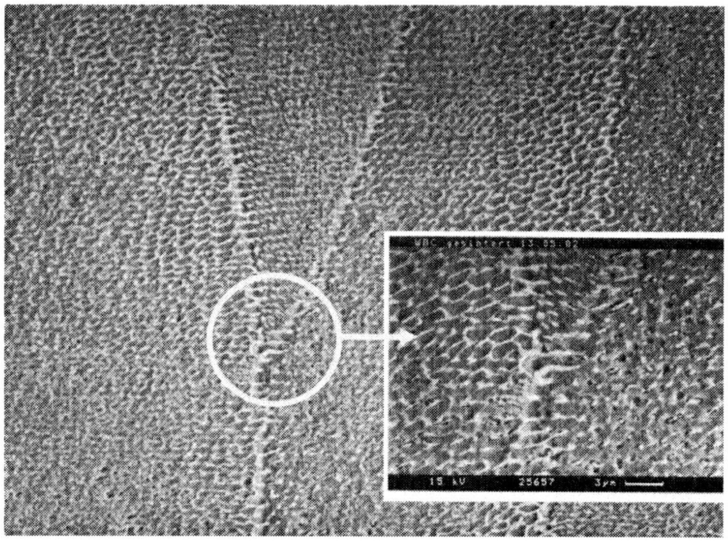

Figure 5. Comparison of the mechanical parameters of Wirobond® C+ and Wirobond® SG. The green bars indicate favorable changes, the red ones unfavorable

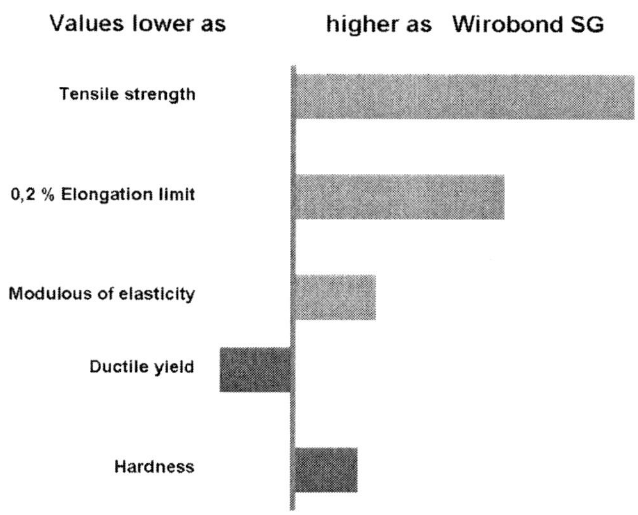

they may also influence the bonding between the metal and the veneering ceramics. The enclosed air will expand strongly during the firing cycles and may cause bubbles in the veneering ceramic, which will lower the strength and aesthetics.

Looking at a conventional cast of Wirobond® SG one can observe several very small bubbles (Figure 6). In the area of a sprueing stud many and also big porosities can be seen. Those may cause problems due to their comparatively large volume. The SLM frameworks made of Wirobond® C+ also reveal porosities but those are in general smaller (Figure 7).

All frameworks reveal porosities, independent if they were cast or produced with the SLM process. The total amount of porosities is far under

1%, or in other words one achieves densities from over 99%.

Another very important property of dental frameworks is the bonding with veneering ceramics. There are several test methods described in literature (Strietzel, 2005). In the international standardization ISO 9693 (DIN_EN_ISO_9693, 2001) the so called "Schwickerath-test", a three point bending test, is defined as a method to determinate the bond strength between alloys and veneering ceramics. The results of a testing with several commercially available veneering ceramics reveal that in every case more than 25 MPa are achieved (Figure 8). Values above this value are regarded as clinical

Figure 6. Cut through an cast four span bridge of Wirobond® SG

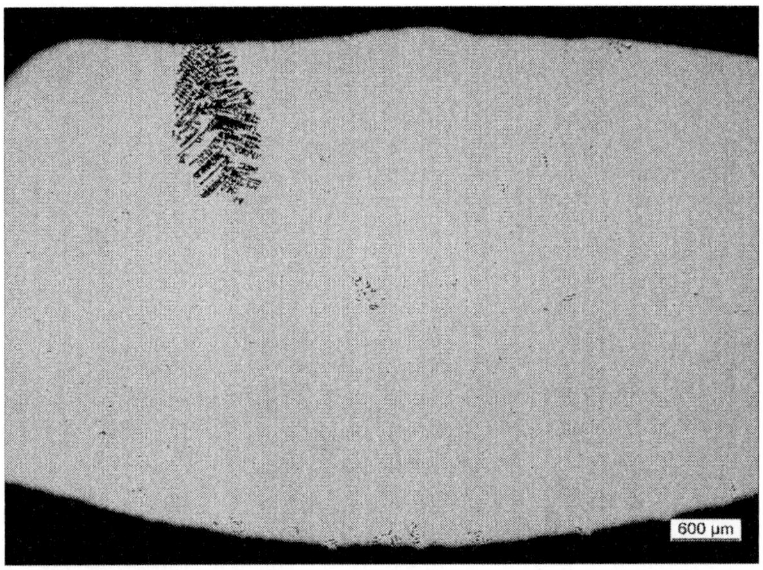

Figure 7. Cut through a four span bridge of Wirobond® C+ produced with the SLM process

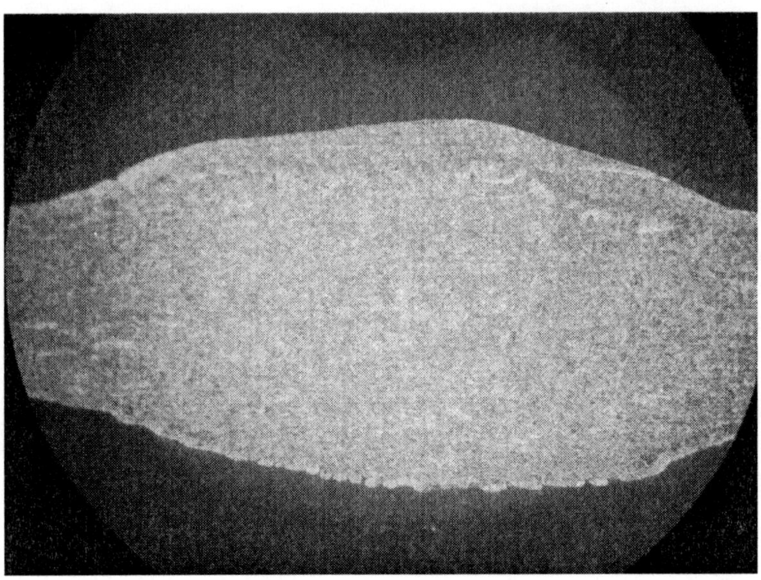

Figure 8. Results of the Schwickerath-Test according to ISO 9693 of Wirobond® C+ with 10 commercially available veneering ceramics

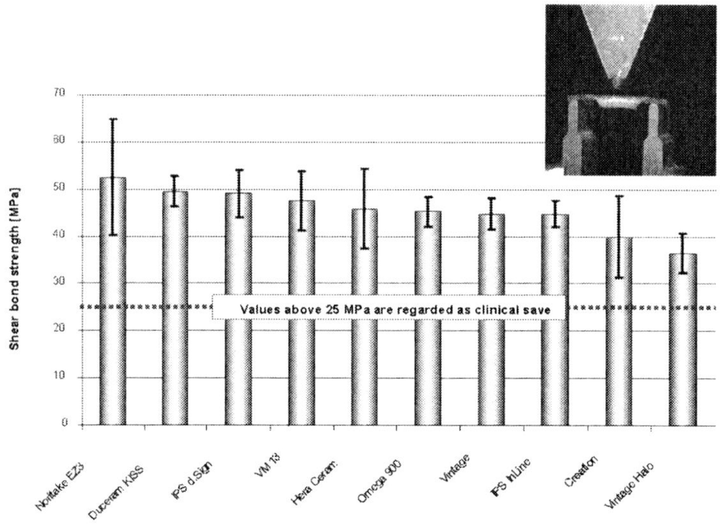

Figure 9. SEM picture of the bonding zone of Bio PontoStar® ++ and a veneering ceramic (Omega 900/Vita company)

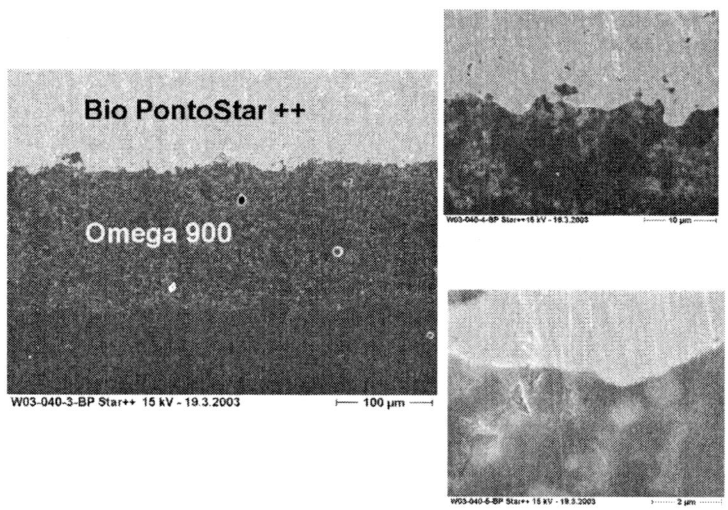

save. The good bonding can also be observed with SEM (Figure 9). There are no cracks or bubbles observable in the bonding zone between the alloy and the veneering ceramic. As an example this is shown for the gold alloy Bio PontoStar® ++ (BEGO Medial company, Figure 9).

The ion release is the key to biocompatibility. The lower the release of ions the lower is the risk of unwanted biological reactions. Besides the composition the manufacturing process is from great importance.

Looking at non precious alloy the chromium content is one of the main parameters for corrosion resistance. The content should be higher than 20% (Meyer, 1977). Besides the electrochemical reaction of the corrosion process there is another origin

Figure 10. Ion releases of Wirobond® SG (cast version)measured in a static immersion test. Given is the sum of released cobalt, chromium, molybdenum, tungsten and silicon ions.

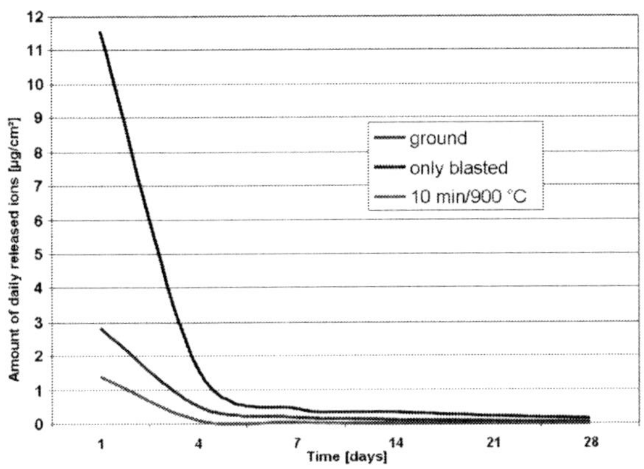

Figure 11. Ion releases of Wirobond® C+ (SLM version) measured in a static immersion test. Given is the sum of released cobalt, chromium, molybdenum, tungsten and silicon ions.

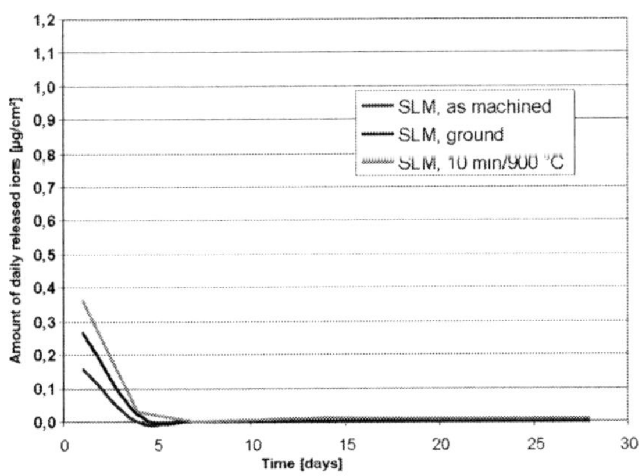

of ions. Oxides formed during the manufacturing process of the ingots for the dental technician and the casting process itself reveals certain solubility. The higher the concentrations of oxides on the surface are, the higher the possible amount of ions due to solution. The sum of corrosion and solubility of formed oxide are the ions released into the oral environment.

Regardless of the surface treatment the ion releases of the SLM test specimen reveals lower ion release in a static immersion test than the cast. In contrast to the static immersion test described in the ISO 10274 (DIN EN_ISO_10271, 2001) the standard by BEGO differs in case of time and amount of the measurement. The standard requires only one measurement after 7 days. In case of the development of new alloys BEGO company measures after 1, 4, 7, 14, 21 and 28 days to get information on the initial and long term corrosion behaviour.

The total ion release of cast alloys are higher than of those fabricated with the SLM technology. In case of the cobalt chromium alloys a daily ion release of 1 - 12 µg/cm² (Wirobond® SG, cast version, different surface conditions) was measured (Figure 10, Figure 11). In contrast thereto 0,3 -, 5 µg/cm² ions were released by the laser molten alloy (Wirobond® C+, different surface conditions). Measured elements were cobalt, chromium, molybdenum, tungsten and silicon. The gold alloys revealed comparable results.

The lower ion releases can be explained by the given argumentation above. What one can see by the SLM specimen is the pure corrosion without the solubility of oxides formed during casting processes.

Due to the low corrosion rates high bio compatibility was assumed. A clinical study (2 year results published) revealed favorable results (Pishwa, Freesmeyer, & Blumenrath, 2007) and confirmed the assumption. Meanwhile several thousand units have been produced without any reports of unwanted biological reactions of the used alloys.

A LOOK IN THE FUTURE

SLM is one technology for the future (Schweiger, Erdelt, & Beuer, 2004). CAD/CAM systems will conquer the dental laboratories in an even higher extent than today. New production processes will be established.

Looking at the SLM process there will be probably a continuous development of new materials. New alloys will come up and maybe it will also be possible to build up ceramics with the SLM technology.

The combination with other technologies will arrive. For example the over press technique is ideal for an automated CAD/CAM process for the crown and bridge technology.

REFERENCES

Andersson, M., Carlsson, L., Persson, M., & Bergman, B. (1996). Accuracy of machine milling and spark erosion with a CAD/CAM system. *The Journal of Prosthetic Dentistry, 76*(2), 187–193. doi:10.1016/S0022-3913(96)90305-4

Becker, F. (2008). Lasersintern versus Gusstechnik. *Dent Lab, 56*(1), 39–48.

Berg, E., Davik, G., Hegdahl, T., & Gjerdet, N. R. (1996). Hardness, strength, and ductility of prefabricated titanium rods used in the manufacture of spark erosion crowns. *The Journal of Prosthetic Dentistry, 75*(4), 419–425. doi:10.1016/S0022-3913(96)90035-9

Bressem, J. (2006). Laserschmelzen. *dent lab, 54*(10), 1337-1340.

Bressem, J. (2007). Laser Melting. *Dent Lab Internat, 3*(1), 29–32.

Cramer von Clausbruch, S. (2003). Zirkon und Zirkonium. *dent lab, 51*(7), 1137-1142.

Cramer von Clausbruch, S. (2006). Zurück in die Zukunft? *dental lab, 54*(9), 1169-1180.

Cramer von Clausbruch, S. (2008). Kopierfräsen als verlässliches Verfahren in der Zahntechnik. *Die Quintessenz der Zahntechnik, 34*(3), 332–342.

DIN_EN_ISO_10271. (2001). *Dentale metallische Werkstoffe Korrosionsprüfverfahren*. Berlin: Beuth Verlag.

DIN_EN_ISO_9693. (2001). *Metall-Keramik-Systeme für zahnärztliche Restaurationen*. Berlin: Beuth Verlag.

Duret, F. (1992). Dental CAD/CAM. *The Journal of the American Dental Association, 123*(6), 11–14.

Duret, F. (1993). The practical dental CAD/CAM in 1993. *J Can Dent Assoc, 59*(5), 445–453.

Duret, F., Blouin, J.-L., & Duret, B. (1988). CAD-CAM in Dentistry. *The Journal of the American Dental Association, 117*(11), 715–720.

Duret, F., & Preston, J. D. (1991). CAD/CAM imaging in dentistry. *Current Opinion in Dentistry, 1*, 150–154.

Eidenbenz, S., & Schärer, P. (1994). Das Kopierschleifen keramischer Formkörper. *Phillip Journal, 11*(3), 91–95.

Eisen, M., & Hinterseher, J. (2008). SLM-Verfahren: Mehr Formgenauigkeit - weniger Eigenspannung. *Zahntech Mag, 12*(10), 626–632.

Gebhardt, A. (2000). *Rapid prototyping: Werkzeuge für die schnelle Produktentstehung* (2. Auflage ed.). München - Wien: Hanser.

Kappert, H. F., & Krah, M. (2001). Keramiken - eine Übersicht. *Die Quintessenz der Zahntechnik, 27*(6), 668–704.

Kirches, M., Pack, N., & Schoofs, R. (2000). Die Komponenten des dualen Legierungssystems Vigo Liberty im Vergleich. *dent lab, 48*(4), 555-564.

Luthard, R., Rudolph, H., Sandkuhl, O., & Walter, M. (2001). Aktuelle CAD/CAM-Systeme zur Herstellung von keramischen Zahnersatz Teil 1: Systeme ohne zusätzliche Sinterung des keramischen Grundmaterials. *Zahnärztliche Welt, 110*(11), 747–754.

Luthardt, R., Rudolph, H., Sandkuhl, O., & Walter, M. (2001). Aktuelle CAD/CAM-Systeme zur Herstellung von keramischen Zahnersatz Teil 2: Systeme mit zusätzlicher Sinterung des keramischen Grundmaterials. *Zahnärztliche Welt*, *110*(12), 797–802.

Meyer, J. M. (1977). Corrosion resistance of nickel -chromium dental casting alloys. *Corrosion Science*, *17*, 971–982.

Negrel, D. (2006). Chromes with CAD/CAM. *The Dental Technician*, *70*, 25–30.

Niemann, P. (2003). Laser-Sinterverfahren in der CAD/CAM-Technik. *Die Quintessenz der Zahntechnik*, *29*(1), 38–42.

Oppacher, R. (2000). Alle guten Dinge sind drei: eine Keramik auf zwei unterschiedlichen Legierungen - erste Erfahrungen mit Vigo Liberty. *Die Quintessenz der Zahntechnik*, *26*(5), 429–438.

Pfeifer, G. M., & Riquier, R. (2006). Outsourcing oder Fertigung? *Die Quintessenz der Zahntechnik*, *32*(12), 1451–1456.

Pishwa, L., Freesmeyer, W. B., & Blumenrath, B. (2007). Verblendkronen aus CAD/CAM-Laser-gesinterten Gerüsten - eine Anwendungsbeobachtung. *Deutsche Zahnarztliche Zeitschrift*, *62*(7), 470–477.

Rekow, D. (1987). Computer-aided design and manufacturing in dentistry: A review of the state of the art. *The Journal of Prosthetic Dentistry*, *58*(4), 512–516. doi:10.1016/0022-3913(87)90285-X

Rekow, E. D. (1991). CAD/CAM in dentistry. *The Alpha Omegan*, *84*(4), 41–44.

Rekow, E. D., & Erdmann, A. G. (1985). Comparison of techniques for aquiring high-precision tree-dimensional computer-based geometric data directly from the human mouth. *Ceramics in Bioengenering*, 139-140.

Rekow, E. D., Erdmann, A. G., & Speidel, T. M. (1985). Computer-Assisted System to Automate Production of Posterior Dental Restorations. *Biostereometrics*, *602*, 204–210.

Rinke, S., Hüls, A., & Chafizadeh, A. (1995). Vergleichende Qualitätsbeurteilung kopiergefräster vollkeramischer Kronen und Brücken (Celay/In-Ceram). *Deutsche Zahnarztliche Zeitschrift*, *50*, 671–673.

Rinke, S., Markgraf, G., Jahn, L., & Hüls, A. (1994). Qualitätsbeurteilung von kopiergefrästen vollkeramischen Kronengerüsten (Celay/In-Ceram). *Schweiz Mschr Zahnmed*, *104*, 1495.

Riquier, R. (2006). Frästechnik versus Lasersintern. *Die Quintessenz der Zahntechnik*, *32*(5), 534–546.

Rudolph, M., Beoeckler, A. F., & Setz, J. M. (2007). Metallkeramikkronen mit lasergeschmolzenem Gerüst: Randspaltmessung und Festigkeitsprüfung - erste Ergebnisse. *Deutsche Zahnarztliche Zeitschrift*, *62*(7), 465–469.

Schweiger, J., Erdelt, K.-J., & Beuer, F. (2004). Rapid Prototyping - Technik der Zukunft? *Dent Lab*, *52*(7), 1109–1118.

Steger, E. (2005). ZirkonZahn für die Grünlingsbearbeitung von Zirkoniumdioxid-Gerüstmaterial. *Die Quintessenz der Zahntechnik*, *31*(6), 624–633.

Strietzel, R. (2004). Herstellung von metallischen Gerüsten mit Hilfe des BEGO Medifacturing Verfahrens. *Die Quintessenz der Zahntechnik*, *30*(4), 406–417.

Strietzel, R. (2005). *Die Werkstoffkunde der Metall-Keramik-Systeme*. München: Verlag Neuer Merkur.

Strietzel, R., & Lahl, C. (2007). *CAD/CAM-Systeme in Labor und Praxis*. München: Verlag Neuer Merkur.

Suttor, D. (2004). Lava zirconia crowns and bridges. *International Journal of Computerized Dentistry*, *7*(1), 67–76.

Völkl, L. (2001). cercon - das CAM-Vollkeramiksystem von Degussa Dental. *Die Quintessenz*, *52*(8), 811–814.

Witkowski, S. (2001). Digitale Workstation und Wachs-Drucker in der dentalen Gußtechnik. *Zahntech Mag*, *5*, 244–247.

KEY TERMS AND DEFINITIONS

Additive (Production): In such a process the workpiece is build up, e. g. by laser melting layer by layer.

Bio Compatibility: A important material property. The incorporated materials should not harm the patient.

Bonding: Ceramic is applied to metallic frame works to improve the esthetics. The connection between metal and ceramic is based on several mechanical (e. g. retention) and chemical (e. g. combined oxiede between c omponents of the alloy and ceramic) mechanism.

CAD: Computer aided design.

CADCast: After a CAD stepp the virtual model is transferred in wax or resin based material which then is casted in a conventional way.

CAM: Computer aided manufacturing

Cobalt Chromium Alloys: In dentistry cobalt chromiuim alloys are used for the production of frameworks for crown, bridges and partial dentures.

Corrosion: Electrochemical process which oxidizes metal to ions.

Grain Size: The powder for the SLM process consists out of particles of different size and geometriy. The average size is important for the precision of the process.

Ion Release: Due to corrosion formed ions, which are released into the saliva (environment).

Milling: With help of rotating instruments surfaces are treated.

Over Press Technique: The veneering of metallic frame works with ceramics is done normally by applying the veneering ceramic layer by layer by the dental technician. A new method is to over press the frame work with ceramic in one step.

Pantograph: Apparatus for copying objects (e. g. keys). Such machines are used in dental technology to produce frame works made out of zirconium dioxide.

Porosites: Defects (e. g. through casting) in the workpiece or blank which can lead to failure when loaded

Powder Management: The metallic powder for the SLM process has to be treated and stored in specific ways to obtain optimal results.

Scanning: A light or laser beam is directed in numerous lines over an object which should be aligned. Through the distortion of the projected line information of the depth is determined. Through mathematical operations the topography of the object is calculated.

SLM: Selective laser melting, a method to produce out of metal powder layer by layer metallic work pieces.

Static Immersions Test: Test specimens are immersed in a corrosion solution for a certain time. Afterward the solution is analysed to determine dissolved ions.

Subtractive (Production): In such a process material is taken away (e. g. by milling, grinding, sparc erosion) from a blank to produce the workpiece.

Sparc Erosion: Due to a high voltage between a metallic blank and a (carbon) electrode sparcs are thrown out which erode the metal.

Titanium: Metal used dentistry for the production of frame works.

Virtual Construction: s. CAD.

Zirconia: See zirconium dioxide

Zirconium dioxide: High-performance ceramics used in dentistry for the production of frame works.

Section 3
3D-Visualization in Oral Diagnosis

Chapter 9
Techniques for the Generation of 3D Finite Element Meshes of Human Organs

C. Lobos
Joseph Fourier University, France

Y. Payan
Joseph Fourier University, France

N. Hitschfeld
Universidad de Chile, Chile

ABSTRACT

The Finite Element Method (FEM) is probably the most used technique to model the mechanic properties of a body. The method needs a subdivision of the body (or domain) to be simulated in simpler geometrical structures. This subdivision is known as a mesh. This chapter gives a short introduction to the FEM, then continues with the most important aspects to consider for choosing a mesh like, element type, quality and node density. Finally this chapter reviews several meshing techniques currently used in the medical-field simulations. The techniques are classified and compared.

INTRODUCTION

Continuum mechanics (CM) is a branch of mechanics that deals with the analysis of the kinematic and mechanical behavior of materials modeled as a continuum, e.g., solids and fluids (i.e., liquids and gases). In a nutshell, CM assumes that matter is continuous (ignoring the fact that matter is actually made of atoms). This assumption allows the approximation of physical quantities over the materials, such as energy and momentum, at the infinitesimal limit. Differential equations can thus be employed in solving problems in CM.

Let Ω be a volumetric domain defined in 3D and P a point inside Ω. A deformation occurs in Ω as external (surface or volumetric) forces f are applied to some P in Ω. If Ω is considered as an elastic body, the deformation is characterized by:

- A displacement vector field u caused by f applied over one or more P.

DOI: 10.4018/978-1-60566-733-1.ch009

Figure 1. Displacement vs deformation. Top, initial system. Bottom left, displacement (a difference regarding the x and y axis). Bottom right. deformation (a difference regarding the r and s axis).

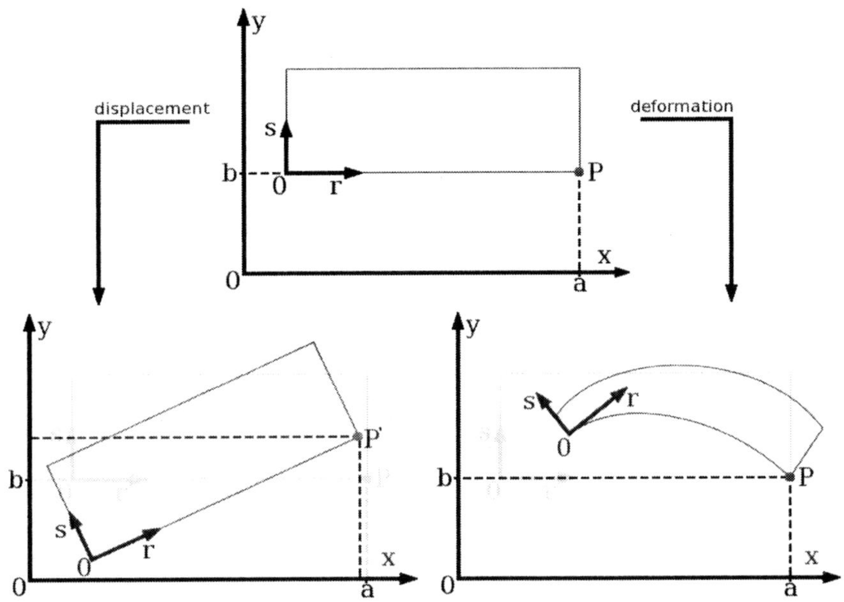

- An internal state of deformation, mathematically defined by a "strain tensor"for each P in Ω.
- The "force reaction" of the body to the external forces; this is mathematically defined by a "stress tensor" for each P in Ω.

The Local Equilibrium of the Medium (LEM) is an expression defined for each P in Ω that links the displacement, the strain and the stress tensor through Partial Differential Equations (PDE). In order to do so, an analytical relationship is assumed between the strain and the stress tensors, known as the constitutive law of the material.

The difference between displacement and deformation is made in function of the Reference System (RS) used to measure each one of them. The first one is made regarding the overall RS. The second one, uses a relative RS associated to the domain. Figure 1 illustrates the initial state of the system at the top; at the bottom left panel a displacement is produced as the coordinates of point P change to P' regarding the x and y axis, however no deformation is presented in the r and s axis. At the bottom right panel the inverse situation is produced as no displacement of P is presented in the x and y axis. In the other hand, point P has a severe deformation regarding the r and s axis.

The strain level measures the domain deformation regarding the relative position of P in Ω. Let vector a be the initial position of P and vector b be the position of P after the deformation in the relative axis: r, s. The strain level is then defined as:

$$\frac{\left\| \|a\| - \|b\| \right\|}{\|a\|}$$

The importance of measuring the strain level is that when it is inferior to 10% the "small strain" hypothesis can be made, which assumes a linear geometrical resolution of the PDEs. Otherwise, a "large strain" framework is necessary, which means a much more complex resolution of the system.

If the constitutive law can be assumed to be linear, another simplification ca be made: an elasticity tensor is computed to link the stress and strain tensors. On the contrary, if a linear law does not account properly for the mechanical behavior of the tissues, a non-linear law can be chosen to account for the hyperelastic behavior of soft tissues (see Bonet and Wood (1997) for more details).

Most of the modeling works proposed in the literature assumed both, the small strain and the linearity of the constitutive law hypotheses. The term "linear elasticity" is then commonly used, i.e. assuming linearity of the geometry and the mechanics. In that case, it can be shown that the constitutive behavior of the material can be characterized by only two parameters: the Young's modulus that depends on the stiffness of the material, and the Poisson's ratio that is related to the compressibility of the material.

Whatever the modeling assumptions are, the PDEs that govern CM cannot be analytically solved over the full domain. They are therefore numerically solved over a piecewise discretization of the domain, usually by means of the **Finite Element Method** (FEM), the Finite Difference Method and the Finite Volume Method. This chapter focuses on the use of FEM since most of the modeling works in the biomechanical field use this method.

The name FEM is due to the principle that the continuous space is subdivided in a finite number of smaller and simpler geometries, namely the elements. This subdivision of the continuous space is called the **mesh**.

CONSTRUCTING THE SOLUTION OF THE FEM

The **Finite Element Method** (FEM) requires the discretization of the spatial domain Ω with "finite elements" interconnected at points called "nodes". The PDE of the CM can then be solved inside each element which geometry is quite simple and regular. For two dimensional problems, triangles and rectangles are commonly used while in three dimensions tetrahedral and hexahedral elements are very popular. As compared to finite difference methods, the finite element mesh may be entirely unstructured, which makes the modeling of complicated and irregular geometries more convenient.

Altogether, the elements should cover the entire domain as accurately as possible. For a given set of boundary conditions (i.e. forces and constraints applied on nodes) and assuming an analytical constitutive law, the unknowns of the systems, i.e. node's displacements, are solved for each element. Then, thanks to interpolation "shape functions" (usually linear or quadratic), displacements, strains and stresses can be computed at each point inside the elements. Because of element interconnections and continuity of the shape functions from one element to another one, the FEM provides solutions of the system inside the full domain.

Figure 2 shows an example of FEM over an arbitrary domain. In this example, an external force f is applied over node A. Node B is considered as fixed (this is an example of constraint applied over a node). The position of the other nodes in the mesh is obtained in function of f and all the modeling parameters in each node (strain, stress and constraints). Finally the position of each point in the domain is obtained by the interpolation function over each element.

GLOBAL MESHING DEFINITIONS

What Is a Mesh?

Several definitions can be found to this question. In this chapter a **mesh** shall be seen as a partition of an arbitrary domain into simpler geometrical objects (or elements). Those elements are compound of nodes, edges, faces and the relations between them.

Figure 2. An example of a deformed domain simulated with the FEM. Left, the initial system. Right, the domain is deformed by the influence of an external force.

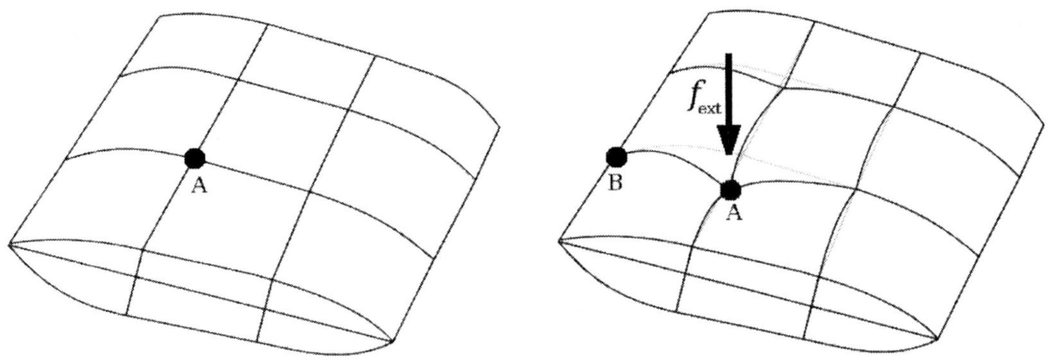

Probably the most common definition is "a mesh is a tessellation of the space", which is equivalent to our definition since a tessellation is a collection of non-overlapping elements that fill a domain.

Achieving this subdivision of the space is not an easy task, therefore many ways to produce this tessellation have been proposed. Sections "mesh adaptation" and "mesh generation" will give a reference over the most popular and useful ones to the medical domain.

What Is a Valid Mesh?

The FEM can be seen as an integration problem (a system of PDE). The computation of this integration is produced over the elements that describe the domain. An element is invalid when the area or volume that it describes is malformed. Two types of malformations can be presented in the mesh:

- **Edge inversion**: This involves several elements and it is produced when the intersection of neighbor elements has a positive volume.
- **Concave element**: This is a local problem and it is produced when one or more faces of the element are concave (this problem cannot be produced in triangle faces).

In both cases, the area or volume described by the elements is artificially increased and do not represents the current state of the domain causing an integration over a "phantom" sub-domain. The case of "edge inversion" is presented in 2D in Figure 3. In this case, the domain is represented by two triangles *t1* and *t2*. Node A, that belongs only to *t1* is dragged into the region defined by

Figure 3. At left a valid 2D mesh. At right an invalid mesh where shaded triangles have a negative area.

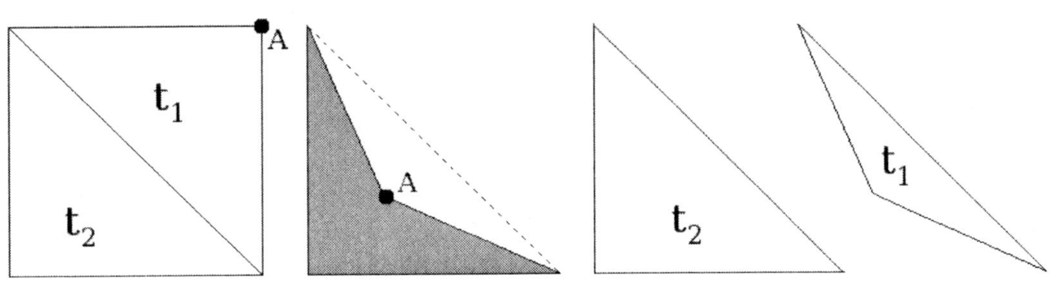

Figure 4. Left, a valid hexahedron. Right, a concave hexahedron considered as an invalid configuration.

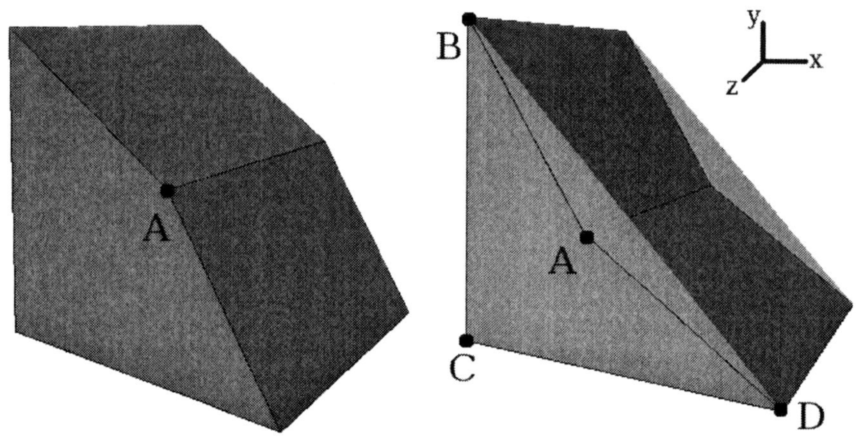

t2. In this new scenario the domain corresponds to the shaded area. If the mesh defined by *t1* and *t2* is used to represent this new state of the domain, the integration should be over *t2 - t1*. However, it occurs over *t2 + t1*.

The same problem can be expanded to 3D with hexahedra. Figure 4 shows an example of a concave hexahedron. A valid hexahedron (left) is transformed by the displacement of point *A* (right) in such a way that it turns into an invalid configuration. The rendering of the hexahedron is shown as a prism (wedge) defined by the triangle *B*, *C* and *D* and its projection through the *z* axis. The final numerical integration occurs over the domain described by this prism (while the actual domain is the concave hexahedron).

The Jacobian matrix of an element can be used to determine if an element is valid or not (this will be shown later).

Note that in the literature, a valid mesh can be also named as a regular mesh (see Luboz, Payan and Couteau, 2001).

What Is a Good Mesh?

Two aspects should be considered to determine if a mesh is good or not. The first has to deal with the representation level of the domain (RLD). This variable is measured as the difference between the areas or volumes of the actual domain and the final mesh.

The second aspect is the quality. The *perfect* element can be described regarding some relations between the angles, edge's length, distance between specific element's points, circumcircle, etc. Unfortunately, no "magic" quality measurement exists for an element, because it depends on the numerical method been used and on the problem being solved.

In the case of tetrahedra, the work of Shewchuk in 2002 is probably the most relevant article concerning mesh quality. Note that in his web page[1] an unpublished article of 66 pages (just about tetrahedrons quality) can be found. The idea of putting a lot of emphasis in quality is because bad quality elements can lead to several computational errors in the simulation.

In order to illustrate some quality measures, let's describe briefly some classical quality criteria, namely the *aspect ratio*, the *warping factor* and the *dihedral angle*.

To obtain the Aspect Ratio (AR) of an element, the distances between element's faces must be computed. The AR for the element is then defined as the ratio between the minimal and the maximal distance. Therefore, an AR = 1 corresponds to an ideal element and as the AR reaches high values, the element becomes increasingly distorted (see Lobos, Bucki, Hitschfeld and Payan (2007) for more details).

The Warping Factor (WF) is a quality measure over the element's faces. For each face, the distances of the face's nodes to an average plane are computed. If all the nodes are co-planar, then the WF is 0 and the face is said to be "perfect". As the WF increases, the quality of the face (thus the element) decreases. Note that WF is out of context for triangle faces as 3 nodes are always co-planar.

The Dihedral Angle (DA) is the angle formed between two planes. Therefore several DA values are computed for each element (all the angles between connected faces). The DA of the element is the "worst" value among all the calculated DA. Note that for each type of element the optimal DA is different: 60° for the tetrahedron and 90° for the hexahedron. Therefore the quality of the element decreases when the "worst" DA of it moves further from the optimal value.

Note that improving some of these quality measures doesn't necessarily produce a "good" element. For example, if only WF and DA are considered as quality measures then the element in Figure 5 (a) would be considered as "perfect". However in terms of AR, this element has a very poor quality. Following the same principle, Figure 5 (b) has a poor DA but a perfect WF and a good AR, and (c) has a poor WF and acceptable DA and AR.

CHOOSING THE TYPE OF ELEMENT

In this section the advantages and disadvantages of using the different types of elements in a mesh are presented. Three categories will be analyzed: tetrahedral, hexahedral and mixed-element meshes. As it will be show in the following sections, most of the meshing techniques proposed in the medical field produce tetrahedral meshes. Some works are done with hexahedra and just a few with mixed-elements.

As this chapter is focused in medical simulations, many works in this field consider deformable domains. A very important work over model deformations has been done by Benzley, Perry, Merkley, Clark and Sjaardema (1995) from the mechanical point of view. This work showed the differences obtained by using tetrahedral or hexahedral meshes in terms of incompressibility and plasticity abilities of each type of element. In this study a simple bar, fixed at one end, with a rectangular cross-section was used to compare the performance of linear and quadratic displacement assumption over tetrahedra and hexahedra meshes. The linear or quadratic property of an element has to deal with the manner to represent their edges and in consequence, the volume the element covers. As Figure 6 shows, in a linear element the edges are represented as an interpolation of the two border points. In the case of quadratic elements, the edges are quadratic functions and therefore an additional middle point is necessary to describe the function. If linear tetrahedra have

Figure 5. Bad elements regarding (a) aspect ratio, (b) dihedral angle and (c) warping factor

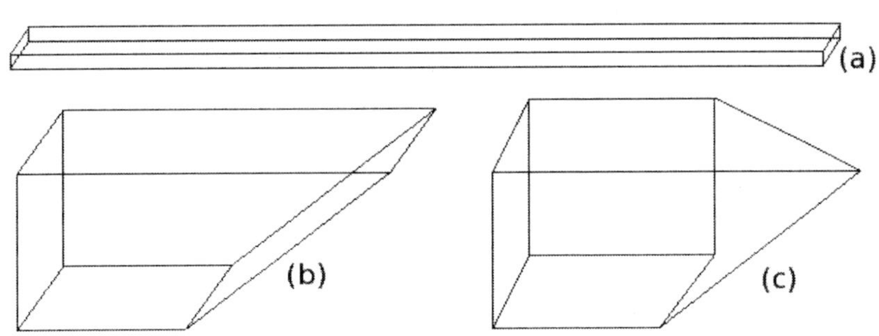

Figure 6. From left to right, linear tetrahedron, quadratic tetrahedron, linear hexahedron and quadratic hexahedron

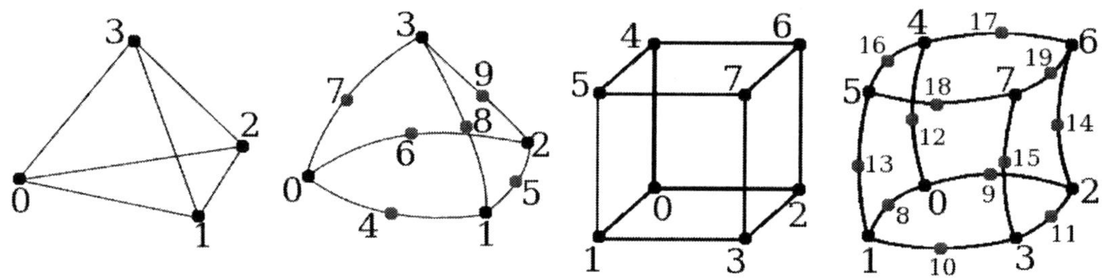

4 points, its quadratic counterpart has the same 4 point plus 6 others located on each edge of it.

The work from Benzley et al (1995) has several important conclusions:

- Linear hexahedrons (LH) can generally deform in a lower strain energy state (i.e. eigenvalues), thus making them more accurate than linear tetrahedrons (LT) in numerous situations.
- The comparison of linear static bending[2] situation indicated that LT models produced errors between 10\% and 70\% in both displacement and stress calculations. Such errors are obviously unacceptable for stress analysis work. On the contrary LH, quadratic hexahedrons (QH), and quadratic tetrahedrons (QT) models all provided acceptable results, even with relatively coarse meshes.
- The linear static torsion problem[3] again showed that the LT element produced errors of an unacceptable magnitude. This problem also demonstrated that, because selective integration is only effective on the bending problem, the LH element, without a significant number of degrees of freedom, produces poor results. Here, as in the previous problem, the QH element is superior.
- Significant information is conspicuous in the nonlinear elasto-plastic calculations. Here, as before, all but LT models are adequate for bending calculations. However, not only LT, but QT models seemed to underperform both LH and QH elements.

As it will be shown, most of the meshes used in medical simulations only consider linear elements. There are just a few works that use quadratic elements, even taking into account that some commercial Finite Element (FE) solvers like ANSYS® are prepared to manage those kinds of elements. In other words, there exist FEM solvers that manage quadratic elements, however and even when this may lead to better simulation results, there are few mesh generators that produce quadratic elements.

Other type of variables can be taken into consideration to choose the elements in the mesh. For example, regarding linear elements, only triangular faces will always be planar. Once again, commercial FE solvers like ANSYS® have specific and well defined thresholds to accept those kinds of elements. Even though making a non-triangle face "more" planar has a solution, this is an extra problem to consider while using other type of element than the tetrahedron (or a dual element taken from it).

Finally, there are some other works that have studied the use of different types of elements (Lobos et al, 2007; Couteau, Payan & Lavallee, 2000). The most global definitions consider tetrahedra, pyramid, prism (wedge) and hexahedra. Two options are possible to consider this kind of meshes:

- A better approximation of the domain in a given region of it. This is the case for meshes that are governed by one type of element, but that prefer in some very specific configurations, to replace bad quality elements with another type of elements.
- Transitions between different levels of refinement. Even though this can be achieved by using just one type of element, some works prefer to include different types of elements during transitions between coarse and refined regions.

The "locking effect" could be another drawback to the use of tetrahedra for quasi-incompressible materials (refer to Hughes (1987) for more details).

IMPORTANT REMARKS OVER MESHING

Validity (or mesh regularity) should be clearly differentiated from the mesh quality. The element's quality optimization[4] involves node displacement. This last procedure might cause neighbor element invalidation. Therefore quality optimization should be always made considering not affecting the validity of the rest of the elements. For instance Figure 7 shows how the displacement of point A could be considered as an action to improve the top left triangle's quality. Unfortunately this causes the invalidation of the two right triangles and makes the entire mesh useless (it cannot be used to produce a simulation with the FEM).

As mentioned before, the representation level of the domain (RLD) is the difference in area or volume between the domain and the final mesh. Another remark can be made relating the RLD and the mesh quality. Figure 8 (a) shows an arbitrary domain. In (b) a tessellation of the domain is presented and the RLD is shown by the shaded regions. In (c) some triangles of (b) were split by the addition of new points which makes the RLD much more precise. In Figure 8 (d) shaded elements correspond to the triangles of (b) that were split resulting in the tessellation presented in (c). As mentioned before, one of the quality measures is the Dihedral Angle (DA) for 3D and just the angle for 2D. If this quality measure is applied to the final mesh in Figure 8 (d) light shaded triangles would be considered as "bad triangles" (because the minimal angle is less than a threshold value) and dark shaded as "good". Following the "angle" quality parameter, the overall mesh quality in (b) would be better than the one presented in (c). Therefore one important remark is that improving the RLD does not necessarily increase the quality of the elements and vice-versa.

As shown through the chapter, several factors must be considered before building a mesh. In particular the following questions should be answered:

- Should we use one type of element or several? which ones?

Figure 7. Right, a valid 2D mesh. Left, an invalid mesh where shaded triangles covers an area that is two times considered in the numerical integration.

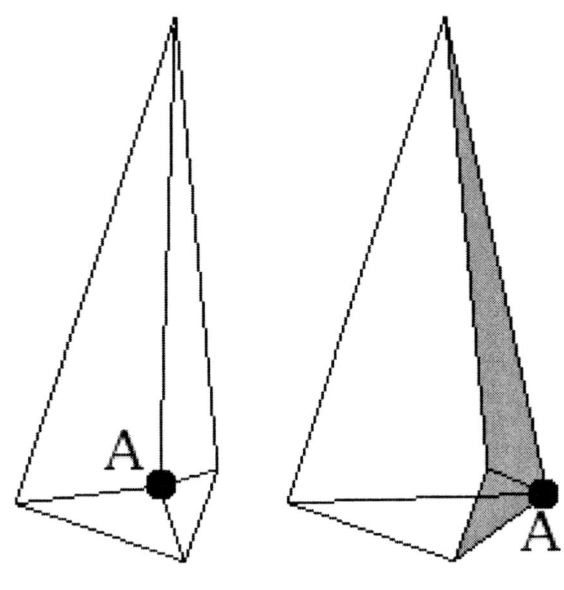

Figure 8. (a) input domain, (b) a mesh of the input domain where shaded regions represents the RLD, (c) some elements of (b) were split which causes an improvement of the RLD, (d) the mesh from (c) where the split triangles from (b) are shaded. The minimal angle quality measure is applied over shaded triangles and light ones are "bad" while dark ones are "good".

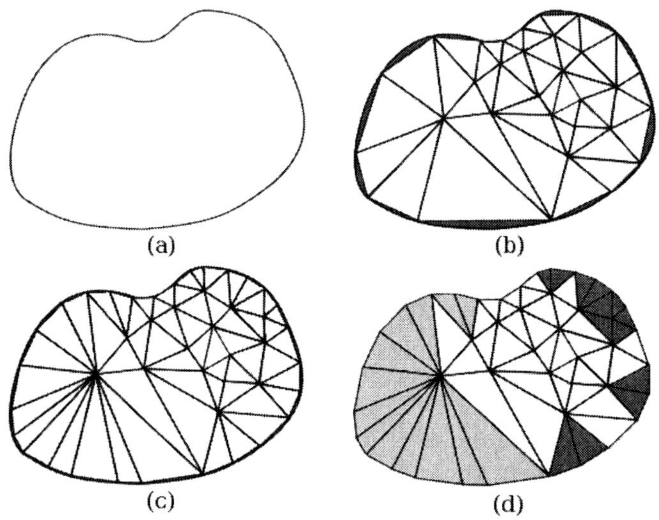

- Is it desirable to count with different levels of refinement through the mesh?
- How quality will be measured?
- How quality improvement will be achieved when necessary?
- How invalid elements will be repaired?

Once answers are provided for those questions, the next step concerns the way the mesh is going to be built.

INPUTS FOR THE GENERATION OF HUMAN ORGANS FE MESHES

In medical applications information concerning the domain to mesh comes from one or more of the following inputs:

- Computed Tomography (CT) images
- Magnetic Resonance Images (MRI)
- Segmented images
- A surface mesh
- A cloud of points
- A pre-generated volumetric FE mesh that describes a generic organ

While CT is more adapted to bone visualization, MRI is better to differentiate soft tissue from an image. Both techniques can be the starting point for the elaboration of a 3D organ geometry. As a person lies in a scanner, several slices of a body region are captured in images. Figure 9 shows how it is possible to build a surface mesh from this set of piecewise 2D images. Pages, Sermesant and Frey (2005) describe one alternative to do the whole process: from image to surface and volume meshes.

A more elaborated input can be the same set of images but with already segmented organs. This process produces a partition of a digital image into multiple regions with objects and boundaries (points, lines, curves, etc) in the images. Several general-purpose algorithms and techniques have been developed for image segmentation. Since there is no general solu-

Figure 9. Left, an example of 2D scan images of the brain. Right, a surface triangle mesh.

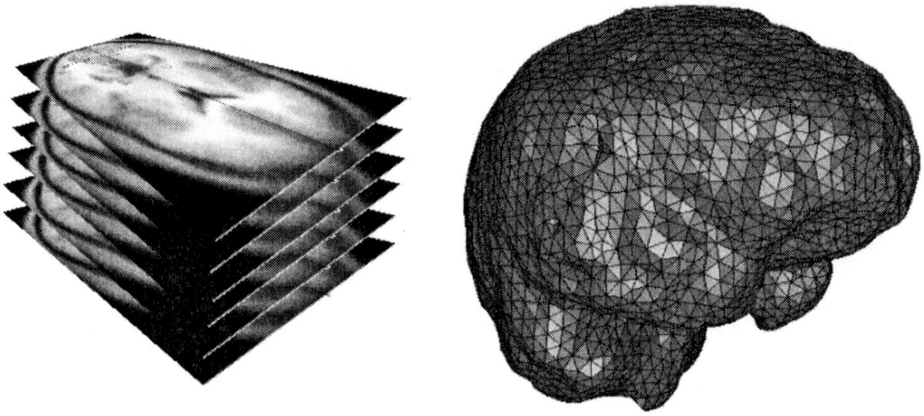

Figure 10. The different alternatives to go from imaging to volume mesh generation

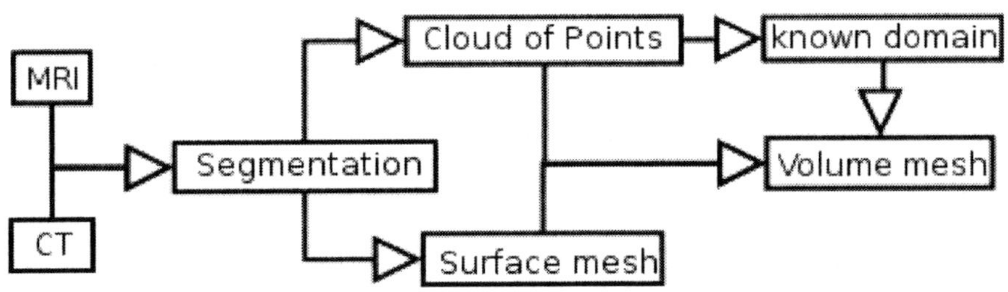

tion to this problem, these techniques often are combined with domain knowledge, i.e. semi-automatic process leaded by the user to identify the target structures.

Subsequently, from the segmented images, a cloud of points can be extracted or a surface model can be constructed. In order to produce a surface mesh, algorithms like the Marching Cubes (Lorensen & Cline, 1987) are very popular (see later for more details).

Most of the meshing techniques that will be explained in further sections start from a surface model of the organ. However one family of meshing techniques does not: a cloud of points is enough as they have additional information on the target organ to mesh (see "mesh registration" section for more details).

Figure 10 shows the different paths to produce a volumetric FE mesh from a set of images and further steps. Note that from a cloud of points, it is also possible to build a triangulation and therefore a surface mesh.

MESHING AND SIMULATION CLASSIFICATIONS

Global Classification of Meshing Techniques

When the geometry to mesh is known a priori there is a substantial advantage because there is more information that can be used. For example, if the target geometry to mesh is a femur, a pre-calculated mesh (ATLAS) that describes a generic femur can be build. Now, to mesh any other femur, only the external surface information of this new target is necessary and by causing nodes displacement over the ATLAS, it is possible to fit the target information. In other words, it is possible to start from a valid pre-defined FE mesh solution and then deform it in order to fit the target's border conditions.

Consider now the case where anatomically malformed femurs have to be modeled. The previous described technique may not work as it is constrained to "small differences" between the ATLAS and the target. If this constraint is not respected, the elements of the resulting mesh can be strongly degenerated or present bad qualities, which will decrease the accuracy of the simulation. Therefore for those types of problems (unknown domain and big changes from one target to another) it is recommended to use other types of meshing techniques.

In most cases those techniques start from an input surface mesh and create a new target-specific volumetric mesh. The other option is to use the surface information to know if a point is outside or inside the geometry boundaries. In those cases, the resulting mesh will not depend on the properties (density, types of elements) of the input surface mesh. This last family of techniques can also be adapted to use a cloud of points instead of a surface mesh; however the resulting mesh can be not so accurate in those zones where point density is not high enough.

Regarding all this, we can now identify two main streams to generate a volumetric mesh:

- **Mesh adaptation:** Those techniques start with a pre-defined FE mesh ATLAS and then, by moving the ATLAS nodes, achieve the representation of a new target domain.
- **Mesh generation:** Those techniques produce an *ad-hoc* volumetric mesh from the specific input domain.

Both streams will be detailed later in the chapter.

Simulation Types

In general, two types of simulations can be distinguished: the ones focused on obtaining fast / interactive results and the ones focused on precise / accurate results. We could also say that some techniques focus on both fast and precise results, but in real practice, most of the times we have to make a choice.

It is very important to mention the differences between fast generation and fast simulation in the meshing field. The first refers to the time needed to produce a mesh. The second refers to the time a numerical framework, like the Finite Element Method (FEM), needs to compute the simulation results.

Regarding the meshes, two aspects must be analyzed. The **quantity of elements** in the mesh is an important variable. The more elements the mesh has, the more the time the FEM needs to produce the simulation results. In the other hand, with more elements it is possible to achieve a better representation of the domain by increasing the quantity of elements in the zone where higher geometry accuracy is required.

The other important variable to achieve a good result is the **quality of the mesh**, however this will increase only the precision of the results. If fast results are required, three options seem possible:

- Fewer elements.
- The use of a cluster of powerful computers with parallel algorithms.
- Some modifications of the FEM with proposals for other modeling and numerical methods (Schwartz, 2001; Picinbono, Delingette & Ayache, 2003; Cotin, Delingette & Ayache, 1996; Nesme, 2008).

Figure 11. The Delaunay property. Left, the property isn't achieved. Right, using the flipping edge technique, the property is satisfied.

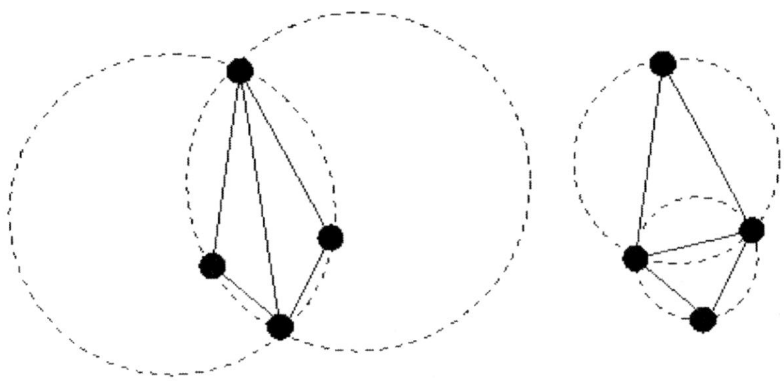

BASIC TOOLS AND PROPERTIES OF MESH GENERATION

Delaunay Property

In 2D, a **Delaunay** triangulation (Delaunay, 1934) for a set *P* of points in the plane is a triangulation *DT(P)* such that no point in *P* is inside the circumcircle of any triangle in *DT(P)* (except for the three points of *P* that conform the triangle). In 3D, the concept remains the same, replacing the circumcircle by the circumsphere. In particular, 2D Delaunay triangulation maximizes the minimum angle of all the triangles in the tessellation.

This is a mathematical property, therefore there is no specific meshing technique associated to it. We can only say that a triangle or a tetrahedral mesh satisfies or not the Delaunay property. In the rest of this chapter, a Delaunay mesh is said to be a mesh that satisfies the above property.

Several meshing algorithms start from the Delaunay mesh because it gives an initial quality value to the mesh. This quality value can be improved by moving, adding or removing some points, achieving a better representation of the input domain.

If a triangle does not satisfy the Delaunay property, the flipping edges technique (see Shewchuk, 1999) can always repair this problem in 2D. This is not true for 3D. Figure 11 illustrates this technique. At the left is a triangulation for a set of points that do not satisfy the property. At the right, the same points are plotted but now with a different triangulation that satisfies the property by changing the common edge of the triangles.

As mentioned before, a Delaunay mesh is a reference in the field of tetrahedral meshing techniques. A lot of works stand over the Delaunay property. However it is very important to mention that the Delaunay property is a "good" starting point but not sufficient to produce quality meshes. Sometimes, a Delaunay mesh can lead to numerical instabilities and that's why it must be refined in order to accomplish other quality constraints. Probably one of the most used refinement technique to produce high quality meshes was proposed by Ruppert in 1995. An implementation, freely available on the web, was implemented by Shewchuk (2002a) in his application Triangle with some improvements over the quality of the output mesh. Just to mention one of this improvements, Miller, Pave and Walkington (2003) continued with the work by improving the triangle's quality in terms of minimal and maximal angle.

To be clear about it, the workflow in most cases is to produce an initial triangle mesh from a cloud of points. The second step is to achieve the Delaunay property for every triangle in the mesh. Finally, the algorithms proposed by Ruppert (1995), Shewchuk (2002a), Miller *et al.*

(2003) and many others, improve the quality of the Delaunay mesh by moving, adding or removing some points.

Grid, Voxel and Octree Meshes

A **grid** (or structured) mesh is a regular tessellation of a given space. It is usually formed using a unique type of elements (squares, rectangles, triangles, etc) that can be:

- Equal in angle: all the elements have the same inner angles but not the same area or volume.
- Equal in area or volume: elements can differ in their inner angles.

A voxel is a small volume element, representing a value on a regular grid in the three dimensional space. This is analogous to a pixel, which represents 2D image data. Voxels are frequently used in the visualization and analysis of medical and scientific data. A voxel mesh is a particular grid where all the elements are hexahedra of the same size.

Voxel meshes are particular useful when the simulation is performed over a 3D imaging exam and virtually all the voxels can be activated. For instance in the context of the brain activity study (functional MRI for example), works like Ashburner and Friston in 2000 and Abell *et al.* in 1999 (just to mention some) allow to identify the regions of the brain that are activated and to compare between different groups of subjects.

In those studies, voxels in the mesh allow to identify not only if there is activity in certain region but also, with a pre-defined scale, the level of activity as Figure 12 shows[5]. Here the level of the mesh refinement is crucial to detect with precision the regions that are activated. In the other hand, there is a direct relation between the number of voxels and the computing time to process the information. Therefore, finding the adequate level of element's density (the size of each voxel) is crucial.

An **octree** is a volumetric mesh and it can be seen as a derivate product of the quadtree in 2D. A quadtree is a tree data structure in which each internal node has up to four children. Quadtrees are most often used to partition a two dimensional space by recursively subdividing it into four quadrants or regions. The regions may be square or rectangular, or may have arbitrary shapes. This data structure was named a quadtree by Finkel and Bentley in 1974.

Figure 13 shows an example of the tree structure for an octree. Every cube (or octant in this case) is divided, when necessary, in 8 new octants. In this figure, the initial octant numbered 1 was divided in the octants from 2 to 9, then the octant numbered 3, was divided in octants from 10 to 17. Octants 8, 9, 16 and 17 are not visible.

To stop the refinement (the subdivision criterion) on a quadtree or octree, there are two options:

- **Geometrical constraint:** Like a minimal distance between octree "surface" points and the actual surface of the domain
- **A level constraint:** Like to reach a maximum number of subdivisions, points or elements in the mesh

Figure 12. An example of a voxel mesh over head MRI. The voxel in this case, measures the level of activity over different zones of the brain.

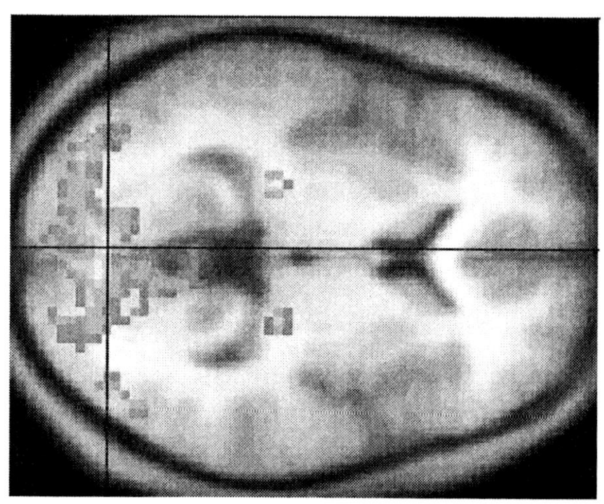

Figure 13. Left, an example of mesh generated with the octree algorithm. Right, the corresponding tree data structure of it.

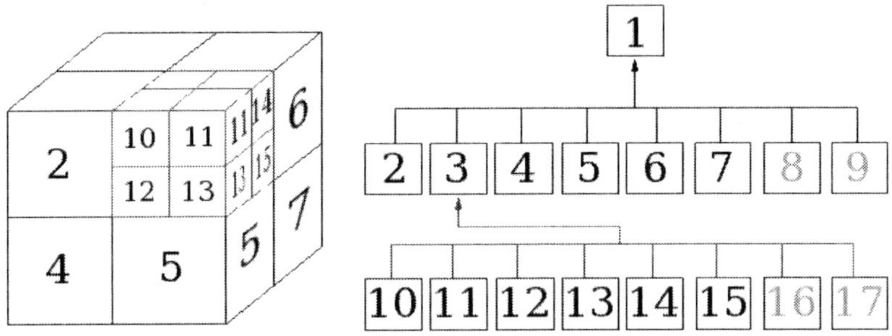

Figure 14. An example of octree mesh from a prostate. At the left the octree mesh is shown in transparent while the input prostate surface mesh is shown in transparent in the right panel.

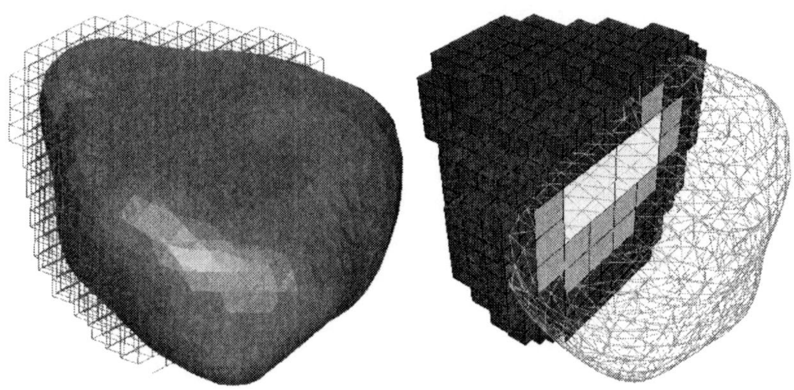

Figure 14 shows an example of octree mesh from a prostate surface mesh. At the left the input surface mesh of a prostate is shown in solid and transparent elements correspond to the octree. Half of the octree mesh has been deleted to show the interior of it. At the right, the same meshes are plotted but now with the input prostate mesh in transparent. Colors in the octree mesh (at the right) show the different sizes of inner elements that can be found. This difference is explained as "big" inner elements don't intersect the input prostate surface mesh and therefore do not continue the splitting process.

The previous description includes the "pure" octree technique, but in order to make this mesh suitable for FEM it is necessary to manage the transitions between coarse and more refined regions. Here three options are possible:

- Manage transitions using only hexahedra (Zhang and Bajaj, 2006)
- Manage transitions using different types of elements (tetrahedra, pyramid and prism or wedge), (Hitschfeld, Navarro and Farias, 2000; Hitschfeld 2005)
- Do not manage transitions and modify the classical FEM (Nesme, 2008)

The two first alternatives use templates (patterns) to identify different types of configuration and add elements avoiding the refinement of the entire mesh to the same level. These two alternatives also need a technique in order to achieve better surface representation, like a projection of all the nodes that reside outside the surface into it. This can lead to distorted elements and has to

Figure 15. The 15 marching cubes patterns. Red points can be inside or outside the target isosurface to represent. The resulting faces will represent the isosurface.

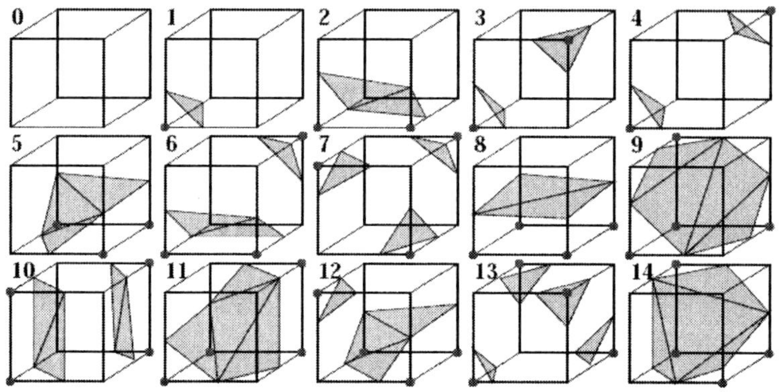

be handled by a reparation algorithm. The other option to achieve surface representation is the largely used marching cube algorithm that will be presented in the next subsection.

The third alternative doesn't need any further changes from the current state of the mesh. The effort must be made over the FEM in order to accept elements with points inserted in their edges. The PhD thesis of Nesme (2008) describes how this can be done.

The Marching Cubes Technique

Marching Cubes is a technique published by Lorensen and Cline in 1987 for extracting a polygonal mesh of an isosurface from a three-dimensional scalar field (sometimes called voxels).

The algorithm proceeds through the scalar field, taking eight neighbor locations at a time (thus forming an imaginary cube), then determining the polygons needed to represent the part of the isosurface that passes through this cube. Since there are 8 points in each cube and every point can be in two states, inside or outside the isosurface, there are $2^8 = 256$ different combinations. However, most of the combinations are topologically equivalent and by applying permutations, rotations and switching states of inside/outside, these combinations can be reduced to 15 patterns as shown in Figure 15.

For the switching states, if there are 7 points inside or just one of the entire cube, the same pattern (number 1) will apply to find the intersection face. Even though this procedure is robust, it doesn't work all the time as it doesn't consider neighboring information. The Marching Cubes technique can produce holes as described and solved by Chernyaev in 1995. These holes are the result of combining two different configurations for neighbors as Figure 16 shows.

Figure 16. Two case of erroneous surface representation, by applying the patterns between two neighbors a hole is produced in the element's shared face. Red points are outside points. Left, pattern 6 and the complement of pattern 3. Right, pattern 3 and its complement.

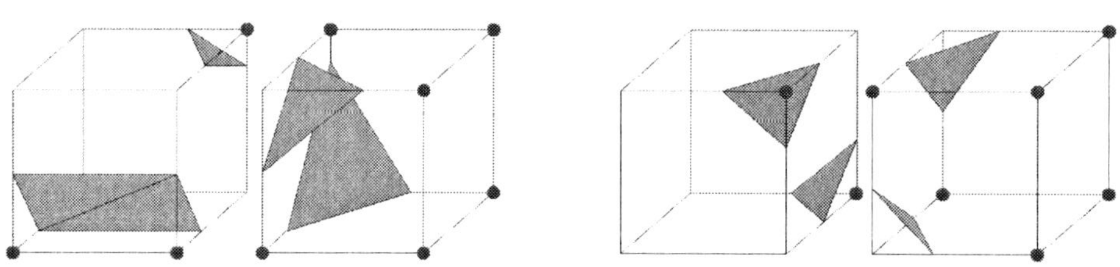

Figure 17. The advancing front technique (a) a portion of a surface mesh with one front to expand, (b) the tetrahedron is created and the new faces can be treated as fronts, (c) another expansion using a recently inserted front and (d) another expansion using already inserted points

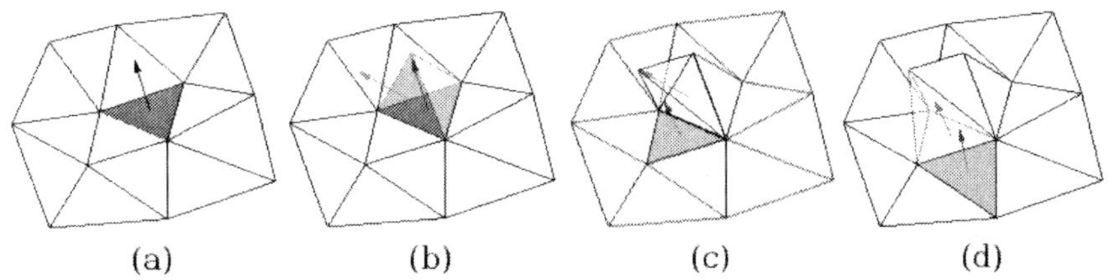

The other option to solve the above problem is to produce a tessellation of the cell into tetrahedra and build the isosurface applying the marching tetrahedra algorithm (Payne & Toga, 1990; Ferrant *et al.*, 1999). This method is similar to marching cubes but based on a tetrahedron instead of a cube. The advantage is that in this case, no hole can be produced. Unfortunately the topology produced by this new process isn't necessarily the same as the one obtained without tetrahedra tessellation (Velasco, Torres, Leon & Soler, 2007).

The Marching Cubes and their improvements are not only used with the voxel meshes, but can be combined with the octree and grid meshes. This is a fast and well studied technique to improve the surface representation of an input domain.

Advancing Front Technique

The **Advancing front** is a 2D and 3D meshing technique that stands from a surface (or in 2D a boundary) representation of the domain. Each face in the surface mesh is considered as a front. The idea is to expand all the fronts into the inner part of the volume until the entire domain is meshed.

Once a front is expanded, it is no longer considered as a front. Finally all shared faces will no more be fronts as they cannot be expanded. The selection of points to create the new faces (thus elements) encourages the use of existing points. Figure 17 illustrates how the advancing front works.

Note that this technique can be adapted to produce any type of elements (tetrahedra, hexahedra and mixed-elements in general: Lobos & Hitschfeld, 2006). Also note that there is no constraint over the technique to insert a new point. There are several advancing front - based techniques and the difference between them is the manner to chose where and when inserting a new point. This last step tries to maximize the quality of the elements in the mesh. As there are several options to measure the quality, this technique has several flavors.

In the next two sections more complex meshing strategies are presented. Several among them, use the techniques described above as a starting point or as part of the meshing process.

MESH ADAPTATION

The Mesh-Matching Algorithm

Couteau *et al.* in 2000 proposed the so called Mesh-Matching (M-M) algorithm. The statement of this work is that building a "suitable" mesh for their purposes is a complex task: count with just a few elements and achieve a "good" domain representation is always a difficult compromise. Therefore in many cases, meshes are built by hand. As this task is time consuming and cannot be done in practice for every patient, the idea is to use a pre-defined FE mesh of the target domain in order to achieve its representation.

Figure 18. The mesh-matching algorithm (a) The ATLAS mesh, (b) the ATLAS and the target surface domain, (c) the matching of ATLAS surface points into the target domain and (d) the final target mesh obtained by applying the transformation function T into the entire ATLAS mesh

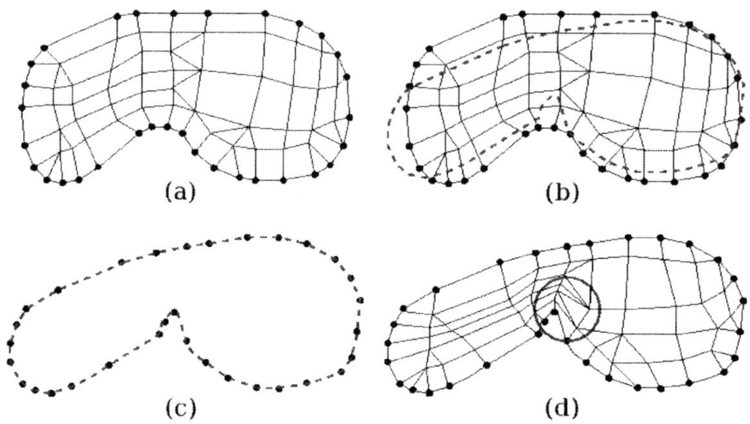

The pre-defined mesh is called the ATLAS. This mesh is, in most cases, built by hand in order to preserve element quality, orientation and density in the desired regions, in terms of what is important for the simulation.

To build a new mesh, target information must be represented with a cloud of points at the surface of the new domain to mesh. Then, a registration process *matches* surface nodes of the ATLAS with the target surface points. The goal of this process is to find a 3D transform *T* that is the combination of a rigid-body transform *RT*, a global warping *W* and local displacement function *S* as follows:

$$T_p = RT \circ W \circ S$$

where *p* is a vector gathering the parameters of *RT*, *W* and *S*. Let $M = M_i$, $i = 1, \ldots, N_1$ and $P = P_i$, $i = 1, \ldots, N_1$ be respectively the ATLAS surface nodes and the target surface points (for example patient data obtained by the segmentation algorithm). The elastic registration algorithm minimizes a least-squares criterion *E(p)* given by:

$$E(p) = \sum_{i=1}^{N_1} \frac{1}{\sigma_i^2} \left[dist(P, T_p(M_i))\right]^2 + R_p$$

where *R* defines a regularization term that is applied to *S* to obtain a smooth displacement function, σ_i^2 is the noise variance of the measurement *i* and *dist* is the distance between *P* and a point M'_i (transformed by *T*).

As *T* is a 3D transformation function, it can be applied to any point in the initial model. When *T* is applied to the internal nodes of the ATLAS, a final 3D target mesh is achieved. The matching of a domain can be seen in Figure 18 where the different steps of the algorithm are shown. Also note that there is a circle in picture (d) of the figure to reflect bad quality elements. This is to reflect that morphing an ATLAS into another domain is not an easy task. The ATLAS must be prepared to confront those types of problems. If in most cases, the target meshes differ a lot from one to another in a specific region, the ATLAS can prevent this type of problems by adding points in those zones.

Another strategy to solve this problem is to use triangles (or tetrahedras in 3D) on those zones. The benefit of this is that contrary to quad (or hexahedra) it is much more difficult to put a triangle or a tetrahedron in an invalid state (concave triangle faces do not exist as in the case of rectangle or hexahedra). Therefore a probably good atlas

Figure 19. An improvement to the ATLAS: using more triangles in complicated zones (left) can improve element quality in the resulting mesh (right)

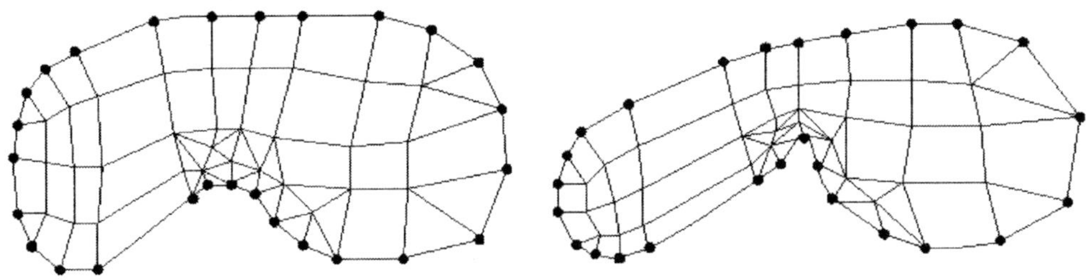

would be the one shown in Figure 19. Note that knowing the zones that deform the most, allows adjusting the number of elements to put in each zone. Therefore, this final mesh represents better the target domain with fewer elements than the resulting one from Figure 18d (as fewer elements are presented in the zones where the deformation is less important).

The M-M algorithm can be used with meshes of any type of elements. In the particular case of Couteau *et al.* (2000), the goal was to obtain femora head meshes and the tested ATLAS was composed of hexahedra and wedges (prisms). In the article, a test over 10 proximal femora is presented. The level of element distortion was satisfactory in comparison to the initial ATLAS.

Meshing 4D Domains

The work of Montagnat and Delingette in 2005 is focused on building *surface models* of 3D domains over time (4D). Despite the surface models (instead of volumetric meshes), this work is important to this chapter as it considers deformable domains through time. But before explaining the 4D technique, lets see the 3D deformable meshes from the same authors in 1998.

The ATLAS mesh (initial model), is a simplex mesh. This mesh can be seen as the dual mesh of a triangulation. Each point of the simplex corresponds to a triangle's centroids[6] in the triangulation as shown in Figure 20 where the simplex mesh is represented by dashed lines. The simplex mesh has some interesting properties like constant connectivity (each point is connected to three others in the discretization), highly deformable, avoiding surface parametrization problems and other properties as mentioned by Delingette (1999).

Back to the work of Montagnat and Delingette in 1998, an analysis of registration techniques *vs* Free Form Deformations (FFD) is made. It mentions the positive and negative aspects of both techniques and finally reports a workflow to merge them. It analyzes the different results obtained by each technique.

There are several types of registration. The basic one is rigid registration, that considers 6 Degrees Of Freedom (DOF). Then, as the number of DOF increases, the registration can achieve a

Figure 20. A triangle mesh and its corresponding simplex mesh (in dashed lines) by the junction of all the triangle's centers

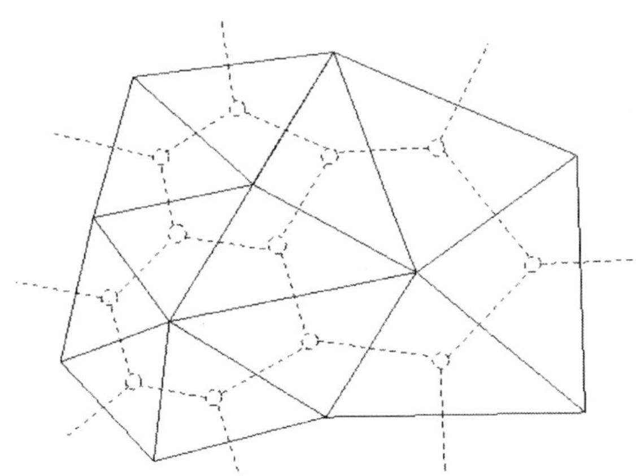

better representation. The authors work shows results with 6,7 and 12 DOF. It also analyzes the result with one registration governed by cubic B-spline.

To couple registration and FFDs, the authors introduce a λ factor that allows the interaction of both registration and FFD. When $\lambda = 0$ the point's displacement has a minimum of DOFs (Registration). As λ approaches to the value 1, the number of DOFs increases. Let V_i^{t+1} be the position of vertex *i* in iteration *t+1*, then the position of any vertex in the mesh can be obtained as:

$$V_i^{t+1} = F(V_i^t, V_i^{t-1}) + \lambda f_i^{FFD} + (1 - \lambda) f_i^{registration}$$

where F is a function of the previous position of the vertex *i*, $f_i^{registration}$ are the forces that control the regular registration and f_i^{FFD} are the forces that control FFD.

With this equation, it is possible to iteratively increase the DOFs. The first "rigid" registration will stop when a threshold of the level of displacement is achieved. Then the DOFs are incremented by the use of λ and the registration continues until the final registration becomes a FFD with cubic B-splines.

The proposed registration hierarchy allows this work to efficiently match one atlas against a cloud of points as some other optimizations are proposed in the article. But going one step further, some organs in the body are important to analyze in motion. Therefore a substantial application of the presented work is to model 3D domains that change with time (4D), as for example: the heart.

The work of Montagnat *et al.* in 2005, first study a set of images that represent the states of the target organ through time. With the ATLAS of the organ, registration matches the cloud of points of the domain in the different states. As the domain changes, the ATLAS changes too and through all the different states, it simulates the motion of the organ.

Mesh Warping

As mentioned by Wolberg in 1998, there are several algorithms to morph an image into another one. One of them is the mesh warping algorithm that was first introduced for a special effect sequence in the movie "Willow" in 1988 by Smythe (1990). It allows producing a smooth transition between two images by using the same mesh in both images and identifies some control points that will lead the transformation.

The work of Castellano-Smith *et al.* in 2001 follows the same principle but produces volumetric meshes. It is strongly based on the 2D image registration proposed by Schnabel *et al.* (2001) that works with grids.

Following the same principle as the one in the previous section, the schema of Schnabel *et al.* (2001) is divided in two steps. First, the global motion is corrected using a rigid (6 DOF) or affine (12 DOF) transformation. The global motion then becomes the starting estimate for the second stage, where the local motion is further modeled using Free Form Deformations (FFD) based on B-splines. The combined motion model can be written as:

$$T(x,y,z) = T_{global}(x,y,z) + T_{local}(x,y,z) \quad (1)$$

with the local motion at each point given by the 3D tensor product of the familiar 1D cubic B-splines. The optimal transformation T is determined by minimizing a registration cost function:

$$C = -C_{similarity}(I_A, T(I_B)) + \lambda C_{deformation}(T) \quad (2)$$

The similarity term maximizes the voxel similarity between the ATLAS image (I_A), and its counterpart in the target image (I_B). The deformation cost term is defined as the 3D equivalent of a thin-plate bending energy in order to maximize the smoothness of the transformation, weighted by a factor λ.

As mentioned in the article, single-resolution FFDs are limited by low mesh resolutions, and may develop folding at high resolutions. Therefore a multi-resolution mesh representation is proposed. Each image is registered several times by using grids of different level of refinements. Note that control points can differ from one grid to another one. After registration, the local deformation of each point in the image volume domain is given by the sum of the local deformations across levels:

$$T_{local}\left(x, y, z\right) = \sum_{h=1}^{H} T_{local}^{h}\left(x, y, z\right) \qquad (3)$$

where each T^{h}_{local} is computed with respect to the B-spline of level h. The use of multi-resolution FFDs avoids the folding problem. Therefore the deformation cost term regularizing the smoothness of the deformation in equation 2 is no longer crucial (λ can be set to 0).

In practice, this technique is applied by Castellano-Smith *et al.* in 2001. In that study, a volumetric ATLAS of the brain is built from a set of MRI and the control points are selected. To build a new brain mesh, it is necessary to count with MRIs of the target (equivalents to the ones from the ATLAS) and to identify the position of the control points. The registration process then matches the ATLAS mesh to the target mesh. Note that the registration provided in the paper is made from a set of 2D images. As their points are correlated to a 3D mesh, it is possible to obtain a 3D mesh as a result.

The big difference between this method and the Mesh Matching (M-M) technique is that it allows identifying inner points to lead the registration. This is very useful to consider the matching of inner structures like in the case of the brain. However, Berar, Desvignes, Bailly and Payan proposed in 2004 a combined approach using the M-M and a multi-resolution grid for matching high resolution ATLAS into low density target data. This was applied to mandible simulation. Another important remark over this last work is that for the definition of control points, they didn't use geometrical points but anatomical ones like the teeth, even though the teeth were not presented in the target model.

Even though the ATLAS can be built with different meshing techniques, it is important to mention that in the work of Castellano-Smith *et al.* (2001), the ATLAS was built from a set of segmented images. Then with a based Marching-Cubes algorithm they produced a surface model of the brain and inner structures. Their paper doesn't give details on the volumetric mesh generation; however it mentions that the final mesh is a tetrahedral mesh of high quality. The last important thing to mention is that they have used quadratic tetrahedra, i.e. 10 nodes.

Finally the differences between this registration process and the one proposed by Montagnat *et al.* (2005) are:

- The type of mesh they use (grid *vs* simplex)
- The first approach uses an iterative strategy where the level of the mesh refinement and the registration are coupled in each iteration
- The entire process is leaded by some specific control points that are added in each iteration

Untangling and Improving Quality After Mesh Adaptation

The accuracy and efficiency of the solution to numerical systems depend on the quality of the mesh. Moreover, in the case of registration techniques, it is possible to compress/stress an element to the point where it becomes folded (i.e. degenerated and therefore invalid for the FEM) as Figure 21 shows. This can occur since the registration techniques do not consider the geometry of the elements in the mesh (the registration is made regarding the points and not the elements).

The workflow of element reparation after registration should be:

Figure 21. A folded face (left) where the dotted line is a diagonal and a folded hexahedron (right) where the dotted lines represent a perfect hexahedron

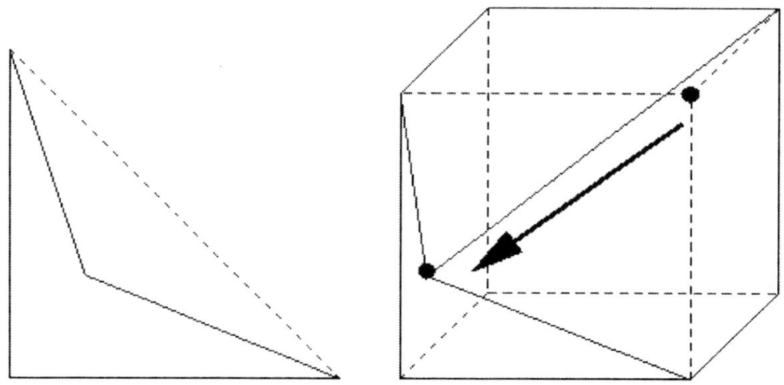

- Make the mesh valid (repair tangle and folded elements) and improve element's quality when possible. In the work of Schnabel *et al.* (2001) presented in the previous subsection, this was done in 2D for each image as the idea of hierarchically increase the refinement level of the mesh[7] avoids the presence of "folded" squares. When passing to the 3D volumetric mesh, this problem was not relevant as the final mesh was tetrahedra-only type. Note that folded faces cannot be produced with triangle faces.

One solution to solve tangled and folded elements was proposed by Luboz et al. (2001, 2005). This work continues the Mesh Matching (M-M) technique presented before as it repairs the invalid elements that are sometimes produced after the registration.

The first step consists in detecting the tangle elements. To do so, the **Jacobian matrix** is used regarding the transformation between the reference and the actual space. This transformation can be computed for any type of element. In particular Figure 22 shows an example for a hexahedron: at the left the reference space R_{rst} and at the right the actual space R_{xyz}. The **Jacobian matrix** for this transformation can be written as:

Figure 22. The reference and actual space from which the Jacobian matrix is calculated. Left, the reference space and right, the actual space.

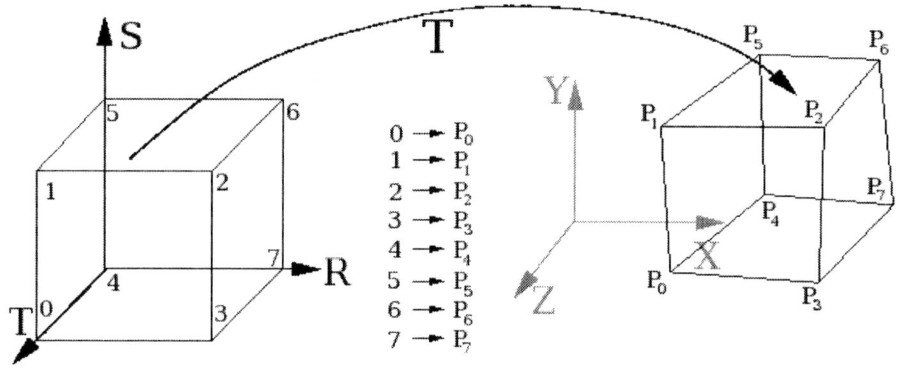

$$J = \begin{bmatrix} J_{xr} & J_{xy} & J_{xz} \\ J_{yr} & J_{yy} & J_{yz} \\ J_{zr} & J_{zy} & J_{zz} \end{bmatrix} = \begin{bmatrix} \sum_i \frac{\partial N_i}{\partial r} x_i & \sum_i \frac{\partial N_i}{\partial r} y_i & \sum_i \frac{\partial N_i}{\partial r} z_i \\ \sum_i \frac{\partial N_i}{\partial r} x_i & \sum_i \frac{\partial N_i}{\partial r} y_i & \sum_i \frac{\partial N_i}{\partial r} z_i \\ \sum_i \frac{\partial N_i}{\partial r} x_i & \sum_i \frac{\partial N_i}{\partial r} y_i & \sum_i \frac{\partial N_i}{\partial r} z_i \end{bmatrix}$$

where N_i are the interpolation shape functions, x_i, y_i and z_i are the actual coordinates and r,s,t are the coordinates in the reference space.

It is possible to compute the Finite Element (FE) if this transformation matrix exists for any element in the mesh. This is equivalent to say that simulation is possible when this matrix is not singular. It is possible to detect singularities by the analysis of the sign of the determinant of *J (detJ)*. By evaluating *detJ* in each vertex of the element, a singularity is presented when not all these values have the same sign (i.e. when a null value is presented somewhere inside the element).

In order to repair those elements, the gradient of the *detJ* is computed. For a distorted element *k*, a displacement $Disp_{k,j}$ for the vertex *j* is proposed as follows:

$$Disp_{k,j} = \sum_i \nabla_j \det J = \begin{bmatrix} \sum_i \frac{\partial \det \mathbf{J}_i}{\partial x_j} \\ \sum_i \frac{\partial \det \mathbf{J}_i}{\partial y_j} \\ \sum_i \frac{\partial \det \mathbf{J}_i}{\partial z_j} \end{bmatrix}$$

where *i* is the vertex index of element *k* that has a negative or nil. The total displacement $Disp_j$ for a given vertex *j* is computed by adding each $Disp_{k,j}$ obtained for every invalid element *k* where the vertex *j* is presented. This displacement vector is then normalized and the final position P'_j for a given point *j* with current position is P_j can be obtained as follows:

$$P'_j = P_j + Disp_j * W_j$$

where W_j is a weight factor chosen to constrain the displacement.

Another approach to solve this problem was proposed by Li and Freitag in (1999). This work intends an optimization approach to untangle (equivalent to solve the folding in 2D) the mesh. It searches to maximize the minimal area or volume of the elements. The first step is to detect tangled elements. This is done by computing the Jacobian sign at each element's vertex. A very important point must be noticed here: the work mentions that an element with one vertex of negative Jacobian can be a valid element. Note that this refers to tangling, i.e., an element can be not tangled having one negative Jacobian vertex. However, this has nothing to deal with the FEM. A negative Jacobian vertex does not allow to compute the FEM, therefore the statement should be: a mesh can be untangled but count with negative Jacobian vertex, however this mesh will not be valid from a FEM point of view as it is not possible to compute a simulation with.

The laplacian smoothing technique (Freitag 1997) consists in positioning each vertex *v* of the mesh in the center of the polygon formed by all the vertex connected to it. This method operates heuristically and does not assure quality improvement over the elements of the mesh; for example it can produce slivers[8]. Therefore, optimization techniques based on some quality measure (dihedral angle, aspect-ratio, etc.) are preferred. Unfortunately optimization approaches have a computational cost much higher than the laplacian smoothing. Therefore a combined strategy is proposed by Freitag (1997). But before going into details it is necessary to introduce two concepts.

The laplacian (a smoothing process) by its own does not consider quality measures. Therefore the first modification is the introduction of a "smart laplacian". This is the typical laplacian smoothing but it will be applied only if the new position for *v* improves the quality of the elements.

Even though it is not presented like this, for understanding purposes let's say that the active value $actVal_v$ corresponds to the worst element quality associated to vertex v, and $actVal_{mesh}$ the worst element quality in the mesh. Now to improve element quality, a user-defined *threshold* value is used and the following iterative algorithms are proposed (each algorithm is independent):

- If $threshold < actVal_{mesh}$ the *smart laplacian* is performed. Otherwise the laplacian is used.
- Apply *smart laplacian* and compute the new $actVal_v$. If $threshold < actVal_v$ repair it using laplacian.
- If $threshold < actVal_{mesh}$ the process is finished. Otherwise apply *smart laplacian* and compute the new $actVal_{mesh}$. If $threshold < actVal_{mesh}$ apply laplacian.
- Compute $threshold = actVal_{mesh} + C$, where C is an arbitrary constant value. Then proceed as the second algorithm (from this list).

Freitag (1997) concludes that all the above algorithms but the third were superior to the *smart laplacian* and optimization approach. However, the third combined approach was the fastest and it also improved the mesh (only with a worst quality than the others but still, better than the input).

MESH GENERATION

Red Green Tetrahedral Meshing Technique

Molino, Bridson, Teran and Fedkiw (2003) have introduced the red green subdivision algorithm. This meshing technique is said to be for modelling highly deformable objects.

The implemented approach starts with a regular octree mesh, i.e. all the octants in the mesh are refined at the same level. Therefore it can be seen as a voxel-based approach but conserving the tree structure of an octree.

Once the desired level of refinement is achieved, each cube is divided in 6 pyramids and each of them in 2 tetrahedrons. As this is done for each hexahedron in the mesh, the global tree structure can be conserved. The difference is that for each leaf in the tree, there will be a reference to the 12 tetrahedrons that replace the original cube.

In order to achieve good surface representation some tetrahedrons must be split. Therefore a pattern that enables tetrahedron subdivision is applied over the regions where more elements are needed. This pattern can be applied recursively over tetrahedra. Those elements are said to be *red* (they can still be refined). However, between refined and not refined regions there must be a consistent transition. In order to avoid propagation of the refinement level, new *green* patterns (see Figure 23) are applied. Those green tetrahedrons cannot

Figure 23. The red green patterns to split tetrahedrons. The standard red refinement (left) and the three green patterns for transitions between regions of different refinement levels (right)

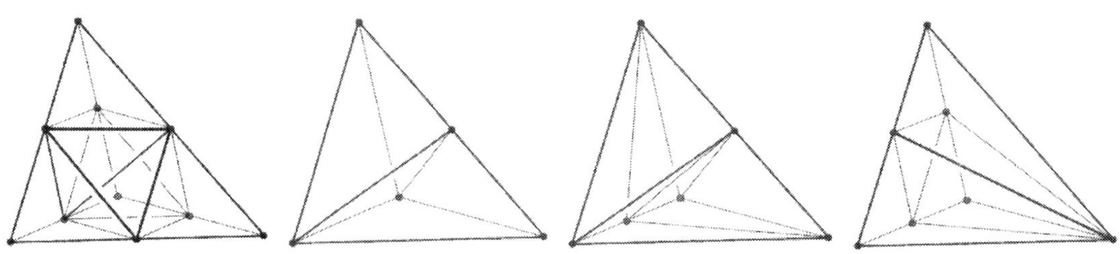

be refined anymore. If for some reason a green tetrahedron must be refined later, it is replaced including his *brothers* with the hierarchical red father (using the tree data structure that enables this process to be fast and robust). Now, with this red tetrahedron the subdivision is applied until the desired element density is achieved.

The red green meshes are desirable because, except for the green tetrahedrons in the transitions, they produce equilateral tetrahedrons (in difference with a pure *Delaunay* approach), avoiding sliver tetrahedra (which increases the level of computation errors in the simulation). It is for this reason that they are said to be optimized for objects that will be highly deformed.

In the context of neurosurgery and brain modeling, Fedorov, Chrisochoides, Kikinis and Warfield in (2005) proposed to use the FEM to project the output mesh of the *red green* algorithm in order to achieve the correct external surface representation. They defined the displacements of the boundary nodes toward the object surface using a distance map, and solved the system with boundary conditions defined by the displacements of the mesh vertices.

Even though the general context of this work is classified under the real-time simulations, the mesh used to carry out the study should be classified as a mesh for accurate simulations. Note that if this work doesn't use parallel computing, the simulation takes one hour or more to be computed.

Marching Cubes with Delaunay-Based Meshes Towards Several Bodies Simulation

The work of Audette, Delingette, Fuchs, Burgert and Chinzei (2007) might be considered as an accurate simulation because it builds detailed meshes for several structures of the brain. However their intention is to produce a realistic simulation of the pitatoria surgery for training purposes. Through virtual reality, this simulation is produced in real-time, therefore it can be considered as part of the real-time simulations.

To simulate the endoscopic pituitary surgery, they produce several non connected triangle surface meshes. Each mesh represents a volumetric or a surface mesh of the head structures like the pituitary gland and the arteries, the cranial nerves, the dura mater, the brain and other pathological structures.

In order to produce those surface meshes they first generate a dense surface mesh of high accuracy and topological fidelity, resulting from the Marching Cubes algorithm. The second step corresponds to a decimation process in order to obtain a mesh of the desired density.

The third step consists in building the simplex mesh of the previous calculated mesh. An optimization process leaded by a balloon force can act over the points of the simplex mesh to cause it to expand until some image-based force halts this expansion. In consequence each dual triangle is reallocated in order to count with edges of equal or locally consistent length. In other words, as the relation between a triangle mesh and the simplex is one-to-one, a displacement over a point in the simplex mesh causes a displacement over the three corresponding points in the triangle. Therefore the optimization over all the simplex points improves the quality of the triangles (as an optimization runs over each triangle's center).

Once all the high quality meshes are obtained, Audette *et al.* (2007) propose to add inner points inside the surfaces that will be modeled as a volumetric object. To do so they use a criterion of "near-equal length of the tetrahedron". Once they have enough inner points the authors proceed to build a Delaunay mesh of it.

Finally, they improve the quality of the mesh by making an optimization over the dihedral angle[9]. They achieve an excellent representation of the inner structures of the brain, allowing via Virtual Reality, the training on pitatoria surgery. This strategy is under the category of Volume generation techniques because even though the authors include the input surface mesh to produce the volume mesh, in a previous step, they regenerate the surface mesh with the Marching Cubes technique. Then they build a new dense surface mesh that soon after is decimated and goes through a quality improvement process.

A previous work by Pages, Sermesant and Frey in 2005, developed a general purpose technique similar to the one above. The goal was to develop an application to go from MRI and CT images to volume meshes. The first step was to achieve image segmentation. As this process is even more complicated when the simulation must consider several sub-structures of the image, they used a user-guided segmentation algorithm. Once the segmented images are produced, the only user interaction is to decide the level of precision the mesh must have. With the segmented images, the marching cubes algorithm is applied to produce an initial surface mesh. Then a bi-laplacian algorithm produced a smooth surface (this step wasn't applied by Audette *et al.* in 2007) to finally proceed with a decimation algorithm to decrease the number of triangles. Now with a "good" quality surface mesh, the inner points are inserted. These new points are inserted regarding the Delaunay property to produce an initial volume mesh. In this work, the quality of a tetrahedron, is defined by $Q = \alpha\rho / h$, where ρ is the inradius, h the largest edge length and α is a normalization coefficient (to get a quality of 1 for a regular element). Following this quality function, an optimization process improves the element's quality by node relocation and face flipping operations.

Variational Tetrahedral Meshing

This work was developed by Alliez, Cohen-Steiner, Yvinec and Desbrun in 2005. It is a general purpose meshing technique starting from a Delaunay mesh. Then the meshes are improved in quality by optimal point insertion in terms of tetrahedral quality.

Concerning the mesh generation, the important constraints to this work are:

- **Count with a fair shape quality measure:** They make a reference to the work of Shewchuk (2002a) and conclude that: "The *radius ratio*, which takes the quotient of inscribed and circumscribed sphere radii (times three for normalization purposes), is a good measure for any kind of degeneracy". This specially avoids the presence of sliver elements.
- **Sizing requirement:** Citing directly from Alliez *et al.* (2005): "Accuracy and efficiency of numerical solvers depend on the local size of tetrahedra. Consequently, a sizing field, prescribing the ideal local edge length as a function of space, must be added". In consequence, a smooth transition between elements of different sizes is necessary to avoid bad dihedral angles.
- **Boundary requirements:** Two options are possible to represent the external surface of the domain to mesh: directly include the input surface mesh in the final output mesh or re-mesh the input domain in order to control its quality and density. The first, of course, achieves perfect surface representation as the Advancing Front algorithm, however as Alliez *et al.* (2005) intend to produce a meshing technique for general purposes, the second option was chosen. In this manner, there is no dependency on the density or quality of the input domain.

Regarding all the above points, Alliez and colleagues (2005) present a Delaunay-based optimization technique, called "Variational Tetrahedral Meshing", to efficiently mesh a bounded 3D domain of arbitrary topology or number of connected components. The base of the algorithm considers optimal surface approximation by the work of Cohen-Steiner, Alliez and Desbrun (2004) and Optimal Delaunay Triangulation by the work of Chen and Xu in 2004. Regarding those techniques the authors propose a simple minimization procedure that alternates global 3D

Delaunay triangulation and local vertex relocation to consistently and efficiently minimize a global energy over the domain. It results in a robust meshing technique that generates high quality isotropic meshes in terms of radius ratios, as well as angles. A notable feature of the method is that it removes slivers (the principal problem of the Delaunay technique already explained) inside the domain. To provide a flexible meshing tool, they also introduce an automatic sizing field construction that guarantees an arbitrary smooth gradation of the mesh together with faithful approximation of the domain boundary.

The authors provided several comparisons with other quality tetrahedral meshing techniques. In all the presented cases their technique gave the highest mesh quality in terms of tetrahedra radius ratios (the one that avoids sliver tetrahedrons and also considers the dihedral angle).

A Brief Remark Concerning Surfaces

As reviewed in the previous works, to get a good representation of the input domain surface is always a difficult task. Many approaches go through high refinement levels to achieve such a good representation and then, by decimation or point reallocation, decrease the number of faces and try to improve their quality.

Another option to improve surface quality is to change the topology of the mesh. This is not exactly decimation as the work of Bunin in 2006 shows. Even though it is focused in 2D, it can be adapted to improve the quality of surface meshes in 3D. The quality improvement over the surface is achieved by removing "bad quality" or "undesirable" sub-domains of the mesh and by re-meshing those zones. Contrary to decimation, this doesn't only change the topology but can also improve the orientation of the elements. In particular this approach improves quadrilateral meshes.

When the focus is triangle surfaces, one remarkable work is the one by Coll, Guerrieri and Sellares in 2006. The algorithm combines different meshing improvements techniques that incrementally modify an initial triangle mesh by local changes. The element insertion or removal is done in such a way that the mesh quality is maintained during the process. The local operations are: deletion, insertion and addition of Steiner[10] points. The overall process goes through a definition of quality zones. Therefore vertices of skinny triangles are forced to those zones. If a vertex must be removed, new vertices are placed in quality zones to improve the overall quality.

Hexahedral Meshes

Unstructured quadrilateral/hexahedral meshes are also an important alternative to simulate applications with the Finite Element Method (FEM). However, it still remains a challenging and open problem to generate adaptive and quality quad/hex meshes directly from volumetric data, such as Computed Tomography (CT) and Magnetic Resonance Imaging (MRI).

The work of Zhang and Bajaj in 2006 goes in this direction. The overall strategy consists of:

- Select a starting level of octree refinement for uniform mesh generation with correct topology, regarding the volumetric data. Produce a representative quad/hex mesh of the input domain.
- Improve the quality of the final elements.

Once an initial octree level of refinement is achieved five patterns enable transitions between refined and coarse regions. Those patterns are applied in function of the vertex signs. This is based on the "dual contouring method" proposed by Ju, Losasso, Schaefer and Warren in 2002. This last method consists in an approximation of the surface by assigning directions to the vertices in all the sections where domain intersection is produced.

Figure 24 shows the contour detection and assigns a sign to each octree vertex regarding the

Figure 24. Extended Marching Cubes and dual contouring (a) octree mesh with domain cutting intersections and the normal of those cutting points, (b) the marching cubes output, (c) the extended marching cubes contour and (d) the dual contour mesh

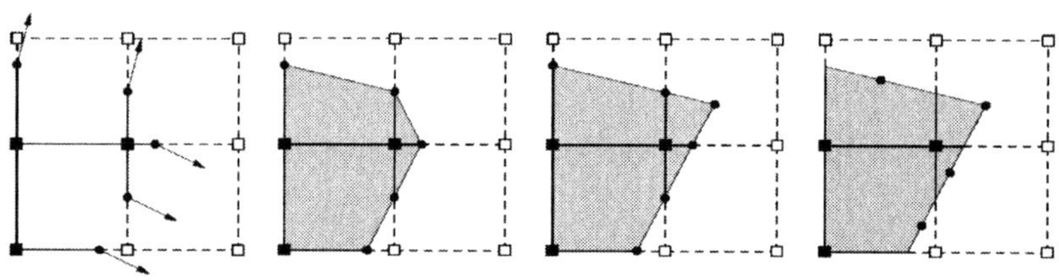

normals of the intersection points. This can be seen in (a) as the black points rest inside the domain. Image (b) represents the output from the marching cubes technique. Image (c) shows the "extended marching cube" (EMC) technique proposed by Kobbelt, Botsch, Schwanecke and Seidel in 2001 and (d) the points of the dual contour regarding the EMC. As the already introduced triangle simplex mesh, here a dual mesh is expanded to a more global concept as it is not restricted to triangles (see Ju *et al.* (2002) for more details).

With all these techniques, the work by Zhang *et al.* (2006) allows to produce quad/hexa meshes that have regions with different levels of refinement and achieve a "good" surface representation. Finally Zhang and Zhao (2007) continues the previous work by adding two new patterns to drastically decrease the number of transition elements between refined and coarse regions.

Table 1.

Meshing Technique	Delaunay	Octree-alike	Marching Cubes
Ruppert (1995)	Ok	-	-
Schewchuk (2002a)	Ok	-	-
Miller (2003)	Ok	-	-
Abell (1999)	-	Ok	-
Ashburner (2000)	-	Ok	-
Finkel (1974)	-	Ok	-
Nesme (2008)	-	Ok	-
Lorensen (1987)	-	Ok	-
Chernyaev (1995)	-	Ok	Ok
Payne (1990)	Ok	Ok	-
Ferrant (1999)	Ok	Ok	-
Velasco (2007)	Ok	Ok	Ok
Couteau (2000)	-	-	-
Castellano-Smith (2001)	-	Ok	Ok
Berar (2004)	-	-	-
Molino (2003)	Ok	Ok	-
Audette (2007)	Ok	Ok	Ok
Pages (2005)	Ok	Ok	Ok
Alliez (2005)	Ok	-	-
Chen (2004)	Ok	-	-
Zhang (2006	-	Ok	Ok

SUMMARY OVER PRESENTED TECHNIQUES

In the two previous sections, several meshing techniques were presented. In the following tables a summary of them is proposed, involving all the relevant aspects of meshing.

Table 1 presents the reviewed techniques regarding the basic and most common meshing techniques and concepts. Note how the Delaunay property is used by all the techniques that produce tetrahedral meshes (see table 2). It is important to mention that not all the techniques produce volumetric meshes. Some of them are used only to achieve a good surface representation. Another important remark is that several techniques

Table 2.

Meshing technique	Tetrahedra	Hexahedra	Mixed-elements
Abell (1999)	-	Ok	-
Ashburner (2000)	-	Ok	-
Nesme (2008)	-	Ok	-
Lorensen (1987)	Ok	-	-
Payne (1990)	Ok	-	-
Ferrant (1999)	Ok	-	-
Velasco (2007)	Ok	-	-
Couteau (2000)	-	-	Ok
Castellano-Smith (2001)	Ok	-	-
Berar (2004)	-	-	Ok
Molino (2003)	Ok	-	-
Audette (2007)	Ok	-	-
Pages (2005)	Ok	-	-
Alliez (2005)	Ok	-	-
Zhang (2006)	-	Ok	-

producing tetrahedra, also use the octree-alike methods to produce a primary tessellation.

Table 2 focuses on the type of element produced by the techniques that generate volumetric meshes. Note how mixed elements meshes are by far the less used.

There are more generation techniques than registration methods as table 3 shows. Note that this doesn't mean that in medical applications, the generation methods are more used than registration techniques. As generation methods tend to solve general problems there is an important global effort to improve them. In the other hand, registration methods are mostly used in the medical field as the difference from one target to another one makes possible to re-use already generated meshes (ATLAS). Registration methods are also largely used in the medical field due to the complexity of the anatomical structures. The goal isn't just to achieve surface representation but also to conserve some element orientation (alienation) regarding sub-structures (like different types of materials, behavior, physical properties, etc).

Also note that several tetrahedral generators improve the quality of the input surface mesh and then continue with some point insertion strategies (using the modified input surface mesh) in order to produce the final volume mesh. In other words, techniques that use the input surface mesh, as the Advancing Front, seem to be "not so used" in the medical field.

CONCLUSION

The goal of this chapter was to show the different possible techniques to produce a suitable mesh for the FEM. Therefore, several related works were omitted as the meshing techniques they used were already explained.

Regarding all the mesh generation techniques presented in this chapter, a workflow for general mesh generation is presented in Figure 25. This is based on the work of Frey (2004). In this picture an example of "isosurface reconstruction" is the Marching Cubes algorithm. The "mesh optimization" with the "geometric constraints" refers to the element deletion or insertion per region in function of the simulation requirements.

Finally, regarding all the adaptation techniques, Figure 26 shows the equivalent workflow

Table 3.

Meshing type	Reviewed works
Registration	Couteau (2000); Montagnat (2005); Castellano-Smith (2001); Berar (2004)
Generation	Alliez (2005); Audette (2007); Molino (2003); Abell (1999); Ashburner (2000); Velasco (2007); Pages (2005); Nesme (2008); Lorensen (1987); Payne (1990); Ferrant (1999); Montagnat (2005); Zhang (2006)

Figure 25. The mesh generation general flow. From image to volume mesh generation based on Frey (2004).

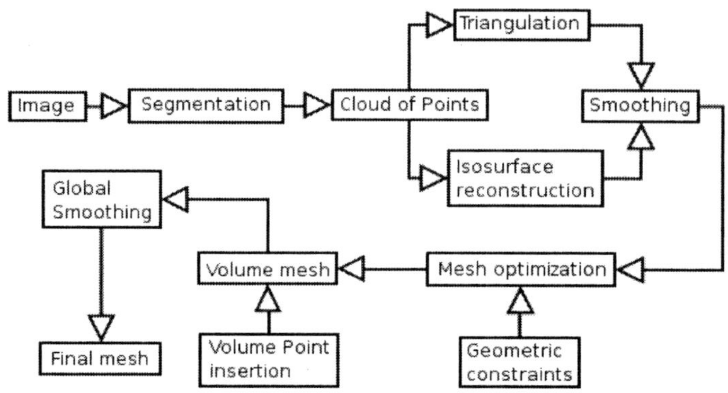

Figure 26. The mesh adaptation general flow. From image to volume mesh generation.

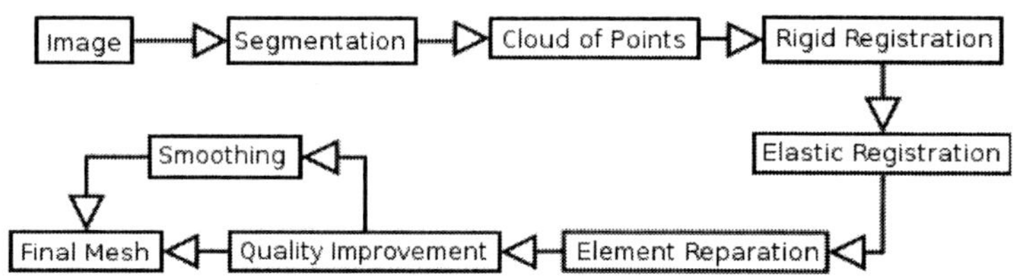

that we propose for a general mesh registration technique. The "rigid registration" can be of different DOF (6,7 or 12) as mentioned above. The "elastic registration" is equivalent to "Free Form Deformation" or "Non Rigid Registration" concepts. The "Element Reparation" corresponds to a re-allocation of the negative Jacobian points and the "quality improvement" needs a measure of quality and then performs an optimization over the elements regarding the selected criterion. Note that a "Smoothing" process is also proposed in order to produce the final volume mesh of the target domain.

ACKNOWLEDGMENT

Financial support by FONDECYT 1061227, ECOS-Sud C06E04 and Plomo Project (TIC Amsud)

REFERENCES

Abell, F., Krams, M., Ashburner, J., Passingham, R., Friston, K., & Frackowiak, R. (1999). The neuroanatomy of autism: a voxel-based whole brain analysis of structural scans. *Neuroreport*, *10*(8), 1647–1651. doi:10.1097/00001756-199906030-00005

Alliez, P., Cohen-Steiner, D., Yvinec, M., & Desbrun, M. (2005). Variational tetrahedral meshing. *ACM Transactions on Graphics*, *24*(3), 617–625. doi:10.1145/1073204.1073238

Ashburner, J., & Friston, K. (2000). Voxel-based morphometry--the methods. *NeuroImage*, *11*(6 pt. 1), 805–821. doi:10.1006/nimg.2000.0582

Audette, M., Delingette, H., Fuchs, A., Burgert, O., & Chinzei, K. (2007). A topologically faithful, tissue-guided, spatially varying meshing strategy for computing patient-specific head models for endoscopic pituitary surgery simulation. *Computer Aided Surgery*, *12*(1), 43–52. doi:10.1080/10929080601167413

Benzley, S., Perry, E., Merkley, K., Clark, B., & Sjaardema, G. (1995). A Comparison of All Hexagonal and All Tetrahedral Finite Element Meshes for Elastic and Elasto-plastic Analysis. In *Proceedings, 4th International Meshing Roundtable* (pp. 179-191).

Berar, M., Desvignes, M., Bailly, G., & Payan, Y. (2004). 3D Meshes Registration: Application to Statistical Skull Model. *Image Analysis and Recognition*, *3112*, 100–107.

Bonet, J., & Wood, R. (1997). *Nonlinear Continuum Mechanics for Finite Element Analysis.* Cambridge, UK: Cambridge University Press.

Bunin, G. (2006). Non-Local Topological Clean-Up. In *Proceedings, 15th International Meshing Roundtable*, (pp. 3-20).

Castellano-Smith, A., Hartkens, T., Schnabel, J., Hose, R., Liu, H., Hall, W., et al. (2001). Constructing Patient Specific Models for Correcting Intraoperative Brain Deformation. In *MICCAI* (pp. 1091-109).

Chen, L., & XU, J. (2004). Optimal Delaunay triangulations. *Journal of Computational Mathematics*, *22*(2), 299–308.

Chernyaev, E. (1995). *Marching cubes 33: Construccion of topologically correct isosurfaces*, (Technical Report CN/95-17).

Cohen-Steiner, D., Alliez, P., & Desbrun, M. (2004). Variational Shape Approximation. In *ACM Transanctions on Graphics (SIGGRAPH)* (pp. 905-914).

Coll, N., Guerrieri, M., & Sellares, J. (2006). Mesh Modification Under Local Domain Changes. In *Proceedings, 15th International Meshing Roundtable*, (pp. 39-56).

Cotin, S., Delingette, H., & Ayache, N. (1996). Real Time Volumetric Deformable Models for Surgery Simulation. *VBC*, (pp. 535-540).

Couteau, B., Payan, Y., & Lavallee, S. (2000). The mesh-matching algorithm: an automatic 3D mesh generator for finite element structures. *Journal of Biomechanics*, *33*(8), 1005–1009. doi:10.1016/S0021-9290(00)00055-5

Delaunay, B. (1934). Sur la sphere vide. *Izvestia Akademii Nauk SSSR . Otdelenie Matematicheskikh i Estestvennykh Nauk*, *7*, 793–800.

Delingette, H. (1999). General Object Reconstruction based on Simplex Meshes. *International Journal of Computer Vision*, *32*(2), 111–146. doi:10.1023/A:1008157432188

Fedorov, A., Chrisochoides, N., Kikinis, R., & Warfield, S. (2005). Tetrahedral mesh generation for medical Imaging. *Insight Journal - MICCAI Open Source Workshop.*

Ferrant, M., Warfield, S., Guttmann, C., Mulkern, R., Jolesz, F., & Kikinis, R. (1999). 3D Image Matching Using a Finite Element Based Elastic Deformation Model. In *Medical Image Computing and Computer--Assisted Intervention (MICCAI)*, (pp. 202-209).

Finkel, R., & Bentley, J. (1974). Quad Trees: A Data Structure for Retrieval on Composite Keys. *Acta Informatica*, *4*(1), 1–9. doi:10.1007/BF00288933

Freitag, L. (1997). On combining Laplacian and optimization-based mesh smoothing techniques, In *Proc. Symp. Trends in Unstructured Mesh Generation*, (pp.37-43).

Frey, P. (2004). Generation and adaptation of computational surface meshes from discrete anatomical data. *International Journal for Numerical Methods in Engineering*, *60*, 1049–1074. doi:10.1002/nme.992

Hitschfeld, N. (2005). Generation of 3D mixed-element meshes using a flexible refinement approach. *Engineering with Computers*, *21*, 101–114. doi:10.1007/s00366-005-0306-x

Hitschfeld, N., Navarro, G., & Farias, R. (2000). Tessellations of cuboids with Steiner points. In *Proceedings, 9th International Meshing Roundtable*, (pp. 275-282).

Hughes, T. (1987). *The Finite element method: Linear static and dynamic Finite element analysis*, (pp. 292-294). Upper Saddle River, NJ: Prentice-Hall.

Ju, T., Losasso, F., Schaefer, S., & Warren, J. (2002). Dual Contouring of Hermite Data. In *ACM SIGGRAPH*, (pp. 339-346).

Kobbelt, K., Botsch, M., Schwanecke, U., & Seidel, H. (2001). Feature-sensitive surface extraction from volume data. In *ACM SIGGRAPH*, (pp. 57-66).

Li, X., & Freitag. L. (1999). *Optimization-based quadrilateral and hexahedral mesh untangling and smoothing techniques*. Tech. Report, Argonne National Laboratory, a contract Laboratory of the United States Department of Energy.

Lobos, C., Bucki, M., Hitschfeld, N., & Payan, Y. (2007). Mixed-element mesh for an intra-operative modeling of the brain tumor extraction. In *Proceedings, 16th International Meshing Roundtable*, (pp. 387-404).

Lobos, C., & Hitschfeld, N. (2006). 3D NOffset mixed-element mesh generator approach, *The 14th International Conference in Central Europe on Computer Graphics, Visualization and Computer Vision (WSCG)*, (pp. 47-52).

Lorensen, W., & Cline, H. (1987). Marching Cubes: A high resolution 3D surface construction algorithm. *Computer Graphics*, *21*(4), 163–169. doi:10.1145/37402.37422

Luboz, V., Chabanas, M., Swider, P., & Payan, Y. (2005). Orbital and Maxillofacial Computer Aided Surgery: Patient-Specific Finite Element Models To Predict Surgical Outcomes. *Computer Methods in Biomechanics and Biomedical Engineering*, *8*(4), 259–265. doi:10.1080/10255840500289921

Luboz, V., Payan, Y., & Couteau, B. (2001). Automatic 3D Finite Element mesh generation: an atlas fitted onto patient data. In *Proceedings of the Fifth international Symposium on Computer Methods in Biomechanics and Biomedical Engineering*.

Miller, G., Pave, S., & Walkington, N. (2003). When and Why Ruppert's Algorithm Works. In *Proceedings 12th International Meshing Roundtable*, (pp. 91-102).

Molino, N., Bridson, R., Teran, J., & Fedkiw, R. (2003). A crystalline, red green strategy for meshing highly deformable objects with tetrahedral. In *Proceedings, 12th International Meshing Roundtable*, (pp. 103-114).

Montagnat, J., & Delingette, H. (1998). Globally constrained deformable models for 3D object reconstruction. [SP]. *Signal Processing*, *71*(2), 173–186. doi:10.1016/S0165-1684(98)00143-1

Montagnat, J., & Delingette, H. (2005). 4D deformable models with temporal constraints: application to 4D cardiac image segmentation. [MedIA]. *Medical Image Analysis*, *9*(1), 87–100. doi:10.1016/j.media.2004.06.025

Nesme, M. (2008). *Milieu mecanique deformable multiresolution pour la simulation Interactive*. Universite Joseph Fourier.

Pages, A., Sermesant, M., & Frey, P. (2005). Generation of computational meshes from MRI and CT-scan data. In *ESAIM: Proceedings*, (pp. 213-223).

Payne, B., & Toga, A. (1990). Surface mapping brain function on 3d models. *IEEE Computer Graphics and Applications*, *10*(5), 33–41. doi:10.1109/38.59034

Picinbono, G., Delingette, H., & Ayache, N. (2003). Non-Linear Anisotropic Elasticity for Real-Time Surgery Simulation. *Graphical Models*, *65*(5), 305–321. doi:10.1016/S1524-0703(03)00045-6

Ruppert, J. (1995). A Delaunay Refinement Algorithm for Quality 2-Dimensional Mesh Generation. *Journal of Algorithms*, *18*(3), 548–585. doi:10.1006/jagm.1995.1021

Schnabel, J., Rueckert, D., Quist, M., Blackall, J., Castellano-Smith, A., Hartkens, T., et al. (2001). A Generic Framework for Non-rigid Registration Based on Non-uniform Multi-level Free-Form Deformations. In *MICCAI*, (pp. 573-581).

Schwartz, J., Langelier, E., Moisan, C., & Laurendeau, D. (2001). Non-linear Soft Tissue Deformations for the Simulation of Percutaneous Surgeries. In *MICCAI*, (pp. 1271-1272).

Shewchuk, J. (1999). *Lecture notes on Delaunay mesh generation.* Technical Report: Department of Electrical Engineering and Computer Science, University of California, Berkeley.

Shewchuk, J. (2002). What Is a Good Linear Element? Interpolation, Conditioning, and Quality Measures. In *Proceedings of the 11 International Meshing Roundtable,* (pp. 115-126).

Shewchuk, J. (2002a). Delaunay refinement algorithms for triangular mesh generation . *Computational Geometry: Theory and Applications*, *22*(1-3), 21–74.

Smythe, D. (1990). *A two-pass mesh warping alogrithm for object transformation and image interpolation*. Tech. Report, ILM Computer Graphics Department, Lucasfilm.

Velasco, F., Torres, J., Leon, A., & Soler, F. (2007). Adaptive cube tessellation for topologically correct isosurfaces. In *Proceeding of the computer graphics theory and applications*, (pp. 220-227).

Wolberg, G. (1998). Image morphing: a surrey. *The Visual Computer*, *14*(8-9), 360–372. doi:10.1007/s003710050148

Zhang, H., & Zhao, G. (2007). Adaptive hexahedral mesh generation based on local domain curvature and thickness using a modified grid-based method. *Finite Elements in Analysis and Design*, *43*(9), 691–704. doi:10.1016/j.finel.2007.03.001

Zhang, Y., & Bajaj, C. (2006). Adaptive and Quality Quadrilateral/Hexahedral Meshing from Volumetric Data. *Computer Methods in Applied Mechanics and Engineering*, *195*(9-12), 942–960. doi:10.1016/j.cma.2005.02.016

KEY TERMS AND DEFINITIONS

Advancing Front: 2D and 3D meshing technique that produce a mesh using the input domain border (2D) or surface (3D).

Continuum Mechanics: Branch of the mechanics that deals with the analysis of the kinematic and mechanical behavior of materials modeled as a continuum.

Delaunay Property: A quality measure over triangles.

Finite Element Method: A numerical integration method that computes an approximated solution over a domain of certain equations that describes the model.

Grid: A mesh where all the elements are of the same type and have the same connectivity.

Jacobian Matrix: A matrix that links an element with an equivalent and 'perfect' one from another reference system.

Marching Cubes: An algorithm to achieve surface representation from an isosurface.

Mesh: The subdivision of the space into simpler elements.

Mesh Adaptation: Deform a given mesh in order to represent another domain.

Mesh Generation: Build a mesh to represent an arbitrary domain.

Octree: A volumetric meshing technique where elements that intersects the surface are split in 8 new hexahedra.

ENDNOTES

1. http://www.cs.berkeley.edu/~jrs/
2. Evaluate linear elements in a single new state after bending the bar.
3. Evaluate linear elements in a single new state after some torsion is applied over the bar.
4. In the meshing field, optimization refers to mesh quality improvement without inserting new nodes.
5. Image taken from wikipedia http://commons.wikimedia.org/wiki/Image:FMRI.jpg with a Public-domain license. Page last visited: July 21, 2008
6. Note that this is different to the *Voronoi diagram*. If not familiar with this last concept, see: http://en.wikipedia.org/wiki/Voronoi
7. Count with several meshes of different levels of detail. For example a grid with 4, 16 and 64 quads.
8. Tetrahedra where all the points tend to be co-planar.
9. The angle formed between two planes.
10. If in a given Delaunay tetrahedralization or triangulation of an arbitrary domain, a new point is inserted in such a way that the entire mesh still satisfies the Delaunay property, this new point is said to be a *Steiner* point.

Chapter 10
Finite Element Analysis and Its Application in Oral Surgery Research

Mercedes Gallas
University of Santiago de Compostela, Spain

ABSTRACT

The Finite Element Method (FEM) is a widely applied mathematical model that permit us to know the biomechanical behavior of the human mandible in various clinical situations under physiological and standardized trauma conditions. The three-dimensional FEM provides to simulate force systems applied and allows analysis of the response of the jawbone to the loads in 3D space. Clinical extrapolations from FEM may not give absolute values but they will provide detailed description of biomechanical pattern and a prediction of regional stresses distribution. This virtual modeling is useful to choose the most efficient localization and design of miniplate osteosynthesis and to test new biomaterials.

INTRODUCTION

The Finite Element Analysis (FEA) is an accepted theoretical technique used in solution of engineering problems specially (used) for problems involving complicated geometries. It can be used to calculate deflection, stress, vibration, buckling behavior and to analyze deflection under loading or applied displaced. It can be employed as well to analyze elastic deformation or "permanently bent out of shape" plastic deformation.

DOI: 10.4018/978-1-60566-733-1.ch010

FEA is a computer-numerical method to obtain a solution to a complex mechanical problem by dividing the problem domain into a collection of much smaller and simpler domains (elements) in which the field variables can be interpolated with the use of shape functions. An overall approximated solution to the original problem is determined based on variational principles. The behavior of an individual element can be described with a relatively simple set of equations. Just as the set of elements would be joined together to build the whole structure, the equations describing the behaviors of the individual elements are joined into an extremely large set of equations that describe the behavior of the whole structure. Therefore in FEA, a structure is modeled with discrete-element mathematical representation by subdividing it into simpler geometric shapes or elements whose apices meet to form nodes. This complex system of points called nodes make a grid called mesh. Each element of the mesh can adopt a specific geometric shape: triangle, square, tetrahedron, ... ; depending on the type of analysis such as two-dimensional and three-dimensional. Each element is defined by a specific internal function. This mesh is programmed to contain the material characteristics and structural properties that defined how the structure will react to certain loading conditions. The elastic constants, Poisson's ratio (ν), Young´s modulus (E) and the material density (ρ) are specified for the modeled material, which each element retaining the material characteristics of the original structure. The assignment of proper material properties to a Finite Element Model (FEM) is the essential step to ensure predictive accuracy. The primary objective of the FEM is to realistically replicate the important parameters and features of the real model. The first step in the creation of a FEM is to describe its geometry in the computer by appropriate software. In general, a FEM is defined by a mesh net-work, which is made up of the geometric arrangement of elements and nodes. Depending on the problem to investigate the numerical representation of the structure under analysis can be achieved either in a two- (2D) or three-dimensionally (3D) ways. As a loading or force is applied, the interconnected elements of mesh start to move. The displacement of nodes is transformed, through calculations, to stress and strain values. The displacements, von Mises stresses and shear stress in different planes could be studied under different and determined situations. Stress distribution was analyzed based on color differences in von Mises equivalent stress.

This process of dividing the whole domain into elements is indispensable in FEA to formulate the solution functions for each finite element and combines them properly to obtain the solution to the whole body. The process of creating the mesh, elements, their respective nodes and defining boundary conditions is denominated "*discretization*" of the problem domain. Stress and strain distribution patterns in a structure depend on its geometry, the boundary conditions and its material properties. The finite element modeling technique offers the advantage of being able to model structures with intricate shapes and indirectly quantify their complex mechanical behavior at any theoretical point. Because the FEM uses the theories of elasticity and static equilibrium, the effects of multiple external forces acting on a system can be assessed as physical events in terms of deformation, stress or strains.

The information needed to calculate stress and displacements in FEM is: the total number of nodal point and element, the elastic modulus and Poisson's ratio for the materials associated with each element, the coordinates of each nodal point, the type of boundary strains and the evaluation of the forces applied to the external nodes with a FEA software and computer. Also FEA provides the possibility to simulate clinical loadings forces (for example: traumatic impact, orthodontic force systems, physiological muscle forces) applied and allows analysis of the response of the bone to these loadings conditions in the three-dimensional space.

In the past four decades, FEA has become an increasingly useful tool in the field of biomechanics and bioengineering. This computer-based numerical technique has proven the most adaptable, accurate, easy and less time consuming process as compared to the other experimental analysis. In spite of certain limitations such as the cost factor and requirement of an expert to operate the analysis, this technique has taken the field of Dentistry to great heights and provided results that could not have been possible with any other technique.

Nevertheless, FEA has important advantages in dental area: it is a noninvasive technique; the actual amount of stress experienced at any give point can be theoretically measured; the tooth, the alveolar bone, periodontal and human craniofacial bones can be modeled and the material properties of these structures can be assigned to the nearest one to can be simulated the oral environment in vitro; the displacement can be visualized graphically; the point of application, the magnitude and direction of a force may easily be varied to simulated the clinical situation; reproducibility does not affect the physical properties of the involved material; and the study can be repeated as many times as the operator wishes. FEA is a powerful contemporary research tool and plenty of scientific literature is available on the study of stress distribution and deformation of anatomical structures affected by three-dimensional stress fields that are difficult to assess otherwise like as a human mandible. However, experimental or clinical confirmation of this theoretical prediction is mandatory to be realized in any FEA simulation study (for detailed review consult Korioth & Versluis, 1997).

The use of this method in the field of Dentistry was started in 1968 when Ledley and Huang developed a linear model of the tooth based on experimental data and on linear displacement force analysis (Ledley & Huang, 1968). The results of this first work gave a relatively simple method for studying the effect of applied forces on actual tooth displacements. This initial lineal model was employed in numerical experiments using various types of applied forces (normal, pathologic and corrective) acting on the upper central incisor (Huang & Ledley, 1969). The FEA employment spreads widely to dental disciplines (oral surgery, restorative dentistry, orthodontic, prosthodontic, dental materials).

The major contribution in mandibular biomechanical field was made by Knoell, (1977) and by Ferré, Legoux, Helary, Albugues, Le Floc'h, Bouteyre, et al. (1985). They reported first three-dimensional finite element model of human mandible bone. Since then, several finite element models of the human mandible bone have been created, either in two-dimension or in three-dimension (for detailed review consult Korioth & Versluis, 1997). J.W. Farah, R.G. Craig, and K.A. Meroueh, (1988) studied the stress and biomechanical characteristics of this anatomical structure. Their two-dimensional finite element model of a mandibular quadrant permitted to examine the stresses and displacements resulting from load placed on the second molar. Even a three-dimensional mathematical model of the human masticatory system, with 16 muscle forces and two joint reaction forces were described. This model allowed simulation of static bite forces and concomitant joint reaction forces for various bite point locations and mandibular positions (Koolstra, van Eijden, Weijs, & Naeije, 1988). The shortcomings of these firsts models were their simplicity. Later on, in the nineties, were capable of modeling the mechanical characteristics of mandible with more realism and accuracy. The mandible model created by T.W.P. Korioth, D.P. Romilly and A.G. Hannam (1992) permitted a realistic approximation to the biomechanical events of the human mandible with the additional ability to predict regional stresses and strains in inaccessible locations. The authors built two three-dimensional finite element models of a human mandible reconstructed from tomographs of a dry dentate jaw. The first model was used for a complete mechanical characterization of physical events. It also provided comparative data for the second model, which had an increased vertical corpus depth. In both cases, boundary conditions included rigid restraints at the first right molar and endosteal cortical surfaces of the articular eminences of temporal bones. Groups of parallel multiple vectors simulated individual masticatory muscle loads were present in these models. The models were solved for displacements, stresses, strains, and forces. In general, the results indicated that principal stresses and strains were highest on the periosteal cortical surface and alveolar bone. The authors performed a validation of their models with in vivo strain data from macaques during comparable biting events, and the predictive strain values were qualitatively similar. Finally they concluded that although the mandible behaved in a beam-like manner, its corpus acted more like a combination of open and closed cross sections due to the presence of tooth sockets.

The principal difficulty in simulating the mechanical behavior of human mandible is the modeling of human mandible bone and its response to applied mechanical forces. Certain assumptions or simplifications need to be make making in the modeling and solving process possible. Some of these necessary assumptions influence the accuracy of the FEA results significantly. In summary, the geometric design (finite element model) and its mechanical properties are determined by the researchers (Figure 1).

Figure 1. Three-dimensional finite element mesh of a dentate human mandible

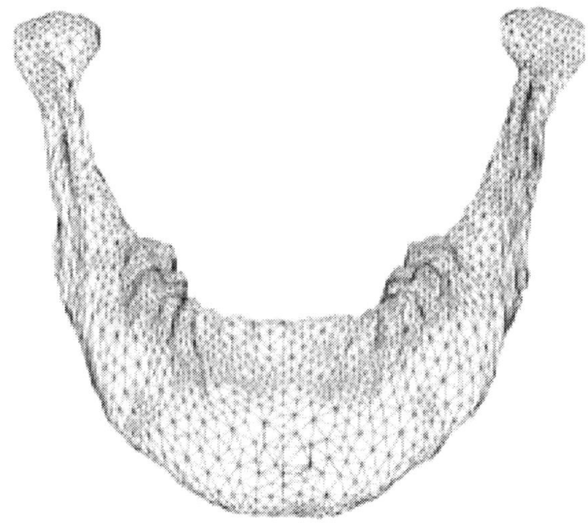

Mandibular bone is a complex biological structure that compromises two different layers, the outer layer being denominated cortical, compact or dense bone; and the inner layer called trabecular, cancellous or spongy bone. In the most reported studies, it is supposed that the mandible had a linearly elastic behavior, and its mechanical properties could therefore be described by specific Young´s modulus (E), Poisson´s ratio (ν) and density (ρ) for cortical and trabecular bone qualities. The material properties were defined according to the experimental data in previous studies from the literature. Early FEA studies ignored the trabecular bone network for example. However, nowadays it is assumed that cancellous bone has a slid pattern inside the inner cortical bone shell. Both bone types are modeled simplistically as linear, homogeneous and isotropic materials but this is not a realistic assumption. To achieve more realistic models the anisotropic and non-homogenous nature of the bone will need to be considered. Besides of this, most FEA studies modeled the mandibular and set the boundary conditions as fixed. Other improvements of FE models are recently possible with the development of digital imaging techniques and specialized software. These technical advances permit us the incorporation of 3-dimensional information data from computed tomography (CT) or magnetic resonance imaging (MRI) into FEA meshes. Zhou, et al. (1999) developed a more realistic three-dimensional mandibular model from transversely scanned CT image data. Although either histological sections, CT or MRI images were used to recreate the surfaces in many of the 3D anatomical models, a close evaluation of their surface representation yielded to sometimes marked geometric inconsistencies, thus necessarily lessening their validity regardless of accomplished model accuracy test. In theses cases, and in accordance with Korioth and Verselius (1997), indirect validation attempts by comparison with data from other basic or clinical studies are mandatory. These experimental validations may help researchers gain useful insight into the potential predictive capabilities of the created models.

The functions of the mastication muscles and the ligaments, functional movement of the temporo-mandibular joints were simulated by means of cable elements and compressive gap elements respectively improving the model mimicry and accuracy. Current FEA programs provide several types of contact algorithms

Figure 2. Von Mises equivalent stress distribution on 3D-FEM of mandible

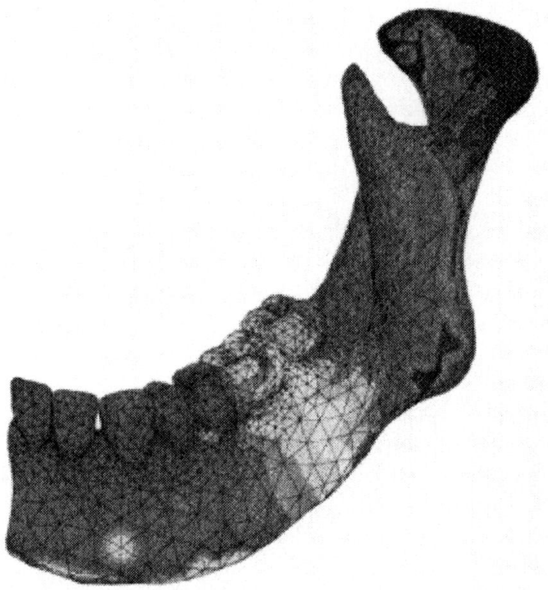

for simulations of contacts. It is therefore now technically more feasible. Loading forces and contact conditions are described in case by case for each analysis. These empirical assumptions allow us to analyze the biomechanical behavior of the object under study (in our case the human mandible) and to determine patterns of biomechanical responses when it is under simulated loads. All of this let us develop an anatomically accurate model. The aim of such research is the determination of stress distribution and improvement of the mechanical strength of this anatomical structure under physiological and standardized trauma conditions or pathological situations. It is important to know that (clinical) extrapolations from mathematical models like FEA may not give absolute values. However, they will provide a detailed and useful description of patterns of biomechanical response. Because all of this, in FE models, some assumptions greatly affects predictive accuracy and it is important noted this subject in the extrapolation of results (Geng, Tan, & Lui, 2001

Therefore, modeling of the mandibular bone is not a trivial task due to their complex 3D geometry, the boundary conditions and the mixture of different load-bearing parts and material properties (Figure 2).

ANALYSIS OF MANDIBLE BIOMECHANIC

The human masticatory system consists of mandible bone which is able to move with respect to the skull and is guide by two temporomandibular joints (TMJs) through activity of the masticatory muscles. The mandible is connected to the skull by TMJs that provide the mandible with a large mobility with respect to the skull (open-close jaw movement, protrusion, retrusion and lateral movements). The articulating surfaces of these joints are incongruent. Between these articulating surfaces is placed an articular disc to decrease the contact pressure by increasing the contact area. Disorders of TMJs are related to overload of the joint due to clenching or trauma. Loads in the TMJ are transferred between the articular surfaces by the TMJ disc. Functional overloading appears to be important in the cascade of events leading to disc displacement and joint destruction in the internal derangement or osteoarthritis (pathological situations). Parafunctions, such as bruxism and prolonged clenching, are ones of the main causes for these overloadings of TMJ.

Analysis of joint load distributions cannot be performed experimentally. Mathematical models of the human masticatory system (including TMJs, disc, muscles and fibroconnective components), have served to predict the loads acting on this human joint. The three-dimensional finite element model simulations of disc movements or TMJ kinetic during jaws opening for example, have been proven to be a suitable tool for approximating the distribution of loads in the structures of the TMJ. Since 1990, many three-dimensional FE models of TMJs, have been reported to probe the biomechanical status in the TMJ (Korioth, Romilly, & Hannam, 1992; Chen & Xu, 1994; Beek, Koolstra, van Ruijven, & van Eijden, 2000, 2001; Tanaka, Rodrigo, Tanaka, Kawaguchi, Shibazaki, & Tanne, 2001). In the early FEA, the material properties of the disc have been assumed to be linear elastic. The disc, however, generally exhibits viscoelastic and poroelastic properties (a rapid deformation upon load application followed by a time-dependent creep or stress-relaxation phase of increasing deformation or reducing stress). These improvements have been incorporated to actual FE models of TMJ (Hirose, Tanaka, Tanaka, Fujita, Kuroda, Yamano, van Eijden, & Tanne, 2006; Tanaka, & Koolstra, 2008). Because through its viscoelastic properties, the articular disc can function as a stress absorber and a stress distributor. Hereby, the disc contributes to prevent excessive stress concentrations in the cartilage and bone components of the joint and the FE models are more exact.

ETIOPATHOGENIC CONSIDERATIONS OF MANDIBLE FRACTURES / ANALYSIS OF MANDIBLE FRACTURES

Mandible fractures are one of the most common facial injuries and account for 23-93% of all facial fractures dependent on surgery. Patients frequently require hospitalization, surgical intervention and extended periods of convalescence. The etiology of mandibular fractures is very variable. There are commonly caused by many human activities: interpersonal violence, assaults, sports, falls, road traffic accidents, industrial accidents, warfare and other causes. The principal fracture areas are located in the condylar necks, the symphysis and the body or the angle of the mandible bone. Despite remarkable progress within the last decade, the treatment of mandibular fractures is still a highly discussed topic in oral and cranio-maxillofacial surgery. The treatment of mandible fractures has made significant advances due to improved understanding of biomechanical principles, progress in biomaterials and surgical techniques applied. The FEA has played an important role in this improvement to permit the analyzing of complex biomechanical behavior of the mandible in the living subjects under realistic clinical situations. Several authors (Korioth & Verselius, 1997; Voo, Kumaresan, Pintar, Yoganandan & Sances, 1996) have reported on the accuracy of FEA in describing biomechanical behavior of bony specimens.

Another application of the FEA is its use as prediction tools for human head injuries caused by falls or traumas. FEA could be useful to assess the possible mechanism for the origin of mandible injuries like this tool has been used for simulating human head injuries caused by car accidents (Raul, Baumgartner, Willinger & Ludes, 2006). Its use in legal medicine appears to be useful for comparing different injuries mechanics. In fact, FE models are considered to be the best and the most powerful tools to investigate the dynamic response of the human head under impact conditions (Raul, Deck, Willinger & Ludes, 2008). Nevertheless, no work has yet been published using FEA for the evaluation of human mandible fractures in forensic cases. Probably the possible traumatologic scenarios are characterized by high variability and complexity.

The principal factors involved in bone fractures are the amount and direction of load, and the biomechanical and anatomical properties of the bone. However, in order to understand the biomechanical behavior of mandible fractures some studies had been published in the dental scientific literature. In 2004, M. Gallas and J.R. Fernández, developed a three-dimensional finite element model of human mandible in order to simulate and analyze biomechanical behavior in two standard trauma situations: a blow in the symphysis region and another one to the body of the mandible. The results of their FEAs indicated that following a blow to the symphysis region,

Figure 3. Stress fields (von Mises norm) after simulated impact on mandibular symphysis

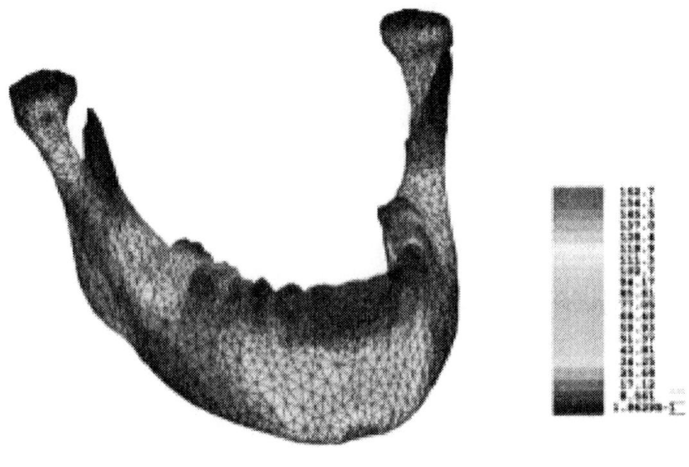

sagitally and perpendicular to the frontal plane with a magnitude of 10^7 N/m^2 lasting for 1s, maximum stress areas were located at the symphysis, (where the impact was produced) and both condylar neck regions and retromolar regions (Figure 3).

In the second case, a blow was simulated to the mandibular body from back to front, upward and perpendicular to transverse plane, the maximum stress areas were located at the ipsilateral body and the ipsilateral condylar neck regions where the impact was simulated and the retromolar region and condilar neck region of the contralateral side of the body of the mandible (Figure 4). This second situation is very common in assaults where the victim attempts to dodge a blow to the face by turning his head away. Subsequently, M. Gallas and J.R. Fernández (2004) described the complex stress distribution in the human mandible and outlined the existence of potentially weak areas in the mandibular geometry (condilar necks and mandibular angles).

The mandibular angle is one of the areas of the mandible that are prone to bone fractures, and in this area the presence of an impacted third molar has been found to be related with increased risk of angle fractures. In the study of H. Takada, S.

Figure 4. Stress fields (von Mises norm) after simulated impact on mandibular body

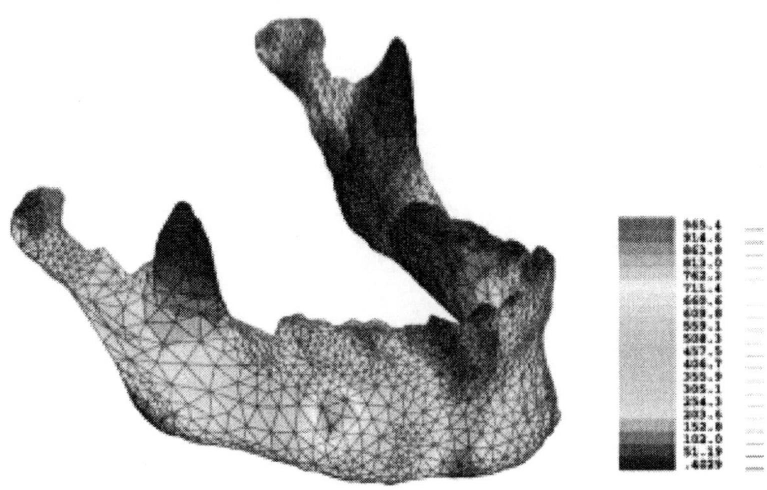

Abe, Y. Tamatsu, S. Mitarashi, H. Saka and Y. Ide (2006), a micro-focused X-ray computed tomography was performed to observe and analyze the three-dimensional bone microstructure of the mandibular angle and FEA was conducted to examine the relationship between angle fractures and the presence or absence of mandibular third molars. Finite element analysis showed that, in the mandible with a third molar, stress was concentrated around the root apex of the third molar, and was transmitted in a direction matching the clinical findings of angle fractures. The results obtained in this study suggest that the presence of an impacted third molar changes the concentration and transmission of stress in the mandible, thus increasing the risk of an angle fracture.

With the rapid advances in computer technology, more sophisticated finite-element models of mandible and simulations could be created (Kober, Stübinger, Hellmich, Sader & Zeilhofer, 2008). This current study is focused on "resimulation" of traumatologic cases given by clinical radiographs by means of finite element method. The mandible was modeled as inhomogeneous and anisotropic and the TMJs were realized as simplified joint capsules, wherein the mandibular condyles are freely mobile with certain limitations. The masticatoy system including the digastrics and the mylohyoid muscles could be activated. The user had the choice of 5 regions on the mandibular surface where the virtual injury can be inflicted. Power and direction of the impact force vector could be set at will. The trauma situations given by radiographs could be "reproduced" by a simulation scenario characterized by high compressive strain at the location of fractures. If masticatory muscles were activated and teeth clenched, the stress/strain profiles were qualitatively changed. The approach may be of benefit for forensic analysis, the model will contribute by elimination of scenarios not matching the given fracture locations. The immediate clinical application of this approach is a better understanding of the injured organ's conditions. It is important to know that fractures of bone as an adaptive biological tissue differ fundamentally from mechanical failure in engineering. Many of trauma simulations showed elevated stress/strain around the fracture, leading to the suggestion of weakened bone there (Kober, Stübinger, Hellmich, Sader & Zeilhofer, 2008).

ANALYSIS OF MANDIBLE FRACTURES TREATMENT

The treatment of fractures of the human mandible does not differ essentially from the treatment of fractures elsewhere in the body. The bone fragments are reduced into a proper position and then immobilized until bony union occurs. Traditionally the treatment of mandible fractures can be divided into open and close techniques. Closed treatment refers to external fixation devices and intermaxillary fixation (IMF). Nowadays open techniques are recognized as the criterion standard for the treatment of mandibular fractures and involve direct exposure of the fracture site and placement of internal fixation to prevent movement of the fracture site. Internal fixation requires the use of bone plates and screws of osteosynthesis to immobilize the mandibular halves relative to each other along the fracture line without need of IMF. There are few experimental studies simulating mandible fractures in a three-dimensional finite element analysis and testing the stability of different methods of osteosynthesis. The research on this subject is limited and these studies are realized in terms of load transfer and stress distribution analysis in the bone and osteosynthesis system and determination of static and fatigue limits for osteosynthesis devices.

FEA models of mandible have previously been developed to aid in the design of devices for treatment choices (Fernández, Gallas, Burguera, & Viaño, 2003). In this work, the mandible fracture was located in the symphsis region and one or two titanium miniplates fixed with monocortical screws were simulated in the complete clinical

Figure 5. 3D-FEM of mandible with miniplates of osteosynthesis

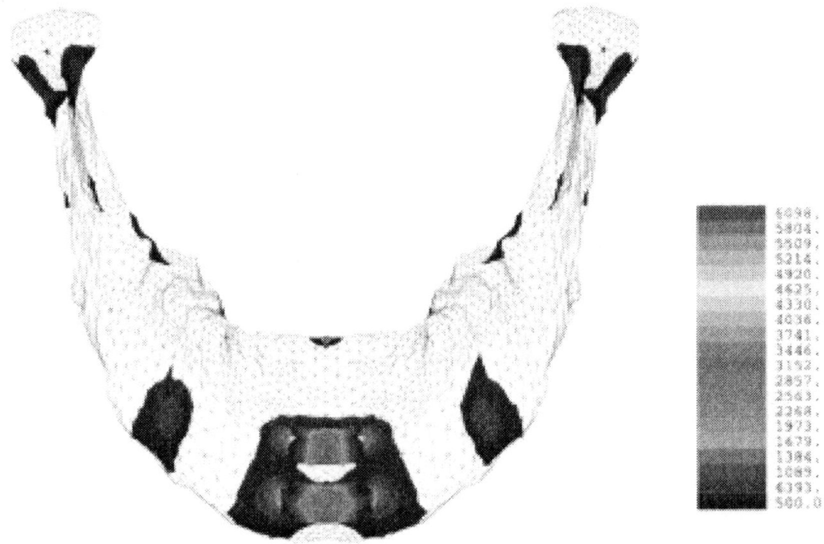

situations (after surgical reduction, post-operatory period and complete healing period). Their study aimed at predicting the stress distribution in the fractures mandible, mainly in the contact area of the miniplates with the cortical mandible bone and in the fractures area regardless of its limitations. Others researchers modeling in FEA a complete human mandible with the objective to compare different styles, shapes and localization of plates used in reduction of a fractured mandible (Lovald, Khraishi, Wagner, Baack, Kelly & Wood, 2006). Inclusive, a 3-D finite-element model was employed recently to formulate biomechanical justification of positioning of different plates to achieve stable fixation (Korkmaz, 2007; Arbag, Korkmaz, Ozturk, & Uyar, 2008). The researchers concluded to provide clinical considerations about miniplates location, orientation or type selection. For example, the miniplates must not be placed inferiorly alone and must be placed as high as possible. Therefore, FEA should permit us to suggest and evaluate new miniplate designs and enable considerable savings to be made in terms of time, material, and animal experiments in the future development of new osteosynthesis materials and surgical techniques (Figure 5).

In this sense, attempts have been made to investigate the biomechanical behavior of the condylar process in cases of mandible bone fractures at different sites (Wagner, Krach, Schicho, Urdt, Ploder & Ewers, 2002). In this case, individual human mandible geometry, the specific bone density distribution and the position and orientation of masticatory muscles were evaluated by performing computed tomography scans and sequential dissection of the cadaver mandible. Three basic loading conditions or bite forces and reaction forces applied to the muscles are simulated too. The authors after investigated the biomechanical properties of the mandible in detail explicitly described the stresses for different common situations proposed the geometrical optimization of titanium condylar process plates in order to achieve sufficient mechanical stiffness. Their results support the use of two plates for osteosynthesis of fractures of the condylar neck in combination with bicortically placed screws. Also the authors pointed out the importance of occlusal protection in particular for patients without full dentition and with an inadequate occlusal relationship in the post-operatory period (Wagner, Krach, Schicho, Urdt, Ploder& Ewers, 2002). Later, in another study have been verified the mechanical stability of a novel condylar process plated designed for the treatment of condylar process fractures instead of the use of two miniplates protocol more expensive and with longer operation times. The researchers conclude that a novel condylar process plates shows results comparable to two miniplates. The postoperative complication rate could be reduced significantly (plates fractures, nerve injury). Their results revealed that the mechanical stability of the novel condylar process plate as expected in a finite element model corresponds well with the clinical outcomes because no fracture of the plates have occurred in retrospective clinical study realized (Seemann, Schicho, Reichwein, Eisenmenger, Ewers & Wagner, 2007).

CONCLUSION

Computer models like FEA are increasingly proving to be an alternative to complicated practically unfeasible or unethical experiments. It is important to know that in FEA, some assumptions considered greatly affect the predictive accuracy of the finite element model and should be taken into account in the evaluation of the results. Clinical extrapolations from mathematical models may not give absolute values but they can provide a detailed description of the distribution and relation of forces and stresses within natural variability.

REFERENCES

Arbag, H., Korkmaz, H. H., Ozturk, K., & Uyar, Y. (2008). Comparative evaluation of different miniplates for internal fixation of mandible fractures using finite element analysis. *Journal of Oral and Maxillofacial Surgery*, *66*(6), 1225–1232. doi:10.1016/j.joms.2005.11.092

Beek, M., Koolstra, J. H., van Ruijven, L. J., & van Eijden, T. M. (2000). Three-dimensional finite element analysis of the human temporomandibular joint disc. *Journal of Biomechanics*, *33*(3), 307–316. doi:10.1016/S0021-9290(99)00168-2

Beek, M., Koolstra, J. H., van Ruijven, L. J., & van Eijden, T. M. (2001). Three-dimensional finite element analysis of the cartilaginous structures in the human temporomandibular joint. *Journal of Dental Research*, *80*(10), 1913–1918. doi:10.1177/00220345010800101001

Chen, J., & Xu, L. (1994). A finite element analysis of the human temporomandibular joint. *Journal of Biomechanical Engineering*, *116*(4), 401–407. doi:10.1115/1.2895790

Farah, J. W., Craig, R. G., & Meroueh, K. A. (1988). Finite element analysis of a mandibular model. *Journal of Oral Rehabilitation*, *15*(6), 615–624. doi:10.1111/j.1365-2842.1988.tb00199.x

Fernández, J. R., Gallas, M., Burguera, M., & Viaño, J. M. (2003). A three-dimensional numerical simulation of mandible fracture reduction with screwed miniplates. *Journal of Biomechanics*, *36*(3), 329–337. doi:10.1016/S0021-9290(02)00416-5

Ferré, J. C., Legoux, R., Helary, J. L., Albugues, F., Le Floc'h, C., & Bouteyre, J. (1985). Study of the deformations of the isolated mandible under static constraints by simulations on physcomathematical model. *Anatomia Clinica*, *7*(3), 183–192. doi:10.1007/BF01654640

Gallas, M., & Fernández, J. R. (2004). A three-dimensional computer model of the human mandible in two simulated standard trauma situations. *Journal of Cranio-Maxillo-Facial Surgery*, *32*(5), 303–307. doi:10.1016/j.jcms.2004.04.008

Geng, J.-P., Tan, K. B. C., & Lui, G.-R. (2001). Application of finite element analysis in implant dentistry: a review of the literature. *The Journal of Prosthetic Dentistry*, *85*(6), 585–598. doi:10.1067/mpr.2001.115251

Hirose, M., Tanaka, E., Tanaka, M., Fujita, R., Kuroda, Y., & Yamano, E. (2006). Three-dimensional finite-element model of the human temporomandibular joint disc during prolonged clenching. *European Journal of Oral Sciences*, *114*(5), 441–448. doi:10.1111/j.1600-0722.2006.00389.x

Huang, H. K., & Ledley, R. S. (1969). Numerical experiments with a linear force-displacements tooth model. *Journal of Dental Research*, *48*(1), 32–37.

Knoell, A. C. (1977). A mathematical model of an in vitro human mandible. *Journal of Biomechanics*, *10*(3), 159–166. doi:10.1016/0021-9290(77)90054-9

Kober, C., Stübinger, S., Hellmich, C., Sader, R., & Zeilhofer, H. F. (2008). Mandibular finite element simulation as a tool for trauma surgery. *International Journal of Computerized Dentistry*, *11*(3-4), 175–181.

Koolstra, J. H., van Eijden, T. M., Weijs, W. A., & Naeije, M. (1988). A three-dimensional mathematical model of the human masticatory system predicting maximum possible bite forces. *Journal of Biomechanics*, *21*(7), 563–576. doi:10.1016/0021-9290(88)90219-9

Korioth, T. W., Romilly, D. P., & Hannam, A. G. (1992). Three-dimensional finite element stress analysis of the dentate human mandible. *American Journal of Physical Anthropology*, *88*(1), 69–96. doi:10.1002/ajpa.1330880107

Korioth, T. W. P., & Versluis, A. (1997). Modeling the mechanical behavior of the jaws and their related structures by finite element (FE) analysis. *Critical Reviews in Oral Biology and Medicine*, *8*(1), 90–104. doi:10.1177/10454411970080010501

Korkmaz, H. H. (2007). Evaluation of different miniplates in fixation of fractured human mandible with the finite element method. *Oral Surgery, Oral Medicine, Oral Pathology, Oral Radiology, and Endodontics*, *103*(6), e1–e13. doi:10.1016/j.tripleo.2006.12.016

Ledley, R. S., & Huang, H. K. (1968). Linear model of tooth displacement by applied forces. *Journal of Dental Research*, *47*(3), 427–432.

Lovald, S. T., Khraishi, T., Wagner, J., Baack, B., Kelly, J., & Wood, J. (2006). Comparison of plate-screw systems used in mandibular fracture reduction: finite element analysis. *Journal of Biomechanical Engineering*, *128*(5), 654–662. doi:10.1115/1.2244575

Raul, J. S., Baumgartner, D., Willinger, R., & Ludes, B. (2006). Finite element modelling of human head injuries caused by a fall. *International Journal of Legal Medicine*, *120*(4), 212–218. doi:10.1007/s00414-005-0018-1

Raul, J. S., Deck, C., Willinger, R., & Ludes, B. (2008). Finite-element models of the human head and their applications in forensic practice. *International Journal of Legal Medicine*, *122*(5), 359–366. doi:10.1007/s00414-008-0248-0

Sakr, K., Farag, I. A., & Zeitonum, I. M. (2006). Review of 509 mandibular fractures treated at the University Hospital, Alexandria, Egypt. *The British Journal of Oral & Maxillofacial Surgery*, *44*(2), 107–111. doi:10.1016/j.bjoms.2005.03.014

Seemann, R., Schicho, K., Reichwein, A., Eisenmenger, G., Ewers, R., & Wagner, A. (2007). Clinical evaluation of mechanically optimized plates for the treatment of condylar process-Fractures. *Oral Surgery, Oral Medicine, Oral Pathology, Oral Radiology, and Endodontics*, *104*(6), e1–e4. doi:10.1016/j.tripleo.2007.07.010

Takada, H., Abe, S., Tamatsu, Y., Mitarashi, S., Saka, H., & Ide, Y. (2006). Three-dimensional bone microstructures of the mandibular angle using micro-CT and finite element analysis: relationship between partially impacted mandibular third molars and angle fractures. *Dental Traumatology*, *22*(1), 18–24. doi:10.1111/j.1600-9657.2006.00368.x

Tanaka, E., & Koolstra, J. H. (2008). Biomechanics of the temporomandibular joint. *Journal of Dental Research*, *87*(11), 989–991. doi:10.1177/154405910808701101

Tanaka, E., Rodrigo, D. P., Tanaka, M., Kawaguchi, A., Shibazaki, T., & Tanne, K. (2001). Stress analysis in the TMJ during jaw opening by use of a three-dimensional finite element model based on magnetic resonance images. *International Journal of Oral and Maxillofacial Surgery*, *30*(5), 421–430. doi:10.1054/ijom.2001.0132

Thresher, R. W., & Saito, G. E. (1973). The stress analysis of human teeth. *Journal of Biomechanics*, *6*(5), 443–449. doi:10.1016/0021-9290(73)90003-1

Voo, L., Kumaresan, S., Pintar, F. A., Yoganandan, N., & Sances, A. (1996). Finite-element models of the human head. *Medical & Biological Engineering & Computing*, *34*(5), 375–381. doi:10.1007/BF02520009

Wagner, A., Krach, W., Schicho, K., Urdt, S., Ploder, O., & Ewers, R. (2002). A 3-dimensional finite-element analysis investigating the biomechanical behavior of the mandible and plate osteosynthesis in cases of fractures of the condylar process. *Oral Surgery, Oral Medicine, Oral Pathology, Oral Radiology, and Endodontics*, *94*(6), 678–686. doi:10.1067/moe.2002.126451

Yettram, A. L., Wright, K. W., & Pickard, H. M. (1976). Finite Element Stress Analysis of the crowns of normal and restored teeth. *Journal of Dental Research*, *55*(6), 1004–1011.

Zhou, X., Zhao, Z., Zhao, M., & Fan, Y. (1999). The boundary design of mandibular model by means of the three-dimensional finite element method. *West China J Stomatol*, *17*(4), 1–16.

KEY TERMS AND DEFINITIONS

Biomechanics: Research field involved in the structural and mechanical behavior of biological systems.

Finite Element Analysis: Mathematical method for solving engineering problems.

Miniplates: A device inserted in the human body to reduce and treat bone fracture.

Poisson's Ratio: A measure of transverse strain against axial strain when uniaxial stress is applied.

Young's Modulus: A measure of the stiffness of an isotropic elastic material. It is also known as the modulus of elasticity, elastic modulus or tensile modulus.

Chapter 11
The Use of Three-Dimensional Reconstructions in the Diagnosis of Impacted Teeth

M. M. Bornstein
University of Bern, Switzerland

P. Pazera
University of Bern, Switzerland

C. Katsaros
University of Bern, Switzerland

ABSTRACT

Numerous efforts have been made towards three-dimensional (3D) radiographic imaging in all fields of dentistry, ranging from oral surgery to orthodontics. Although computerized tomography (CT) has been available for quite some time now, its use in dentistry has always been limited because of cost, access, and dose considerations. In orthodontics, diagnosis and treatment planning has been based traditionally on 2D imaging, mainly cephalometric and panoramic radiographs. The introduction of cone-beam computed tomography (CBCT) represented a true revolution in dento-maxillofacial radiology, and a shift from 2D to 3D data acquisition, image reconstruction, and visualization. Therefore, CBCT has now been introduced in different areas of orthodontic diagnostic procedures and treatment planning: Evaluation of cleft palate patients, airway and soft tissue analysis, temporomandibular joint morphology assessment, diagnosis of bony asymmetry, localization of impacted teeth and detection of resorption of adjacent teeth. This book chapter gives an overview of the current literature regarding the present use of CBCT in the localization of impacted teeth for orthodontic purposes. The potential, advantages and disadvantages in the diagnosis of impacted teeth will be discussed, also using case examples from the clinical practice.

DOI: 10.4018/978-1-60566-733-1.ch011

INTRODUCTION

The incidence of fully impacted teeth is reported to vary between 5-20% in the general population (Grover & Lorton L, 1985, Frank, 2000). The overwhelming majority of impacted teeth involve third molars, followed by maxillary canines and mandibular second premolars. While most of the other teeth in the upper and lower jaws can also be affected, the incisors and first molars in the mandible are very rarely impacted (Grover & Lorton L, 1985, Dachi & Howell 1961).

A special category of impacted teeth are supernumerary teeth that can be present in various forms and in any region of the mandible or maxilla, but have a predisposition for the anterior maxilla (Scheiner & Sampson, 1997). The prevalence of supernumerary teeth in the permanent dentition has been reported to be between 0.1% and 3.8% (Rajab & Hamdan, 2002, Schulz et al., 2009). The most widely accepted pathogenetic theory is that the tooth bud splits into two (dichotomy) equal or different-sized parts, developing into two teeth of normal size, or one normal and one dysmorphic type, as a result of local, independent, conditioned hyperactivity of the dental lamina (Taylor, 1972). Supernumerary teeth can occur as single, multiple, unilateral or bilateral entities in one or both jaws and are classified according to location-related, size-related or shape-related characteristics (Ooshima et al., 1996).

Principally, the treatment of impacted teeth is based on four concepts: observation, intervention, relocation or extraction (Frank, 2000, Kokich & Mathews, 1993). Observation implies no treatment for a specific period of time. This time period can be further subdivided in a preimpaction and postimpaction phase. Trained dentist are therefore able to either predict tooth impaction (during the preimpaction observation period) or anticipate pathological sequelae associated with impacted teeth (in the postimpaction observation period). Intervention involves orthodontic procedures to establish adequate space in the dental arch that enables eruption. Theses procedures are often performed in combination with removal of hard- and soft-tissue obstructions form the eruption path of the impacted teeth (Ohman & Ohman, 1980, Shapira et al. 1996). Relocation implies active orthodontic movement of the impacted teeth or even surgical reposition (autotransplantation; Schatz & Joho, 1994). Finally, if impacted teeth cannot be repositioned in the alveolar process using treatment strategies mentioned above, their removal might be indicated.

In orthodontics, three-dimensional (3D) structures have been routinely analyzed using on two-dimensional (2D) imaging. Besides conventional intraoral radiographs, cephalometric imaging and panoramic views were applied on a routine basis for diagnostic and treatment planning purposes (Hechler, 2008). To diagnose and to locate impacted teeth accurately, periapical and occlusal radiographs were the radiographic methods of choice for decades. Orthodontists have used the tube shift technique to compare two periapical radiographs taken at different beam angles to determine the facial/oral position of impacted teeth, and also to base surgical and/or orthodontic treatment planning upon. Although the „same lingual, opposite buccal“ rule is helpful in determining whether the impacted tooth is positioned buccal or oral to the roots of the neighbouring teeth, it has clear limitations when assessing the exact angulation of the impacted tooth and possible crown/root proximities with or without resulting root resorptions. (Jacobs, 1999).

Although computerized tomography (CT) has been available for quite some time, its use in dentistry has always been limited because of cost, access, and exposure to radiation (White & Pharoah, 2008). The introduction of cone-beam computed tomography (CBCT) represented an important new development in dento-maxillofacial radiology, and precipitated a shift from two- to three-dimensional data acquisition, image reconstruction, and visualization. In contrast to conventional CT scanning, CBCT imaging captures the object to be evaluated as the radiation source falls onto a two-dimensional detector. This difference allows a single rotation of the radiation source to capture an entire region of interest. For cone-beam imaging, multiple basis projections form the projection data from which orthogonal planar images are secondarily reconstructed (Scarfe & Farman, 2008). For conventional CT, multiple slices (an therefore rotations round the scanned object) are stacked to obtain a complete image (Scarfe & Farman, 2008, Kau et al., 2005).

In comparison to computed tomography (CT), CBCT has several advantages, the most important being less radiation administered to the patient. Imaging with the NewTom QR-DVT 9000 resulted in an effective absorbed dose ranging from 19.9–77.9 μSv (Ludlow et al., 2003), compared to a range of 6.2-22 μSv for panoramic views, and 314 μSv for conventional CT scans. In a recent study evaluating the effective dose for the CBCT device used in the present study (Hirsch et al., 2008), 20.02 μSv were measured for a limited field of view (FOV) of 4x4 cm, whereas 43.27 μSv were detected for a larger FOV (6x6 cm). Therefore, a smaller FOV should always be used when possible, thus adhering to the ALARA (as low as reasonably achievable) principle (McCollough et al., 2009).

In dentistry, CBCT has been used for diagnosis and treatment planning in implant dentistry (Spector, 2008), caries diagnosis, for the detection and characterization of bony aspects of periodontal disease (Tyndall & Rathore, 2008) as well as in endodontics. Especially for the diagnosis of endodontic pathology, CBCT has demonstrated important advantages over conventional intraoral radiographs. Lofthag-Hansen et al. (2007) compared PA radiographs and limited CBCT for detection of apical pathology in maxillary molars and premolars and in mandibular molars. The study demonstrated that 38% of the lesions were undetected by PA radiography, despite the fact that an additional PA radiograph was taken from a different angle. These findings were confirmed in a recent study by Low et al. (Low et al., 2008), in which 34% of roots with periapical lesions were only detected on CBCT images.

In orthodontics, CBCT has been introduced in different areas: Evaluation of cleft palate patients, airway and soft tissue analysis, temporomandibular joint morphology assessment, diagnosis of bony asymmetry, localization of impacted teeth – mostly canines (Hechler, 2008) and root resorption of adjacent teeth. The present book chapter gives an overview of the current literature regarding the present use of CBCT in the localization of impacted teeth for othodontic purposes. Potential, advantages and disadvantages in the diagnosis of impacted teeth will be discussed using case examples from the clinical practice.

IMPACTED CANINES

The incidence of impacted upper permanent canines within the general population is approximately 1.5 – 2% (Thilander & Jakobsson, 1968), with up to 85% of these being palatal impactions (Ericson & Kurol, 1987). Management of this condition is possible using several approaches. Initially, a comprehensive evaluation must be done to assess whether space is available in the arch or can be made available for alignment of the impacted canine. Other important factors to address before a treatment strategy can be chosen, are patient age, degree of oral hygiene, suitability of the first premolar to replace a permanent canine, length of orthodontic treatment and costs of the planned therapy. Treatment options for patients with a permanent canine impacted in the hard palate comprise: (Grover & Lorton, 1985) interceptive removal of the deciduous canine; (Frank, 2000) no treatment, but with periodic evaluation for pathologic changes; (Dachi & Howell, 1961) surgical removal of the impacted canine and prosthetic replacement; or (Scheiner & Sampson, 1997) surgical exposure of the canine and orthodontic alignment (Ericson & Kurol 1988, Bishara, 1992, Motamedi et al., 2009).

The treatment planning with and without three dimensional imaging was investigated recently in a study using computerized tomography (CT) (Bjerklin & Ericson, 2006). The treatment plans of 43.7% of the treated children were modified when 3D data became available to the orthodontists. Of the patients with root resorptions on the incisors adjacent to retained canines, more than half (53.8%) of the treatment plans had to be altered. These results can be extrapolated to CBCT, but with the big advantage of lower radiation exposure.

To illustrate the diagnostic advantages of CBCT two cases with impacted canines and a similar indication are presented:

Figure 1 show the detail of two panoramic radiographs of patients with one (a) and with two (b) not erupted maxillary canines. Both radiographs show root proximity and an unclear root resorption status of adjacent teeth (image a: upper left lateral incisor, image b: both upper central incisors). For this reason CBCTs (Accuitomo®, images c-j; field of view / FOV both 6x6 cm) were performed. In case 1 a massive apical resorption of the upper left lateral incisors was present (images c,e,g,i). In case 2 no tooth resorption of the upper incisors by the two impacted canines could be detected (images d,f,h,j).

Figure 1. Suspicion of root resorption of incisors by impacted canines

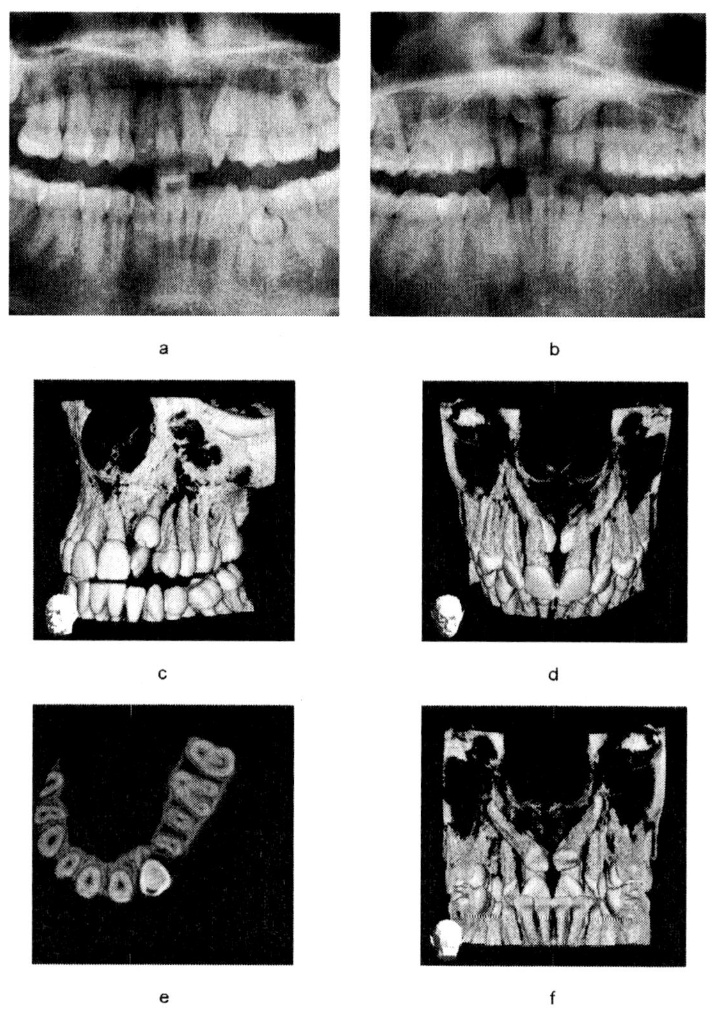

Figure 2. Impaction of two incisors due to a supernumerary tooth

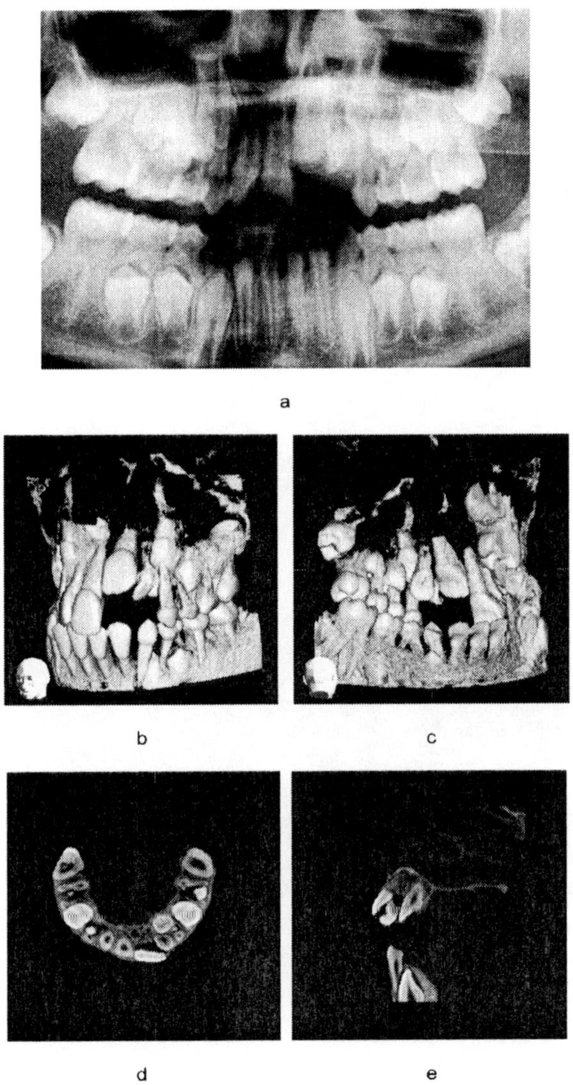

MAXILLARY CENTRAL INCISORS

There are several etiologic factors associated with the impaction of a maxillary incisor, which may be grouped into two categories. The presence of an odontoma or midline supernumerary tooth (mesiodens), which are most commonly found in the premaxillary area, provide a physical obstruction, hence, resulting in a disturbed tooth eruption. The second cause relates to previous trauma to the deciduous teeth, often in the very young child, which may result in dilaceration of the permanent successor and, with it, impaction (Chaushu et al., 2009). Resolution of the problem requires a combination of surgical exposure and orthodontic traction, both of which may cause incidental damage to the affected teeth and to the supporting structures. The different methods of exposure have been shown to affect the quality of the periodontal and esthetic outcome of the treated case to a greater or lesser extent, and the manner in which the exposure is executed may also have an influence (Chaushu et al., 2002). In this respect, the exact 3D mapping of the region is very important.

Figure 2 (a) shows an OPT of a 9-year-old girl with two not erupted upper central incisors. Although the OPT shows a supernumerary tooth its spatial position is not clearly defined on this traditional 2D x-ray. After performing a CBCT (Accuitomo®; FOV 6x6 cm, images b-e), the 3D image and the individual slices showed a clear picture of the position of the teeth: the supernumerary teeth upper left lateral incisor is located in the middle of the alveolar process between the upper left central incisor and the deciduous upper left canine, buccally of the upper left lateral incisor. The root formation of the supernumerary tooth is not complete.

Figure 3 (a) shows an OPT of an 8-year-old boy with a not erupted upper left central incisor. After a trauma in the early childhood the upper left central incisor never erupted. Because the OPT neither clearly showed the 3D position of the tooth nor showed the root shape and formation status, a CBCT (Accuitomo®; FOV 6x6 cm, images b-f) was performed. The 3D image and the individual slices showed the exact position of the upper left central incisor together with its crown-root angulation and root development status. They also show the degree of displacement of the missing incisor.

Figure 3. Impaction after a trauma in the early childhood

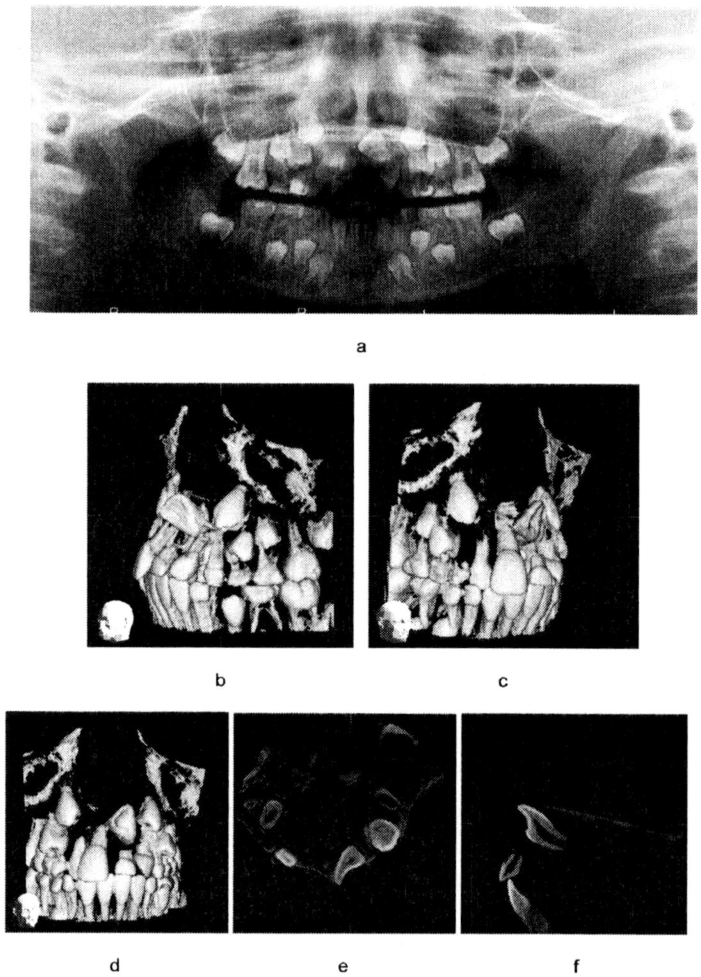

MANDIBULAR AND MAXILLARY SECOND PREMOLARS

Lower second premolars account for approximately one fourth of all impactions, excluding the third molars, with the overall frequency for lower premolar impactions being 0.2-0.3% (Colett, 2000). Aetiological factors for premolar impaction appear to include arch length deficiency, ectopic position of the tooth germ, obstacles to eruption such as an ankylosed primary molars, the presence of supernumerary teeth or odontomas, and genetic factors. Conservative management with exposure of the crown has been advocated (Ohman & Ohman, 1980, Jacobs, 1987). In some cases, orthodontic traction and repositioning may be indicated.

Figure 4 (a) shows an OPT of a 13-year-old boy with two impacted supernumerary maxillary premolars. Resorption signs of the adjacent could be excluded. A CBCT (Accuitomo®; FOV 6x6 cm, images b-f) allowed us to examine the position of the supernumerary premolars and the integrity of roots of the adjacent teeth: on the right side the supernumerary premolar was located between the roots of the two other premolars, in the middle of the alveolar process, on the left side it was buccally ectopic. There were no signs of root resorption on any of the adjacent premolars.

Figure 4. Impaction of supernumerary maxillary premolars

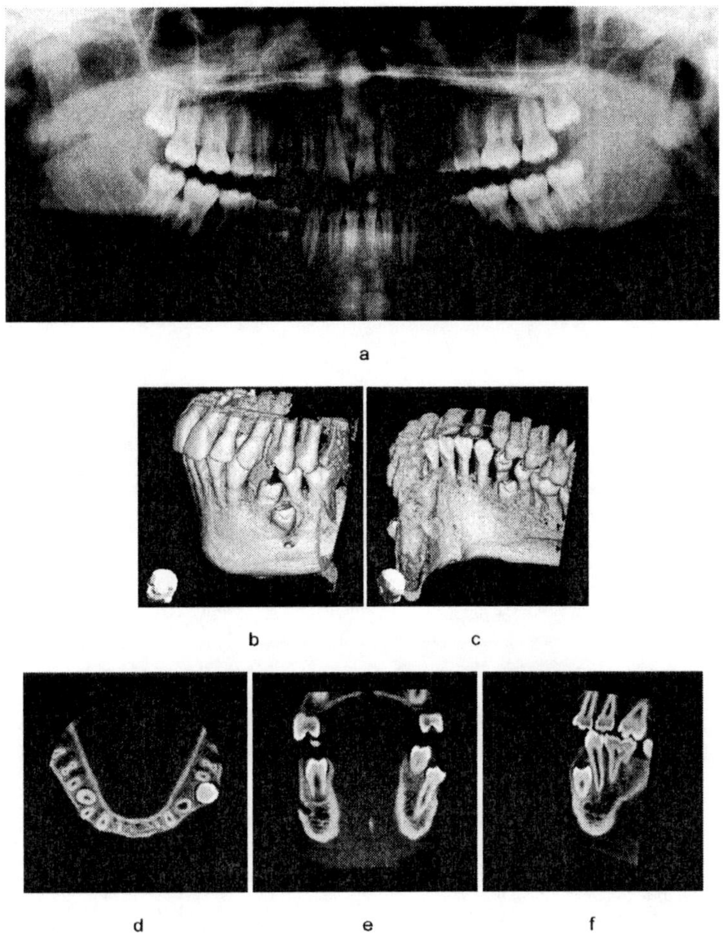

As with mandibular premolars, the most common reason that maxillary second premolars become impacted is due to loss of space in the dental arch following early extraction of deciduous second molars and the subsequent drifting of the adjacent teeth (Becker, 2007). Often, the crown of the premolar is deflected palatally, and palpable on the palatal side of the alveolar process.

Figure 5 (a) shows an OPT of a 11-year-old girl with multiple agenesis of teeth together with two not erupted upper left premolars. The 2D image shows the impaction but does gives no information about the exact 3D position of the two left upper premolars. The CBCT (Accuitomo®; FOV 4x4 cm, images b-e) allowed us to examine the exact 3D configuration of teeth: both teeth are distally angulated, the most anterior premolar is located on the buccal aspect of the maxilla, the more distal premolar on the palatal aspect. Root formation is not competed and there are no signs of root resorptions on any of the involved teeth.

MANDIBULAR AND MAXILLARY SECOND MOLARS

Molars can also become impacted and malpositioned. In the case of second molars, possible causes often lie in an ectopically positioned adjacent third molar, or second molar follicles that are inexplicably tipped in an oblique or horzontal orientation Other proposed causes of second-

Figure 5. Impaction of two maxillary premolars

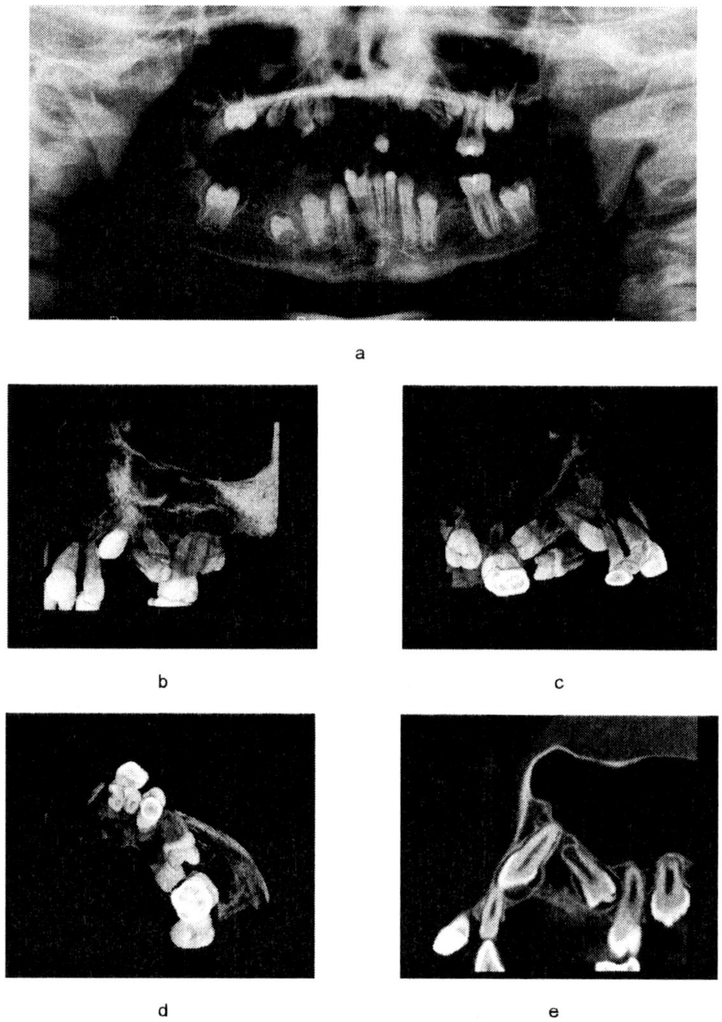

molar impaction include delayed emergence of the second premolars, premature primary molar extraction, ankylosed primary molars, dentigerous cysts, and competition for space by the third molar and odontomas (McAboy et al., 2003). Treatment options for impacted second molars include surgical extraction, surgical uncovering with orthodontic-assisted eruption and surgical uprighting (Frank, 2000).

Figure 6 (a) shows an OPT of a 13-year-old girl with two not erupted upper right molars. Again, this 2D view does not allow us to determine neither the cause of retention nor the exact 3D position of both teeth, nor any possible root resorption. It just shows the displaced first upper right molar and an impacted upper right second molar. An CBCT (Accuitomo®; FOV 6x6 cm, images b-e) was performed. The 3D reconstruction and the individual slices show the buccal root displacement and the mesial inclination of the impacted upper right first molar together with a root proximity between the roots of both molars. No root resorption can be observed on any of the involved teeth (acknowledgement Dr. S. Wahlen, Münsingen).

Figure 6. Impaction of two maxillary molars

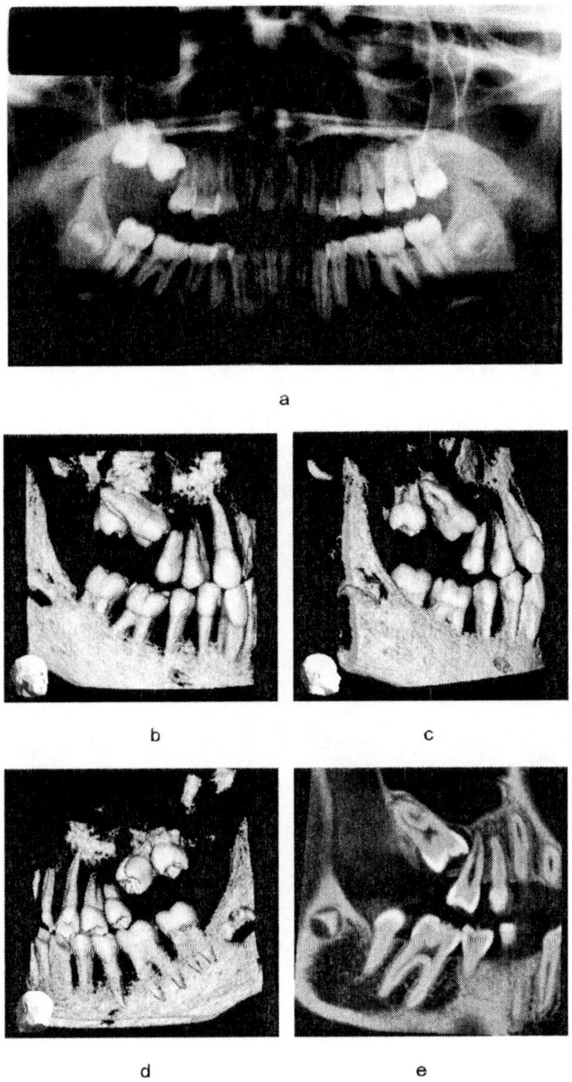

CONCLUSION

The introduction of cone-beam computed tomography represents an important step forward in dento-maxillofacial radiology. Especially for the exact localization of impacted teeth and the subsequent treatment planning, 3D images broaden our diagnostic horizon by providing a clear picture of the clinical situation that is not achievable by traditional x-ray techniques. Nevertheless, because of its higher radiation exposure, CBCTs should be only used in selected cases with a clear indication when other, lower dose images do not provide the decisive information that might improve a treatment plan. If, in the future, the radiation dose can be reduced to a level that is comparable to that of a set of traditional x-rays used in orthodontic planning, CBCT devices have the potential to become the only x-ray data acquisition machines in an orthodontic office.

REFERENCES

Becker, A. (2007). *The orthodontic treatment of impacted teeth,* (2nd Ed.). Hampshire, UK: Thompson Publishing Services.

Bishara, S. E. (1992). Impacted maxillary canines: a review. *American Journal of Orthodontics and Dentofacial Orthopedics, 101,* 159–171. doi:10.1016/0889-5406(92)70008-X

Bjerklin, K., & Ericson, S. (2006). How a computerized tomography examination changed the treatment plans of 80 children with retained and ectopically positioned maxillary canines. *The Angle Orthodontist, 76*(1), 43–51.

Chaushu, S., Brin, I., Ben-Bassat, Y., Zilberman, Y., & Becker, A. (2002). Periodontal status following surgical-orthodontic alignment of impacted central incisors with an open-eruption technique. *American Journal of Orthodontics and Dentofacial Orthopedics, 122,* 9–14.

Chaushu, S., Dykstein, N., Ben-Bassat, Y., & Becker, A. (2009). Periodontal status of impacted maxillary incisors uncovered by 2 different surgical techniques. *Journal of Oral and Maxillofacial Surgery, 67,* 120–124. doi:10.1016/j.joms.2008.08.012

Colett, A. R. (2000). Conservative management of lower second premolar impaction. *Australian Dental Journal, 45,* 279–281. doi:10.1111/j.1834-7819.2000.tb00264.x

Dachi, S. F., & Howell, F. V. (1961). A survey of 3, 874 routine full-month radiographs. II. A study of impacted teeth. *Oral Surgery, Oral Medicine, and Oral Pathology*, *14*, 1165–1169. doi:10.1016/0030-4220(61)90204-3

Ericson, S., & Kurol, J. (1987). Radiographic examination of ectopically erupting maxillary canines. *American Journal of Orthodontics*, *91*, 483–492.

Ericson, S., & Kurol, J. (1988). Early treatment of palatally erupting maxillary canines by extraction of primary canines. *European Journal of Orthodontics*, *10*, 283–295.

Frank, C. A. (2000). Treatment options for impacted teeth. *The Journal of the American Dental Association*, *131*, 623–632.

Grover, P. S., & Lorton, L. (1985). The incidence of unerupted permanent teeth and related clinical cases. *Oral Surg Oral Med Oral Pathol, 59*, 420-425. Hechler, S.L. (2008). Cone-beam CT: Applications in orthodontics. *Dental Clinics of North America*, *52*, 809–823.

Hirsch, E., Wolf, U., Heinicke, F., & Silva, M. A. (2008). Dosimetry of the cone beam computed tomography Veraviewepocs 3D compared with the 3D Accuitomo in different fields of view. *Dento Maxillo Facial Radiology*, *37*, 268–273. doi:10.1259/dmfr/23424132

Jacobs, S. G. (1987). The surgical exposure of teeth – simplest, safest and best? *Australian Orthodontic Journal*, *10*, 5–11.

Jacobs, S. G. (1999). Radiographic localization of unerupted maxillary anterior teeth using the vertical tube shift technique: the history and application of the method with some case reports. *American Journal of Orthodontics and Dentofacial Orthopedics*, *116*, 415–423. doi:10.1016/S0889-5406(99)70226-X

Kau, C. H., Richmond, S., Palomo, J. M., & Hans, M. G. (2005). Three-dimensional cone beam computerized tomography in orthodontics. *Journal of Orthodontics*, *32*, 282–293. doi:10.1179/146531205225021285

Kokich, V. G., & Mathews, D. P. (1993). Surgical and orthodontic management of impacted teeth. *Dental Clinics of North America*, *37*, 181–204.

Lofthag-Hansen, S., Huumonen, S., Gröndahl, K., & Gröndahl, H. G. (2007). Limited cone-beam CT and intraoral radiography for the diagnosis of periapical pathology. *Oral Surgery, Oral Medicine, Oral Pathology, Oral Radiology, and Endodontics*, *103*, 114–119. doi:10.1016/j.tripleo.2006.01.001

Low, K., Dula, K., Bürgin, W., & von Arx, T. (2008). Comparison of periapical radiography and limited cone-beam tomography in posterior maxillary teeth referred for apical surgery. *Journal of Endodontics*, *34*, 557–562. doi:10.1016/j.joen.2008.02.022

Ludlow, J. B., Davies-Ludlow, L. E., & Brooks, S. L. (2003). Dosimetry of two extraoral direct digital imaging devices: NewTom cone beam CT and Orthophos Plus DS panoramic unit. *Dento Maxillo Facial Radiology*, *32*, 229–234. doi:10.1259/dmfr/26310390

McAboy, C. P., Grumet, J. T., Siegel, E. B., & Iacopino, A. M. (2003). Surgical uprighting and repositioning of severely impacted mandibular second molars. *The Journal of the American Dental Association*, *134*, 1459–1462.

McCollough, C. H., Primak, A. N., Braun, N., Kofler, J., Yu, L., & Christner, J. (2009). Strategies for reducing radiation dose in CT. *Radiologic Clinics of North America*, *47*, 27–40. doi:10.1016/j.rcl.2008.10.006

Motamedi, M. H., Tabatabaie, F. A., Navi, F., Shafeie, H. A., Fard, B. K., & Hayati, Z. (2009). Assessment of radiographic factors affecting surgical exposure and orthodontic alignment of impacted canines of the palate: A 15-year retrospective study. *Oral Surgery, Oral Medicine, Oral Pathology, Oral Radiology, and Endodontics*, *107*, 772–775. doi:10.1016/j.tripleo.2008.12.022

Ohman, I., & Ohman, A. (1980). The eruption tendency and changes of direction of impacted teeth following surgical exposure. *Oral Surgery, Oral Medicine, and Oral Pathology*, *49*, 383–389. doi:10.1016/0030-4220(80)90279-0

Ooshima, T., Ishida, R., Mishima, K., & Sobue, S. (1996). The prevalence of developmental anomalies of teeth and their association with tooth size in the primary and permanent dentitions of 1650 Japanese children. *International Journal of Paediatric Dentistry*, *6*, 87–94.

Rajab, L. D., & Hamdan, M. A. (2002). Supernumerary teeth: review of the literature and a survey of 152 cases. *International Journal of Paediatric Dentistry*, *12*, 244–254. doi:10.1046/j.1365-263X.2002.00366.x

Scarfe, W. C., & Farman, A. G. (2008). What is cone-beam CT and how does it work? *Dental Clinics of North America*, *52*, 707–730. doi:10.1016/j.cden.2008.05.005

Schatz, J. P., & Joho, J. P. (1994). Indications of autotransplantation of teeth in orthodontic problem cases. *American Journal of Orthodontics and Dentofacial Orthopedics*, *106*, 351–357. doi:10.1016/S0889-5406(94)70055-9

Scheiner, M. A., & Sampson, W. J. (1997). Supernumerary teeth: a review of the literature and four case reports. *Australian Dental Journal*, *42*, 160–165. doi:10.1111/j.1834-7819.1997.tb00114.x

Schulz, M., Reichart, P. A., Stich, H., Lussi, A., & Bornstein, M. M. (2009). Bilateral malformation of maxillary third molars. *Oral Surgery, Oral Medicine, Oral Pathology, Oral Radiology, and Endodontics*, *108*, e25–e31. doi:10.1016/j.tripleo.2009.04.017

Shapira, Y., Borell, G., Kuftinec, M. M., Stom, D., & Nahlieli, O. (1996)... *The Journal of the American Dental Association*, *127*, 1075–1078.

Spector, L. (2008). Computer-aided dental implant planning. *Dental Clinics of North America*, *52*, 761–775. doi:10.1016/j.cden.2008.05.004

Taylor, G. S. (1972). Characteristics of supernumerary teeth in the primary and permanent dentition. *Dental Practitioner and Dental Record*, *22*, 203–208.

Thilander, B., & Jakobsson, S. O. (1968). Local factors in impaction of maxillary canines. *Acta Odontologica Scandinavica*, *26*, 145–168. doi:10.3109/00016356809004587

Tyndall, D. A., & Rathore, S. (2008). Cone-beam CT diagnoistic applications: caries, periodontal bone assessment, and endodontic applications. *Dental Clinics of North America*, *52*, 825–841. doi:10.1016/j.cden.2008.05.002

White, S. C., & Pharoah, M. J. (2008). The evolution and application of dental maxillofacial imaging modalities. *Dental Clinics of North America*, *52*, 689–705. doi:10.1016/j.cden.2008.05.006

KEY TERMS AND DEFINITIONS

Cephalometric Radiograph: A cephalometric radiograph is a 2D lateral x-ray of the head used in orthodontics and maxillofacial surgery for examining and quantifying the relationship between anatomical structures. The relationship between radiograph source, subject, and film are standardised.

Cleft Lip and Palate: Cleft lip and/or cleft palate are variations of a congenital deformity caused by abnormal facial development during pregnancy. Cleft lip or palate occurs in one of 600-700 births and is treated by a specialized team consisted of many medical disciplines (surgeons, ENT doctors, orthodontists, speech pathologists, dentists etc.). Depending on the severity, patients with a cleft lip and palate remain in treatment from birth till the end of growth at an age of about 20 years.

Computerized Tomography (CT): Computerized tomography is an imaging technique often used in medicine employing imaging by sections (tomography) created by computer that can generate a volumetric (3D) representation of structures of the inside of an patient from a big number of two-dimensional x-ray images taken around a single axis of rotation. The volume data can also be reformatted in different planes. In traditional CT scanners just one slice at a time was acquired by an one dimensional array of detectors exposed by a rotating x-ray source while the patient remained static. In modern multislice CTs (MSCTs) up to 64 arrays of dedectors are used mounted on a rotating gantry while the patient is moved axially at a uniform rate. This helical scan method reduces the x-ray dose to the patient required for a given resolution while scanning more quickly. Modern machines can produce an image of an organ less than a second.

Cone-Beam Computed Tomography (CBCT): Cone-beam computed tomography is an imaging technique often used in dentistry, where the x-ray source produces a cone-shaped x-ray beam. Its difference to MSCT is that it captures the whole image in one sweep, instead of capturing every individual slice separately. One of the major advantages of CBCT in dentistry is the reduced radiation when compared with MSCT scans.

Field of View: The Field Of View (FOV) is the size of an area being imaged. This expression is often used in association with CT or CBCT.

Impacted Tooth: When a tooth fails to emerge, or emerges only partially, at the moment it physiologically should, it is considered to be impacted. The most common impacted teeth are the wisdom teeth (third molars).

Panoramic Radiograph (OPT): A panoramic radiograph or orthopantomogram (OPT) is a x-ray of the upper and lower jaw that shows a two-dimensional view of a half-circle from ear to ear. The panoramic image has important distortions because the vertical and the horizontal magnification vary differently along the image.

Radiation Dose: Radiation dose can be measured in different units, but the amount of damage to living tissue by ionizing radiation is related to the amount of energy deposited. This is called the absorbed dose. A usual unit of absorbed dose is the gray [1 Gy = 1 J/kg], which represents the amount of radiation required to deposit 1 joule of energy in 1 kilogram of matter. Equal doses of different types or energies of radiation cause different amounts of damage to living tissue. For example, 1 Gy of alpha radiation causes about 20 times as much damage as 1 Gy of x-ray radiation. Therefore an equivalent dose was defined to give an approximate measure of the biological effect of radiation. It is calculated by multiplying the absorbed dose by a weighting factor that is different for each type of radiation. The Sievert (Sv) is the unit of equivalent dose. Although it has the same units as the Gray [J/kg], it measures the dose of a given type of radiation in Gy that has the same biological effect on a human as 1 Gy of x-rays radiation. The 'background' dose of natural radiation in Switzerland is about 1.6 mSv per year. A dental low-dose CBCT delivers a dose to a patient of 20-60 μSv per scan.

Root Resorption: Root resorption is the breakdown or destruction of a root or parts of a root of a tooth. It can vary in severity from microscopic evidence of pits in the root surface to a complete resorption of a root. Deciduous root resorption is a natural process which allows exfoliation of the primary teeth to make way for the secondary teeth. Root resorptions of secondary teeth might be a consequence of trauma, teeth erupting in the path of the root or orthodontic treatment among others.

Supernumerary Tooth: A normal human permanent dentition has 32 teeth including 4 third molars (= wisdom teeth). Sometimes extra teeth are present and called supernumerary teeth. Dental X-rays are often used to diagnose supernumerary teeth. The most frequent supernumerary teeth include mesiodens, which is a mal-formed tooth that is located between the maxillary central incisors. Supernumerary teeth are more common in the permanent dentition.

Chapter 12
Accuracy of the First Integrated Cone-Beam System for Computer Aided Implantology

Timo Dreiseidler
University of Cologne, Germany

Jörg Neugebauer
University of Cologne, Germany

Lutz Ritter
University of Cologne, Germany

Daniel Rothamel
University of Cologne, Germany

Robert A. Mischkowski
University of Cologne, Germany

Jochim E. Zöller
University of Cologne, Germany

ABSTRACT

The aim of the chapter is to give a complete survey of Computer Aided Surgery (CAS) systems in dental implantology from the different 3D visualization technologies to the different available approaches for implant planning data transfer to the corresponding anatomical patient's sites. Focus will be on the illumination of advantages and disadvantages for the different systems components. Further on, the diagnostic value, radiation dosages to the patient, availability and costs as well as the transfer accuracy results for the investigated system will be discussed.

DOI: 10.4018/978-1-60566-733-1.ch012

ACCURACY OF THE FIRST INTEGRATED CONE-BEAM SYSTEM FOR COMPUTER AIDED IMPLANTOLOGY

Since 1997 different approaches for computer-assisted surgery (CAS) and computer aided dental implantology (CAI) are available. These systems comprise different technologies for three-dimensional (3D) visualization of the patient´s anatomy and visualization software capable of virtual dental implant position planning. The artifice of registration is the key for transferring the virtually planned implant positions to the corresponding patient´s anatomical sites on basis of different navigation technology approaches.

Visualization

Since the introduction of the cone-beam (CBCT) technology (Mozzo, Procacci, Tacconi, Martini, & Andreis, 1998), 3D visualization in dental medicine mainly was available by computer-tomography (medical CT) and magnetic resonance imaging (MRI). Nowadays, mainly 3D CBCT and medical CT data sets are utilized for visualization of the patient´s anatomy, making diagnosis and virtual dental implant position planning. Both image modalities have their distinct advantages and disadvantages. Beside the operational availability and the device costs, the main impact for evaluating these technologies in terms of dental implant planning are diagnostic value of the achieved data sets, as well as the radiation dosages to the patient.

High diagnostic values of the achieved data sets result from highly accurate visualization of all important anatomical structures of the facial skull. Concerning the geometric accuracy of 3D medical CT and CBCT data sets our investigations proved highly effective linear and volumetric measurement opportunities (Mischkowski, Pulsfort et al., 2007). For comparison purposes linear and volumetric phantoms as well as dried human skulls equipped with gutta-percha-points in prefabricated drill holes were exactly measured and scanned with a CBCT scanner (GALILEOS, Sirona Dental Systems, Bensheim, Germany) as well as a 6-detector row medical CT scanner (SOMATOM Sensation 6, Siemens Medical Solutions, Erlangen, Germany). On basis of 100 linear as well as 25 volumetric measurements the accuracy for both investigated technology in contrast to the real distances and volume could be described. We could prove that there was no significant difference in the measurement accuracy between the two investigated visualization technologies. The investigated linear deviations ranged in the area of 1%, the volumetric deviations turned out to range around 5% from the real values. Similar errors also were reported for different CBCT systems by other investigators.

Besides the geometric accuracy also the visualization quality for the important anatomical structures in pre-surgical dental implant planning play an extremely important role. To establish a basis for weighing the potential diagnostic and therapeutic benefits of 3D CBCT data sets in contrast to digital orthopantomography (PT) and medical CT, we performed an investigation comparing the visualization quality of different anatomical structures important for pre-surgical dental implant planning (Dreiseidler, Mischkowski, Neugebauer, Ritter, & Zöller, 2009). This study compared the visualization properties of the general image quality, the mandibular canal, incisive foramen, mental foramen, temporo-mandibular joint (TMJ), the bony nasal floor, maxillary sinus floor, the implant region its bone borders and adjacent teeth. Analysis was performed on an implant group and a control group. The implant group consisted of twenty-seven patients receiving a single pre-implantologic CBCT scan as well as a post-OP follow-up digital PT. In the control group 29 patients received both medical CT and CBCT diagnosis. Significant superior imaging quality in contrast to PT imaging could be approved for

CBCT imaging in the implant group. In contrast to this, no significant difference could be assessed between CBCT and medical CT visualization quality for the investigated anatomical structures in the control group.

Finally, the radiation dosages from the above mentioned 3D imaging devices have to be considered critically. Concerning the effective dosages a pretty rough estimation is that CBCT investigations have five-time higher radiation dosages than PT investigations and that medical CT investigations also have five-time higher radiation dosages than CBCT investigations. However, this statement has to be further critically analysed.

Ludlow and Ivanovic 2008 (Ludlow & Ivanovic, 2008) found a huge broadband of effective radiation dosages emitted to the patient in dependence to the applied CBCT device ranging from 68 μSv up to 1073 μSv for a single CBCT scan. In contrast to this digital PT imaging ranges in the area of 25 μSv and medical CT visualization of the facial skull emits 860 μSv to the patient.

The main reasons for the strongly varying radiation dosages from the different CBCT devices are the CBCT scan volume sizes, also referred to as field of view (FOV) and resolution. Further the applied CBCT detector technology and the settings for tube voltage and x-ray current intensity can strongly influence the radiation dosages of a CBCT scan.

FOV sizes from different CBCT devices can cover small regions hardly covering the molar region of a jaw quadrant to FOV sizes covering the complete skull including facial skull and neurocranium. Generally there is a progressive correlation between volume size and radiation dosage emitted to the patient.

The CBCT volume resolution is an important influence factor on the diagnostic value of the visualization also contributing to the image quality of the reconstructed visualization planes. Higher volume resolutions contribute to higher information degrees necessitating higher or denser amounts of radiation penetrating through the FOV.

For the applied technologies in CBCT imaging we mainly have to differentiate flat panel detectors from image intensifiers. Flat panel detectors more and more are replacing the image intensifiers due to their physically flatness and advantageous attributes of reducing veiling glare and pincushion or s-shaped distortions. On the other hand image quality from flat panel detectors can suffer from excessive lag and ghosting, decalibration and defaulting pixels. The so called detective quantum efficiency (DQE) of a detector is an objective measure of how the available signal-to-noise ratio is degraded by the imaging system with respect to the spatial frequency of the input signal. Since the spatial frequency of the x-rays is a manner of their energy the DQE also describes the ability of a system to transfer x-ray signals into exploitable visualization information.

The DQE can become calculated with respect to the visualization systems (u) modulation transfer function (MTF) and the noise power spectra of the input X-radiation (W_{in}) and of the linearised detector output signal (W_{out}) by following equation:

$$\text{DQE}\ (u) = \text{MTF}^2(u) \cdot \frac{W_{in}(u)}{W_{out}(u)}$$

The MTF (Figure 1) is a quantitative measure for the image quality of a visualization system stating its ability to transfer contrast from the specimen to the intermediate image plane at a specific resolution. The MTF is also defined as ability of a visualization system to display contrast in dependence to the spatial frequency.

Comparing DQE from image intensifiers and flat panel detectors state higher DQE levels for low x-ray dosages to image intensifiers (Koch et al., 2001). This means that image intensifiers reach their most favorable signal-to-noise ratio with lower radiation dose than flat panel detectors. This physical attribute refers to a higher effectiveness for the visualization of lower energy x-rays and therefore contribute to potential lower radiation dosages for image intensifier based CBCT sys-

Figure 1. Illustration of the modulation transfer function (MTF). In the left picture area the transfer from a certain object (line pattern) to a corresponding picture by an imaging system is visualized. In contrast to the object, the resulting pictures shows blurring at the changes from black to white. The middle area of the illustration shows the mathematical modulation of the original object and the picture. Optimally for any imaging system would be a 100% contrast maintenance from the object to the corresponding picture. In reality the contrast fades from clear black/white boarders to a constant grey shade (zero contrast) in dependence with spatial frequency (line pairs per mm) of the object. This phenomenon is depicted in the right part of this illustration as the modulation transfer of line pattern. Adapted from Wikipedia source.

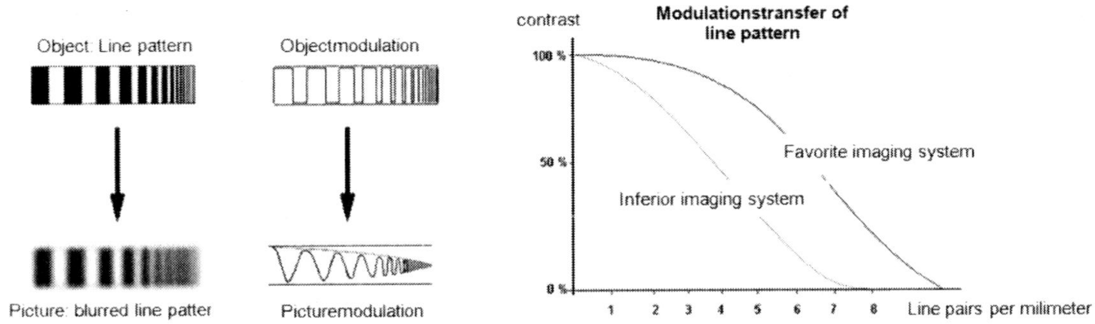

tems. Image intensifiers and flat panel detectors both have limited resolution capabilities of ~3 line pairs / mm. Since both technologies right now have their advantages and disadvantages none can be considered thoroughly advantageous over the other. However, especially flat panel detectors constantly become evolved for optimization of DQE and other attributes (Kuhls-Gilcrist et al., 2008) so that in future they might be considered generally advantageous over image intensifier systems.

The technical settings for image taking like tube voltage and x-ray current intensity also have a major impact on the image quality on the one side and also hardly affecting the effective radiation dosages of a scan on the other side. So generally, settings have to be chosen wisely to show a sufficient net benefit between radiation dosage and image quality.

Not only CBCT radiation dosages can vary significantly. Also for medical CT investigations a huge broadband of different radiation dosages can be found. Special low-dose protocols in dental medicine have been established and investigated to reduce radiation dosages to the patient (Harris et al., 2002; Rustemeyer, Streubuhr, & Suttmoeller, 2004). These protocols mainly contribute to the technical image taking settings for tube voltage and x-ray current intensity, scan time reduction, medical CT slice thickness and optimisation of the FOV size, also referred to as collimation. These low-dose protocols can lead to decreased image quality and diagnostic value of the medical CT investigation.

The correct choice of the 3D imaging device for CAS in dental implantology has to respect two major and some minor important aspects. The major important aspects are radiation dosage and the achieved image quality and diagnostic value from each investigation. Of minor importance are reflections about imaging device costs and operational availability.

From ancient x-ray times there is the basic demand that the radiation exposure should always obey the ALARA principle (as low as reasonable achievable) and therefore should show a sufficient net benefit, weighing the total potential diagnostic or therapeutic benefits it produces (Harris et al., 2002). From the investigations of Ludlow and Ivanovic (Ludlow & Ivanovic, 2008) we know that that generally we can prefer some of the investigated CBCT devices over medical CT investigations in terms of the radiation dosages. From our investigations we can state that the image quality and diagnostic value for high contrast structures of CBCT data sets are comparable with medical CT data sets.

CBCT devices in contrast to medical CT devices can be operated by dentists in their own practice and their device costs contribute to a rough tenth compared to medical CT devices.

Summarizing the above mentioned information prefers well-reflected 3D CBCT over medical CT imaging for computer aided implantology (CAI). However, not all of the available CAI systems on the marked right now are similarly good compatible with CBCT and medical CT data sets, which has to be discussed later.

Visualization Software

The visualization software of CAI systems should be intuitive, well-arranged and capable of virtual implant placement within in patient´s data sets. Dental implant position planning optimally can become adapted to the anatomical situation of the patient for maximal surgical safety and implant positioning improvement, as well as achievement of optimal aesthetical and long-time results in implant dentistry. Following the approach of back-ward planning also enables to align the virtual dental implant positioning with a prosthetic proposal to be visualized in the 3D examinations.

To visualize a prosthetic proposal patients have to wear radio-opaque scan-stents during the scanning procedure. These scan-stents ideally represent the prosthetic wax-up transferred to the scan-stent via vacuform-procedure with barium-sulphate acrylic resin in the prosthetic dental crown positions. Most commonly, software-solutions are independent to any kind of visualization technology necessitating the user to deal with the im- and export of medical data sets, most often formatted as DICOM (Digital Imaging and Communications in Medicine) data sets.

Registration and Navigation Technologies

For conversion of the virtual dental implant position planning certain navigation technology has to be utilized. The suggested solutions mainly comprise real-time tracking systems sumable as dynamic or active systems, as well as static surgical drill templates also referred to as passive systems.

Dynamic/Active Systems

The dynamic or active systems work on basis of a direct match from the real patient position in the operation room (OR) to his own 3D radiological data set. Besides magnetic approaches these dynamic systems most commonly utilize optical infra-red cameras for fiducial-based registration. This approach requires the patient to wear fiducial makers in the exact same position during the 3D scan as well as during the surgical procedure in the OR. The infrared camera directly can capture the fiducial-marker positions on the patient within in OR and set them in context to their position in the corresponding data set. Also surgical instruments are equipped with those fiducial markers and therefore can become real-time tracked in the OR and translated into virtual surgical instruments within the patient´s 3D data set. The fiducial-based marker registration therefore enables to lead the real surgical instruments to the patient´s anatomical sites and simultaneously indicating their exact positions as virtual analogues within the 3D data set on a computer screen.

One of the first dynamic systems for dental implant placement is the robodent system. During the implant insertion procedure the surgeon has to align the real burr position with the virtually planned implant axes. A visualized guiding system helps to optimally adapt the angulations of the surgical drill. As disadvantages of these systems a high technical effort in combination with high expenses can be mentioned. Additionally the

Figure 2. This alignment illustrates the conversion of virtual dental implant positioning within a CBCT data set (left) into the corresponding surgical templates achieved by the modulation of the original scan-stent the patient wore during the CBCT investigation (right). (© 2009, SICAT Company. Used with permission.)

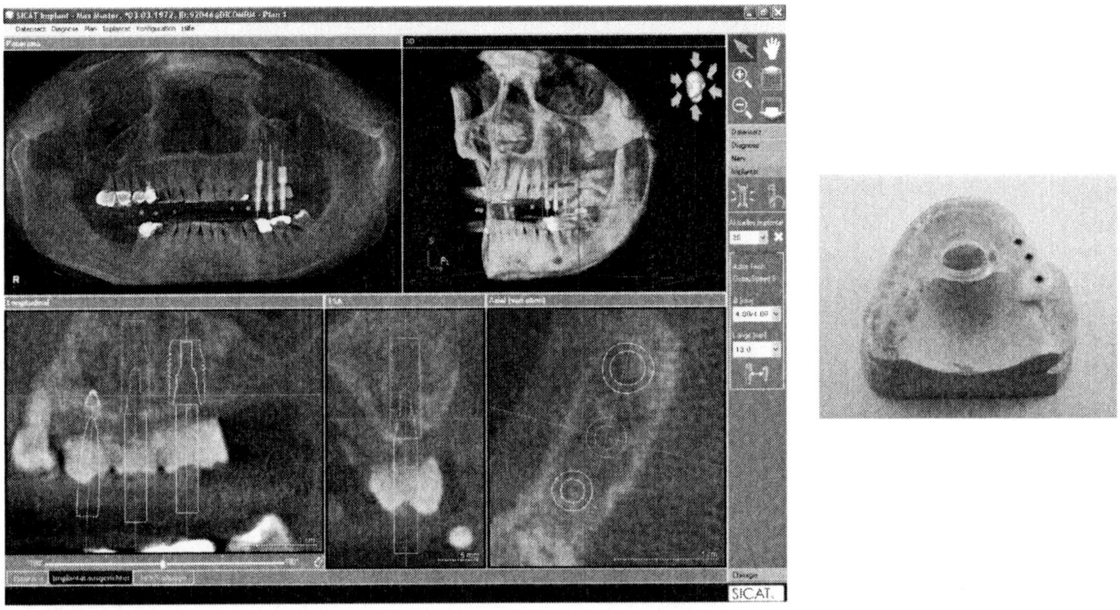

achieved accuracy for implant placements highly depends on the user's experience but can achieve the same accuracy levels than those described for static systems (Widmann & Bale, 2006), a topic that will be closer looked at in later sections of this chapter.

Since there is no real guidance, random influence factors like trembling of the surgeons hand cannot substantially become eliminated. On the other hand, due to the missing guidance, individual adaption to patient specific restrictions like small stoma is easier to cope with than for static systems. Further on, the dynamic systems are more appropriate for situations were template-mounting is imprecise or not achievable without further ado, for instance in edentulous patient´s.

The achieved ground precision from these systems is often described in terms of the so called as target detection error (TDE). The TDE can be described as linear deviation in x-, y- and z- direction between a virtual position and the corresponding anatomical position. For instance, if the surgeon sets a probe tip on a cuspid tip, also the virtual probe tip should correlate with the exact position within the 3D data set. Deviations are described as TDE´s. Our investigations could describe similar TDE´s for the active systems no matter which 3D visualization from medical CT, CBCT and MRI was applied (Mischkowski, Zinser et al., 2007). So basically the active systems for CAI are flexible to the applied 3D visualization technology.

Static/Passive Systems

The static or passive systems comprise different surgical template groups. Generally these templates result from the virtual dental position planning data and either become centrally manufactured by stereolithographic rapid-prototyping (RP) procedures (i.e. SurgiGuide, NobelGuide) or on basis of modulation of fiducial-marker equipped scan-stents, patients wore during the 3D radiological diagnosis (see also figure 2).

Figure 3. From left to right, computer-numerically-controlled (CNC) milling machine in full view, middle) Close-up of a scan-stent affixed in CNC milling machine, right) close-up of the transfer process of the virtual dental position planning data to the corresponding scan-stent sites. (© 2009, SICAT Company. Used with permission.)

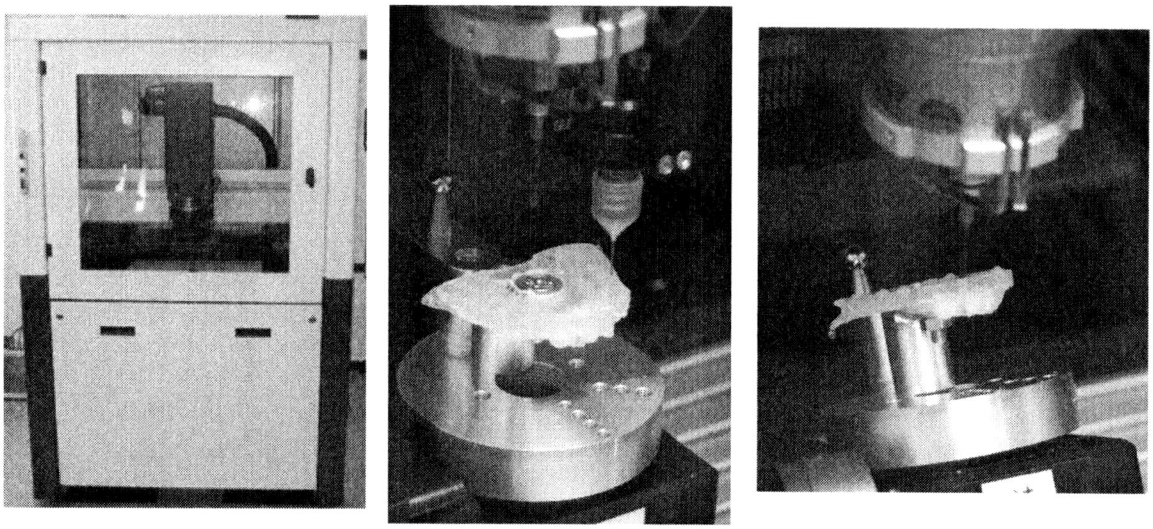

The group of templates based on modulated scan-stents further can become sub-divided. So, modulation either can take place manually by dental technicians utilizing certain coordinate transfer tables for conversion of the virtual planning (Bredent, Med3D, IVS solutions), or alternatively by the aid of computer-numerically-controlled (CNC) milling machines (Figure 3) after computerized registration (Galileos Sytem/Sicat).

The SurgiGuide System (Materialise, Leuven, Belgien) was the first commercially available rapid-prototyping CAI system on the market. For the stereo-lithographic procedure surface data of bone and teeth have to be calculated on basis of the different grey values within the 3D data sets. This procedure is called segmentation and a necessary precondition for the RP-based surgical template production. For a proper separation of soft and hard tissues for segmentation, the distribution of grey values should show a clear threshold within the 3D data sets, which is almost only true for medical CT and more restricted for CBCT data sets. Since the proper differentiation of grey values between soft and hard tissues for segmentation often is difficult in CBCT data sets these RP-based CAI systems are rather optimized for medical CT visualization.

For the non-rapid-prototyping templates vectors will be calculated on basis of the virtual implant positioning and the positions of the fiducial-markers. After registration of the scan-stents in terms of the exact fiducial marker positions these vector data serve for conversion of the planning data to corresponding drill-hole positions within the later surgical guide originating from the scan-stent. Either the dental technician with the aid of one of the above mentioned coordinate transfer tables or CNC milling machines directly after detection of the fiducial marker positions then will bore vector correlates into the scan-stents. After insertion of titanium sleeves for safe burr guidance into these bore holes, the original scan-stent becomes the final surgical template. Since there is no 3D data segmentation necessary for these non-RP templates, medical CT and CBCT datasets similarly good can become utilized.

Advantageous for the static / passive systems are lower initial expenses and easier handling in contrast to the active systems. Especially if the surgeon used to work with conventional dental-technicians drill-templates before, the established work-flow for implant insertion can become completely maintained. Disadvantageous for the static systems often can be the restricted space in the posterior molar regions leading to insertion problems of the surgical drill into the leading titanium sleeve. For edentulous situations surgeons have to deal with inaccurate placements on the soft-tissue or otherwise have to deal with bone-mounted stereolithographic templates or temporary implant insertion for secure mounting of the scan-stents during the radiological examination as well as the surgical procedure.

However, the most important attribute of the CAI systems is the accuracy level from virtual dental implant planning to their conversion. While some authors suggest higher accuracy levels for the static template systems other claim for similar application accuracies between static and dynamic systems. In this context especially the vast variety of study designs, measurement strategies and different vendors' soft- and hardware solutions hamper objective comparison opportunities. Generally the stated mean accuracy deviation level for the different systems mainly varies between 0.2 and 3 mm (Widmann & Bale, 2006). Especially for non-experienced users deviations are higher and within the millimetre range for dynamic systems (Birkfellner et al., 2001), whereas these discrepancies are lower and in the sub-millimetre range for static templates or for experienced users of dynamic systems (Fortin, Champleboux, Bianchi, Buatois, & Coudert, 2002).

In the following section of this chapter we focus on our actual investigations on the accuracy level for the transfer of virtually planned implant positions to their conversion. For this investigation the Galieos-System (Sirona, Bensheim, Germay) was utilized. This system is the first integrated system for CAI treatment offering the complete work-flow from CBCT data acquisition, virtual dental implant position planning to the corresponding surgical template conversion. So, virtual dental implant planning directly can be performed with the device accompanying visualization software and without the drawback of time-consuming DICOM data ex- or import. Since surgical template production is based on a non-RP CNC milling procedure, no data segmentation is necessary.

Presented data are already published (Dreiseidler et al., 2009).

The study was carried out to detect the accuracy for the above mentioned CAI-System. The study consists of two major parts:

a) The system inherent accuracy was investigated utilizing the vendors surgical guides in addition with the vendors titanium sleeves for pilot drilling.
b) To investigate the accuracy for fully guided implant insertions, vendors' surgical guides were combined with the Nobel Guide RP sleeves and the corresponding NobelGuide surgical kit. So, an demand the vendor inserted the Nobel Guide RP sleeves into the surgical guides in correspondence to the virtual implant positioning planning data. Accuracy was investigated in terms of the measurement for different linear and angle deviations between virtually planned and the resulting burr-hole and dental implant positions.

MATERIALS AND METHODS

For the accuracy evalutation of the Galileos-System, the vendor work-flow protocol meticulously was followed (Figure 4).

In the first step after the clinical diagnosis, a plaster cast for each treatet jaw will be manufactured due on an alginate impression taking. On basis of the plaster cast the dental technician can manufacture scan-stent adapted to the patient´s anatomical situation. To achieve an optimal

Figure 4. Illustration of the work-flow for the investigated CAI system involving the interaction of the patient, the surgeon, the dental technician and the manufacturer. While the clinical and radiological examination of the patient as well as the surgical procedure belongs to the surgeon the dental technicians responsibility belongs to a proper scan-stent production. The conversion of the planning data to the scan-stent is within the duty of the systems vendor. (© 2009, SICAT Company. Used with permission.)

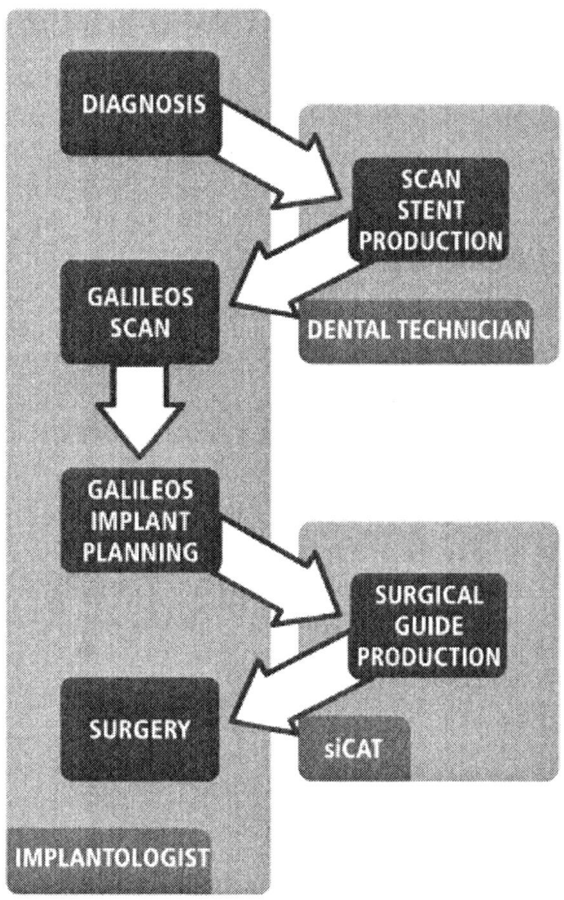

scan-stent, the dental technician has to generate a prosthetic wax-up on the patients plaster cast. A vacuforming procedure has to be carried out to create a denture mounted stent. Prosthetic teeth have to be eliminated and substituted with barium-sulphate containing methacrylic material. For registration purposes, the vendor of the system distributes acrylic registration plates each including 6 glass-ball markers of 3 mm in diameter. With glue-fixed connection of one of these registration plates to the occlusional plane, the stent becomes the scan-stent which the patient necessitates to wear during the CBCT scan with the Galileos CBCT device. In beforehand, a perfect fit to the patients anatomy can clinically estimated by placing the scan-stent in the patient´s mouth. There must be no jiggling and a unique and reproducible fitting situation is a necessary precondition for the later achievement of highly accurate dental implant placements. With such a fitting scan-stent the CBCT investigation then can be executed. The corresponding 3D data set will be visualized by the CBCT device accompanying visualization software showing the patients anatomy and the scan-stent with the six fiducials and the radio-opaque prosthetic crown positions. Now, with respect to the backward planning concept, dental implant positions can become optimized to both, patient´s anatomy as well as the later prosthodontic solution. Since the applied technology is an open-source approach, surface data from different vendors implant products can be chosen from a data-bank and virtually placed with optimal adaption ability for implant length and diameter. After finishing the planning procedure, software will guide through a brief surgical template order menue in order to create a CD-Rom with the patient´s data set in addition with the implant position planning data and to print an oder form. CD-Rom, order form and the scan-stent than has to be send to the vendor. The implantologist in return will receive the ready surgical template after execution of the CNC-based milling procedure at the vendors site. On basis of this surgical template with titanium sleeves in the corresponding positions to the planned implant positions, the surgeon´s drills can become guidedly inserted into the patient´s anatomy. While choosing from different sleeve systems during the order process, surgeons can choose between mere pilot drill guidance or full guidance systems for implant insertion like the NobelGuide sleeves.

For the actual investigation, instead of real patients, patient equivalent partially edentulous anatomical models (Bredent, germany) were utilized. In order to be able comparing pre-surgical virtual planning data to the post-OP results, also these anatomical models were equipped with a total of six glass ball markers with 3 mm in diameter for later registration purposes. Apart from that the vendors protocol accurately was followed (Figure 5).

Plaster casts as well and a scan-stents for each anatomical model were manufactured due to the above mentioned describtion. These scan-stents firmly were adapted to the anatomical models after controlling that there was no jiggling and a definite and reproducible scan-sent fit. These arrangements were accurately placed and scanned with the GALILEOS CBCT Scanner. The utilised CBCT technique described elsewhere corresponds to the principle set-up (Mozzo, Procacci, Tacconi, Martini, & Andreis, 1998; Ziegler, Woertche, Brief, & Hassfeld, 2002) with the following specific developments: During a single scan of 14 seconds duration, the x-ray generator and a 2D detector in oppositional alignment rotate around the patient´s head. Scanning parameters constantly were 85 kV and 28 mAs. The reconstructed 3D volume had a size of 15 cm in all three dimensions. Visualizations were performed with 512^3 pixels and a volxel size of 300 x 300 x 300 µm.

Datasets of the scanned anatomical models in addition with the scan-stents were visualized utilizing the device accompanying visualization software (SICAT, Bonn, Germany). For assessment if the system inherent accuracy for guided pilot drills 30 pilot drill positions of 10 mm length and 2 mm in diameter were planned for 6 patient equivalent anatomical models respecting the emulated anatomical situation as well as the prosthetic proposal. Corresponding to the planning data, surgical templates were consecutively equipped with SICAT titanium sleeves with 5 mm in height and 2 mm internal diameter dedicated to guide the 2.0 mm pilot drill within the simulated surgical procedure and the anatomical models.

For the assessment of the completely guided surgical implant insertion a total of 24 implant positions were planned for Brånemark MKIII Groovy implant dummies (Nobel Biocare, Göteborg, Sweden) of 3.75 mm in diameter and 13 mm in length in 4 patient equivalent models. Corresponding to these planning data for fully guided implant insertion assessment, surgical templates later consecutively became equipped with Nobel Guide RP sleeves (Nobel Biocare, Göteborg, Sweden) with an internal diameter of 4.1 mm and 3.5 mm in length into the templates.

Due to the above mentioned work-flow, scan and planning data were stored on CD-Rom and in addition with the scan-stents and plaster models sent to the vendor (Sicat, Bonn, Germany). For template fabrication a computerized numerically controlled (CNC) milling machine was utilized. For a proper transfer of the generated implant planning data from the software to the corresponding positions within the scan-stent registration procedure was carried out on basis of the six fiducials within the registration plate of the scan-stent. For this registration exact locus detection within the data sets as well as hardware fiducial locus detection on basis of a high accuracy coordinate measuring device was carried out. In cognition of these data, a match of the virtual scan-stent position to its real position within the CNC milling machine became possible and the virtual vectors from the planning data were converted into mill hole positions within the scan-stent. The above mentioned titanium sleeves then became inserted in the exact position of the milled holes. Stents then were slightly modulated in terms of a reduction from unnecessary methacrylate. Now the scan-stents were completely converted into the surgical templates in concordance with our virtual planning data.

On basis of these templates the surgical procedure for the 30 pilot drill positions, as well as 24 fully guided dental implant insertions were car-

Figure 5. Depiction of the investigation workflow with patient equivalent anatomical models. a) plain patient's equivalent model, b) prosthetic wax-up on patient equivalent model, c) visualization and dental implant planning in the CBCT data set of an anatomical model with scan-stent in well-defined position, d) surgical template with NobelGuide sleeves inserted in correlation to the virtual dental implant position planning, e) conversion of the virtually planned dental implant positions in the patient equivalent model. (© 2009, University of cologne, Author.)

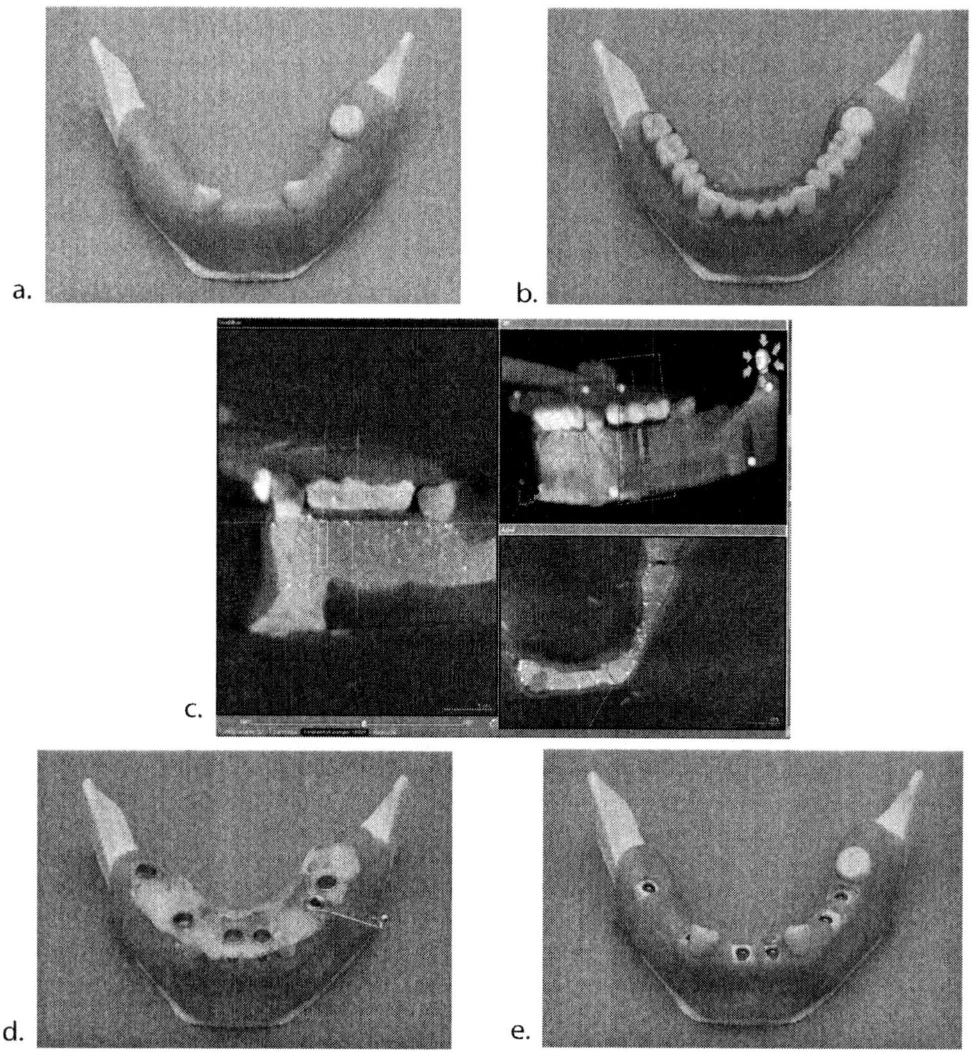

ried out. In this context, the gingival masks of the patient equivalent models were partially removed according to positions determined by the surgical template. The surgical procedure was performed on basis of a mobile surgical assembly (Fa. Sirona, Bensheim, Germany) consisting of an electronic system (SiroTorque L), an electric motor (EL 1) and a handpiece (Sirona Implant 20:1).

In concordance with the titanium sleeves and for the assessment of the system inherent accuracy a pilot drill (Friadent, Mannheim, Germany) of 2 mm in diameter and a work piece length of 18 mm was utilized for pilot drilling. In concordance with the marks on the pilot burs drill-hole depths of approximately 10 mm were achieved.

For the assessment of fully guided implant insertion, the corresponding NobelGuide surgical kit was utilized in accordance with the exact vendor´s protocol.

In this context the NobelGuide RP sleeves in the first step were utilized with a guided start drill of 2.0 mm in diameter and 10+ (7-18 mm) in length in addition with the so called guided drill guide. The latter mentioned guided drill guide basically is the necessary link between the inner diameter or the PP sleeves and the outer diameter auf the pilot drill. So the drill guide within the RP sleeves fill the empty space between sleeve and drill and exactly centres the pilot drill within the PR sleeve to aim in the correct vector due to the original planning data. In the same manner also the expansion drill holes were carried out with 2.8 mm and 3.4 mm diameter twist drills and the corresponding guided drill guides. In a last step before the actual implant body insertion a guided screw tap (Ø 3.75mm, 7-13 mm) again fully guided was utilized for tapping the achieved drill holes. All the above mentioned twist drills were utilized in combination with the corresponding drill stops affixed in the 13 mm position corresponding to the planned implant body length. Implant bodies were template-guided inserted through the RP sleeves on the systems corresponding implant mount with a ratchet.

After each drilling step, burr canals were cleansed from drill shavings and again scanned with the CBCT device, so that every single step from pilot drill over the expansion drills and the final implant positioning could become evaluated in the further investigation process.

For the actual accuracy evaluation again a registration procedure had to be performed but this time on basis of the fiducials which were attached to the patient equivalent anatomical models. Since these fiducials were in the exact same position during the time of virtual dental implant planning and after the surgical procedures, the virtual planning data could be transferred to the post-surgical CBCT scans. This registration and data transfer then enabled to compare the alignment of the planning data with the actual outcome situation.

Now, the horizontal, vertical and angle deviations for drill holes and implant positions in contrast to the virtually planned positions were could become assessed (Figure 6).

Horizontal deviations at the crestal and apical end, as well as angle deviations were measured for the SICAT sleeves pilot drill positions in terms of the ground accuracy evaluation of the system. Since no vertical stop control of the pilot drill was performed for this investigation branch, vertical deviations only were assessed for the Nobel Guide fully guided implant insertion.

In terms of the actual measurement-workflow in a first step, a second virtual implant cylinder was aligned with the post-surgical drill hole or implant body position. In Afterwards each single investigation position was selected and visualized in the implant aligned view enabling for virtual rotation around the central axis for the selected planned implant position. While rotating around the axes of the virtual planning data cylinder, the visualization plane showing the biggest deviation between planned and executed cylinder could be visualized. In this context, the above mentioned deviations could exactly be measured from the central axes of both, the virtual planning cylinder and the secondary placed outcome cylinder.

Statistical analysis of the extracted data were calculated by the two-sided independent T-Test between the pilot drill positions in the first branch of this study describing the systems ground accuracy. Further on, the one-way ANOVA for variance analysis between the groups form pilot drill over the expansions to the final implant body position within the second branch of the study for evaluation of the fully guided implant insertion was utilized. Finally, the two-sided paired T-Test analysis was carried out to calculate if there is a significant difference between the apical and crestal horizontal deviations.

Acquired data were saved and edited in Excel (Microsoft Corporation, Redmond, USA) and calculated with SPSS 13.0 (SPSS Inc, Chicago, USA).

RESULTS

First branch of this analysis for evaluation of the system inherent ground accuracy for pilot drilling with the SICAT sleeves (n = 30) showed mean horizontal deviations for the achieved 10 mm pilot drill holes of 150 ± 120 µm at the crestal and 400 ± 120 µm at the apical measurement position. The averaged deviation for the measured angles between planned and executed implant positions was 1.18 ± 0.55 degrees.

For the second branch of the study evaluating the fully guided implant insertion with the Nobel Guide sleeves (n = 24) for the achieved 13 mm pilot drill (Ø 2 mm) an averaged deviation of 205 ± 132 µm at the crestal and 438 ± 278 µm at the apical end in the horizontal plane could be detected. In the vertical plane these value was 204 ± 156 µm for the apical end. Averaged axes deviations of 1.04 ± 0.7 degrees could be detected.

For the Ø 2.8 mm guided twist drill within the branch of fully guided implant insertion evaluation averaged deviations corresponded to 238 ± 142 µm at the crestal and 441 ± 238 µm at the apical end in the horizontal plane, as well as 200 ± 111 µm at the apical end in the vertical plane. Axes deviations with an average of 0.89 ± 0.49 angle degrees could be detected.

Burr holes from the Ø 3.4 mm guided twist drill deviated 240 ± 124 µm at the crestal and 416 ± 165 µm at the apical end in the horizontal plane, as well as 225 ± 109 µm at the apical end in the vertical plane. Axes deviations between planned and executed position ranged around 0.81 ± 0.35 angle degrees.

Finally, deviations between the planned and executed implant position after fully surgical indirect guidance with the surgical templates were assessed. In this context the inserted implant body's (Brånemark MKIII Groovy, Ø 3.75 mm, 13 mm length) showed averaged linear deviations of 217 ± 99 µm at the crestal and 343 ± 146 µm at the apical end in the horizontal plane, as well as 254 ± 204 µm at the apical end in the vertical plane. The measured angle deviations ranged around 1.09 ± 0.51 degrees.

The highest investigated linear deviation here was 990 µm for the horizontal apical deviation of the pilot drill hole for the NobelGuide sleeve system.

For statistical comparison purposes the two-sided T-Test was performed to calculate significance level between the pilot drill position accuracy of the two branches. So, piloting burr holes was compared between the Sicat pilot drill sleeves and the NobelGuide sleeves showing no significant deviation differences in the horizontal plane at the crestal ($p = 0.1$) and apical ($p = 0.29$) measuring position, as well as for the angle deviations ($p = 0.39$). Summarizing this that the accuracy of conversion from virtual position planning to pilot burr hole position was similar for both investigated sleeve systems.

To compare the accuracy amongst the different diameter burr hole positions and final dental implant placements, the grouped ANOVA calculation was performed, showing no significant deviation differences in the horizontal plane at the crestal ($p = 0.72$) and apical ($p = 0.36$) measuring position, in the vertical position at the apical end ($p = 0.59$), as well as for the angle deviations ($p = 0.23$). As a result of that one can state, that the same accuracy level could be achieved for each of the single preparation steps from pilot drill to final implant insertion.

Finally another calculation was performed to figure out, weather generally the crestal linear deviations were higher than the apical linear deviations. In this context, the two-sided paired T-Test was carried out between the apical and crestal horizontal deviation for each all positions. Results confirmed crestal horizontal deviations to be highly significant ($p < 0.0001$) smaller than the apical horizontal deviations. A result that will further be discussed in the following.

DISCUSSION

Technical Discussion

Each investigation has its restrictions. Measurement results in this study are to some degree compromised by the technical limitations as well as the applied study model inherent limitations. These limitations to some degree hamper the validity of the absolute distance and angle values and have to be discussed here.

The most important thing is to look at the limitations of the measurement procedure. The validity for the measured distances and angles mainly can be compromised by the CBCT visualizations detail accuracy and software-inherent measuring accuracy and the potential error in fiducial marker registration.

Measurement Validity: CBCT Visualizations Detail Accuracy

The detail accuracy of the visualized CBCT data sets mainly is a product of three major important parameters: The modulation transfer function (MTF) and the volumes voxel size in addition to the tri-linear interpolation algorithm of grey values between the voxels. The meaning of the MTF in addition with the DQE already was explained within the introduction of this chapter.

A pretty rough landmark for visualization limitations is the resolution of the CBCT data sets. In this study, visualization was carried out on basis of a voxel size of 300 µm in each direction.

The tri-linear interpolation algorithm of grey values between the voxels enables to calculate grey values "between" the voxels, when the magnification of the visualization exceeds the data set resolution. Due to the 3D geometric alignment of the voxels the tri-linear interpolation of grey values enables to visualize details also in the dimension smaller than the resolution or voxel size respectively.

These circumstances reduce the detail accuracy for the here applied CBCT system to approximately 100-150 µm. This circumstance also can be supported by our clinical experience that also the periodontal ligament (PDL) is generally visible in real patient´s CBCT data performed with the Galileos CBCT device. PDL space is known to range between 100 -250 µm. For structures below this dimension of approximately 100-150 µm borders begin to blur for the visualization with the applied CBCT technology. For the measurements of this study these limitations of the detail accuracy partially were coped with planning additional position cylinders in alignment with the post-surgical positions so that distance deviations could be measured based on the exactly displayed central axes of both, the original planning data and the executed positions (figure 6). Although the most feasible and appropriate solution for compensation of limited detail visualization, this solution goes along with a certain error-proneness since aligning the visualized drill holes with a corresponding cylinder is a manual procedure whose accuracy depends on the observers exactitude. For the actual study this potential error-proneness was compensated by accurate complete circumferential 3D diagnosis of the correct position alignment and assumption of the highest deviations in doubtful cases.

Measurement Validity: Trueness of Software-Based Measurements

Concerning the trueness of the software-based measurements for the applied CBCT technology, as mentioned above, former investigations already approved deviations of less than 1% between real distances and the corresponding distances in the 3D data sets (Mischkowski, Pulsfort et al., 2007), so that reliable data can be expected to be measured in this study.

Figure 6. CBCT data set from a maxilla model. Within the CBCT data set the virtually planned implant position (white cylinder) and the template guided surgically converted 3.4 mm expansion drill hole are visible. For superior visualization and measurement opportunity the drill hole position was aligned with a virtual orange cylinder. Measurements were executed between both cylinder´s central axes for horizontal, vertical and angle deviations. (© 2009, University of cologne, Author.)

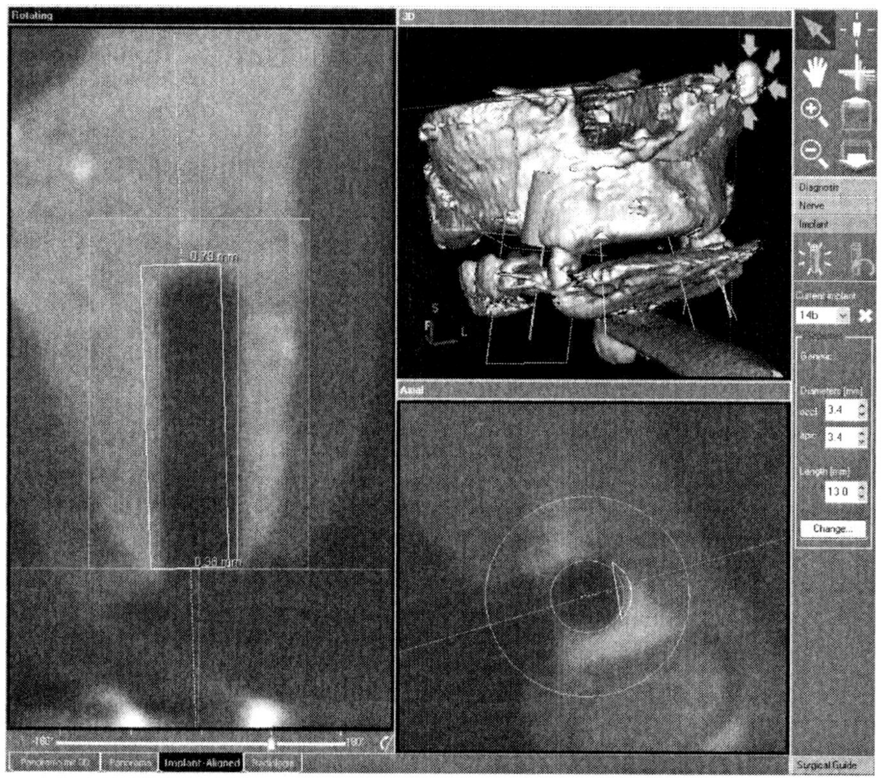

Measurement Validity: Potential Error in Fiducial Marker Registration

This chapter will be discussed in context with the following chapter on possible reasons for the observed accuracy deviations.

Each CAS system for dental implant planning contains its specific error sources. In the following passage reasons for the observed accuracy deviations between planned and converted implant positions will be discussed.

For a systematic discussion of this topic, the potential error sources will be diverted into the groups of intrinsic (technical) and extrinsic (non-technical) errors.

Extrinsic error sources contribute to the proper surgical application of the templates and therefore are affected by the manufacturer of the scan-stent, the surgeon as well as the patient during the surgical procedure.

Extrinsic Error: Scan-Stent Production

For the scan-stent production the crucial demand is to achieve a unique and reproducible fitting-position in the patient´s mouth. Only if this precondition is achieved, the scan-stent for the pre-surgical planning procedure will fits in the exact same position when converted into the corresponding surgical. Deviations of the stents position during the scanning procedure and the surgical treatment on the contrary will lead to inaccurate implant placements.

Extrinsic Error: Template Application

A general contempt of the vendor´s optimized specific work-flow protocol as well as a major patient incompliance during the surgical procedure can lead to any level of inaccuracy during dental implant insertion. Since the actual analysis was basically a model study, template application easily could be adapted to an optimal workflow leading almost to extinction of these potential template application errors. The artificial bone material of the patient equivalent anatomical models applied in this study to some degree was softer than real patient bone, especially if compared with a class one cortical mandible bone. Therefore, the artificial bone possibly deflected the drills to a minor degree than on a real patient´s bone. For the applied study model, there were no patient specific restrictions on the surgical procedure like patient trembling or limited access due to restricted stomata.

The intrinsic error sources for the investigated technology are mainly limitations that origin from impreciseness's of the registration procedures as well as the surgical template manufacturing. In this context it becomes clear, that the operator of the system has no real influence on these intrinsic errors.

Intrinsic Errors: Registration

The main weak-point of surgical template production is the transfer of virtual planning data to corresponding drill sleeve positions within the template prone to fiducial registration error (FRE) for software and fiducial localization error (FLE) for hardware registration (Birkfellner et al., 2001). This classification contributes to the fact that the registration procedure aims for perfect alignment of the virtual fiducial positions with the actual real positions. As above mentioned within the description of the registration procedure virtual fiducial positions have to be detected by software approaches in the 3D reconstructed CB data set. In this context, again the limited visualization accuracy of these data sets potentially can compromise the accurate position detection. The corresponding detection error corresponds to the FRE. The potential error level of this detection is smaller than the limitation of the visualization, since the geometry of the fiducial markers is a predictable variable (here a perfect spherical glass ball marker with 3 mm in diameter) which due to the tri-linear interpolation algorithm described above highly accurate can be matched with the visualized fiducial marker position. In the actual study software-based FRE to our experience is less than 60 μm provided that the spherical fiducials were clearly visualized. This potential FRE has to be doubled for the studies investigations due to the fact that software registration here was necessary two times for data assessment: One for the transfer of planning data to the surgical template and one additional registration for transferring the planning data to the postoperative control CBCT data set.

The FLE in contrast to this refers to the actual real 3D position detection of fiducials by the coordinate measuring device. This measuring device allows precise measurements with a nominal vendor accuracy of 2.5 μm.

The image quality of the CBCT data sets in addition to this can hamper the CAS system´s accuracy as well. As mentioned above, a proper visualization of the fiducial markers is necessary precondition for accurate software position detection and low FRE levels. The fiducial visualization and registration potentially can become hampered if motion or massive metal artifacts are present or if fiducials are not proper located in the primarily reconstructed volume (FOV) from the CBCT data set. Motion artifacts can result from patient movement due to lack of compliance or inappropriate fixation while running the radiological investigation. Metal artifacts can results from metal-dense tooth restorations. In the actual study, patient equivalent models were accurately placed within the FOV and no metal artefacts were present.

Intrinsic Errors: Surgical Template Manufacturing

The accuracy results for the surgical template manufacturing process is a product of the above mentioned extrinsic scan-stent production and a proper registration with low FRE and FLE in combination with the CBCT data sets visualization quality. These three aspects already have been discussed in the earlier sections of this chapter.

For a summarized quantitative determination of the template production accuracy after registration and conversion, as well as quality control purposes the vendor of the applied technology in this study routinely calibrates the templates on basis of the coordinate measuring machine for interpolation of the expected implant positions and compares them with the virtual implant positions. Quality control here was considered granted if virtual interpolated deviations from the template analysis were below 500 μm at the crestal and apical end for the virtual planned positions.

Further Influence Factors on the Accuracy Level

Some further uncategorized aspects with potential impact on the measured systems accuracy have to be discussed here like the passive guidance of the drill through a titanium sleeve. Also surgical templates with optimal fitting between the guiding sleeves and the pilot drill reduce the degrees of freedom of the surgeon to a minimal level there still has to be a minimal degree of freedom between drill and sleeve to guarantee rotational drill movements. Hence, a minimal leap of diameter has to be present between the drill and the guiding sleeves. Our own measurements on basis of a high accuracy measuring device showed differences of approximately 60 μm between the outer diameter of the utilized Friadent drills and the inner diameter of the SICAT sleeves. A small lee-way space between a sleeve and the basis of a drill can lead to higher deviations at the tip of the drill due to the theorem of intersecting lines. In this context, the apical and crestal horizontal deviations were statistically analyzed in this study. The assumption in this context was that a typical criterion of passive CAI systems are higher deviation rates between planned and converted positions at the apical in contrast to the crestal end. This assumption for the first time could be statistically approved by significantly higher deviation rates at the apical end of drill hole and implant position in the paired T-Test analysis. In contrast to this, for dynamic systems similar deviation rates at each point of drill holes potentially have to be expected since no passive guidance is present here.

DISCUSSION OF THE RESULTS

With respect to all the above mentioned error sources, accuracy deviations of up to 500 μm technically had to be expected for the investigated template solution if the extrinsic error sources were kept within a minimal level. In this context the investigated accuracy here optimally reflects these theoretical considerations while referring to the minimal and the lowest technically possible error level.

A slight difference could be detected for pilot burr positioning between the two investigated sleeve systems but without reaching significance level. However, the slightly but not significantly higher deviation values for the NobelGuide system may contribute to the fact that drill holes were approximately 3 mm deeper (13 mm burr holes) than the pilot burrs accomplished with the Sicat system (10 mm pilot burr holes). As mentioned above and corresponding to the theorem of intersecting lines possible deviations of a drill tip increase with the distance to the guiding sleeve.

Further on, there were always two lee-way spaces present for drill procedure with the NobelGuide system in contrast to only one leeway-space for the Sicat system. So, while the drill directly was guided through the Sicat titanium sleeve, there was one leeway-space between the twist drill and the guided drill guide as well as an additional one between the guided drill guide and the inner diameter of the RP NobelGuide sleeves. Assuming that the summarized lee-way space of the NobelGuide system is higher than the measured single lee-way space of 60 μm for the Sicat system, one also has to expect higher potential deviation rates at the apical tip of a fully sleeve inserted drill.

Many different CAI systems have been investigated utilizing a vast diversity of study designs and measuring protocols (Birkfellner et al., 2001; Fortin, Champleboux, Bianchi, Buatois, & Coudert, 2002; Hassfeld & Muhling, 2000; Ruppin et al., 2008; Sarment, Sukovic, & Clinthorne, 2003; Widmann & Bale, 2006). Most favourable mean deviation results range below 500 μm in horizontal and vertical dimension, as well as 1° angle deviation between planned and executed implant position.

For the investigated technology here, the tested accuracy corresponds to these most favourable results of alternative systems. On the other hand comparing results from different studies is the real crux due to missing standardized evaluation methods and different study designs with different measurement validities. Different radiographic imaging modalities also can have an impact on measurements validity and registration accuracy since their resolution and detail accuracy can fairly vary. A closer look on medical CT protocols and nominal resolutions of CBCT data sets can illuminate the potential measurement validity.

Further on, one must not forget that most of these study results like the actual one were generated under optimized model conditions. In this context especially the patients influence factors like mentioned in the "extrinsic errors" section are more or less completely faded out.

CONCLUSION

Accuracy analysis of guided implant insertion with the first integrated CBCT system for computer aided implantology resulted in highly precise conversion levels which can compete with the most favourable accuracy results published for CAI systems so far. The systems ground accuracy could be maintained if SICAT´s surgical templates were combined with the surgical set of the Nobel Guide system for fully guided implant insertion. Maximal linear deviations of 990 μm were detected so that a minimal security distance of 1 mm has to be claimed to any important anatomical structure during virtual implant positioning.

However, these results provide that the manufacturer's workflow is meticulously followed, i.e. optimal scan-stent fitting, CBCT scan image quality is not hampered by motion or metal artifacts, no significant patient specific influence on the surgical procedure due to trembling or stoma limitations. In-vivo studies are necessary to investigate the accuracies of the different CAS systems in clinical routine where settings are not always optimal. Assuming that further failure sources can result from in-vivo application of the investigated system here, the necessary security distance should generously exceed the above mentioned 1 mm.

REFERENCES

Birkfellner, W., Solar, P., Gahleitner, A., Huber, K., Kainberger, F., & Kettenbach, J. (2001). In-vitro assessment of a registration protocol for image guided implant dentistry. *Clinical Oral Implants Research*, *12*(1), 69–78. doi:10.1034/j.1600-0501.2001.012001069.x

Dreiseidler, T., Mischkowski, R. A., Neugebauer, J., Ritter, L., & Zöller, J. E. (2009). Comparison of Cone-Beam Imaging with Orthopantomography and Computerized Tomography for Assessment in Presurgical Implant Dentistry. *The International Journal of Oral & Maxillofacial Implants*, *24*(2), 216–225.

Dreiseidler, T., Neugebauer, J., Ritter, L., Lingohr, T., Rothamel, D., & Mischkowski, R. A. (2009). Accuracy of a newly developed integrated system for dental implant planning. *Clinical Oral Implants Research*, *20*(11), 1191–1199. doi:10.1111/j.1600-0501.2009.01764.x

Fortin, T., Champleboux, G., Bianchi, S., Buatois, H., & Coudert, J. L. (2002). Precision of transfer of preoperative planning for oral implants based on cone-beam CT-scan images through a robotic drilling machine. *Clinical Oral Implants Research*, *13*(6), 651–656. doi:10.1034/j.1600-0501.2002.130612.x

Harris, D., Buser, D., Dula, K., Grondahl, K., Haris, D., & Jacobs, R. (2002). E.A.O. guidelines fo the use of diagnostic imaging in implant dentistry. A consensus workshop organized by the European Association for Osseointegration in Trinity College Dublin. *Clinical Oral Implants Research*, *13*(5), 566–570. doi:10.1034/j.1600-0501.2002.130518.x

Hassfeld, S., & Muhling, J. (2000). Comparative examination of the accuracy of a mechanical and an optical system in CT and MRT based instrument navigation. *International Journal of Oral and Maxillofacial Surgery*, *29*(6), 400–407. doi:10.1016/S0901-5027(00)80069-7

Koch, A., Macherel, J. M., Wirth, T., de Groot, P. M., Ducourant, T., Couder, D., et al. (2001). *Detective quantum efficiency of an x-ray image intensifier chain as a benchmark for amorphous silicon flat-panal detectors* (Vol. 4320).

Kuhls-Gilcrist, A., Yadava, G., Patel, V., Jain, A., Bednarek, D. R., & Rudin, S. (2008). The Solid-State X-Ray Image Intensifier (SSXII): An EMCCD-Based X-Ray Detector. *Proc Soc Photo Opt Instrum Eng*, *6913*, nihpa68284.

Ludlow, J. B., & Ivanovic, M. (2008). Comparative dosimetry of dental CBCT devices and 64-slice CT for oral and maxillofacial radiology. *Oral Surgery, Oral Medicine, Oral Pathology, Oral Radiology, and Endodontics*, *106*(1), 106–114. doi:10.1016/j.tripleo.2008.03.018

Mischkowski, R. A., Pulsfort, R., Ritter, L., Neugebauer, J., Brochhagen, H. G., & Keeve, E. (2007). Geometric accuracy of a newly developed cone-beam device for maxillofacial imaging. *Oral Surgery, Oral Medicine, Oral Pathology, Oral Radiology, and Endodontics*, *104*(4), 551–559. doi:10.1016/j.tripleo.2007.02.021

Mischkowski, R. A., Zinser, M. J., Ritter, L., Neugebauer, J., Keeve, E., & Zoller, J. E. (2007). Intraoperative navigation in the maxillofacial area based on 3D imaging obtained by a cone-beam device. *International Journal of Oral and Maxillofacial Surgery*, *36*(8), 687–694. doi:10.1016/j.ijom.2007.04.001

Mozzo, P., Procacci, C., Tacconi, A., Martini, P. T., & Andreis, I. A. (1998). A new volumetric CT machine for dental imaging based on the cone-beam technique: preliminary results. *European Radiology*, *8*(9), 1558–1564. doi:10.1007/s003300050586

Ruppin, J., Popovic, A., Strauss, M., Spuntrup, E., Steiner, A., & Stoll, C. (2008). Evaluation of the accuracy of three different computer-aided surgery systems in dental implantology: optical tracking vs. stereolithographic splint systems. *Clinical Oral Implants Research*, *19*(7), 709–716. doi:10.1111/j.1600-0501.2007.01430.x

Rustemeyer, P., Streubuhr, U., & Suttmoeller, J. (2004). Low-dose dental computed tomography: significant dose reduction without loss of image quality. *Acta Radiol*, *45*(8), 847–853. doi:10.1080/02841850410001402

Sarment, D. P., Sukovic, P., & Clinthorne, N. (2003). Accuracy of implant placement with a stereolithographic surgical guide. *The International Journal of Oral & Maxillofacial Implants*, *18*(4), 571–577.

Widmann, G., & Bale, R. J. (2006). Accuracy in computer-aided implant surgery--a review. *The International Journal of Oral & Maxillofacial Implants*, *21*(2), 305–313.

Ziegler, C. M., Woertche, R., Brief, J., & Hassfeld, S. (2002). Clinical indications for digital volume tomography in oral and maxillofacial surgery. *Dento Maxillo Facial Radiology*, *31*(2), 126–130. doi:10.1038/sj.dmfr.4600680

KEY TERMS AND DEFINITIONS

CAI (Computer Aided Implantology): Summarization for computerized applications in pre-implantologic diagnosis, treatment planning and/or therapy.

CAS (Computer Aided Surgery): Summarization for computerized applications in pre-surgical diagnosis, treatment planning and/or therapy.

CBCT (Cone-Beam Computer Tomography): Radiologic method to acquire 3D data sets.

CNC-Machine (Computerized Numerical Control Machine): Devices utilizing modern guidance electronic for automated high-precision manufacturing.

DICOM (Digital Imaging and Communications in Medicine): Standard formatting for the management of medical imaging.

DQE (Detective Quantum Efficiency): Objective measure of how an available signal-to-noise ratio is degraded by a radiological imaging system with respect to the spatial frequency of the input signal. Therefore also describing the ability of a system to transfer x-ray signals into exploitable visualization information.

FOV (Field-of-View): Area or volume that is covered and correspondingly visualized by a radiological diagnosis device.

MTF (Modulation Transfer Function): Quantitative measure for the image quality of a visualization system defined as ability to display contrast in dependence to the spatial frequency.

RP (Rapid Prototyping): Automatic construction of physical objects using solid freeform fabrication.

Chapter 13
Imaging in Periodontology: 2D versus 3D Visualization Techniques

B. Vandenberghe
Katholieke Universiteit Leuven, Belgium

O. Nackaerts
Katholieke Universiteit Leuven, Belgium

ABSTRACT

Periodontal disease is the most common oral disorder in the elderly population. Early detection of bony and soft tissue support changes is therefore crucial in relation to the prevention of tooth loss and/or the patient's general health. Unfortunately, the current diagnostic tools for accurate assessment of this periodontal status have shown several limitations. Most image analysis tools are based on 2D images, while bone remodelling is a 3D process. At present, Cone Beam Computed Tomography (CBCT) has become a powerful diagnostic tool in dentistry. This chapter will bring an overview of 2D and 3D visualization methods of the periodontal tissues and their pathologic manifestations like infrabony craters and furcation involvements. The diagnostic use of 2D radiographic projections, image filtering and subtraction will be compared to the use of 3D cross-sections and the image analysis tools for 3D visualization and/or follow-up of bony changes.

IMAGING IN PERIODONTOLOGY: 2D VERSUS 3D VISUALIZATION TECHNIQUES

In this chapter, image analysis tools in the field of periodontology will be described for both two-dimensional and three-dimensional radiographic modalities. First, the current concepts in the diagnosis of periodontal diseases will be outlined with emphasis on the radiographic examination, which plays a crucial role in the detection of alveolar bone loss. The following section will thus cover traditional two-dimensional modalities, which are the most common used in dental practice. Because of their inherent limitation of projecting structures in two dimensions, advanced imaging tools will be explored and a need for 3D imaging will be underscored. Finally, a new three-dimensional imaging modality in periodontal imaging will be introduced. Visualization and interpretation techniques using

DOI: 10.4018/978-1-60566-733-1.ch013

this cone beam computed tomography (CBCT) will be complemented with more advanced applications where 3D volume rendering and image registration of clinical data may change the face of periodontal diagnosis.

INTRODUCTION TO PERIODONTAL DISEASES

Periodontal disease is the leading cause of tooth loss in the elderly population and shows an increasing incidence with age. It consists of several disorders of the periodontium, including gingivitis and periodontitis, which represent chronic infectious diseases. The presence of certain bacteria initiate plaque and calculus formation supra- and subgingival, affecting the soft tissues surrounding the teeth and causing inflammation. This gingivitis associated with bleeding of the gums, can progress to periodontitis when soft tissue attachment loss and/or supporting bone loss is seen. This results in pocket formation between the teeth and the remaining soft tissues or bone (see Figure 1) and may affect one to all teeth and eventually, when left untreated, lead to tooth loss.

Figure 1. The two main topographic manifestations of alveolar bone loss. (A) Incisor and premolar radiographs revealing an overall horizontal breakdown of bone. The distance from the CEJ (white line) to the actual bony crest (red line) is larger than 1.5mm (the green line should be the healthy bone level) and appears similar for all teeth. (B) The radiograph of the maxillary molars reveals a non-uniform pattern of bone loss. Note that actual bone levels are difficult to assess because of radiographic superposition of the bony structures.

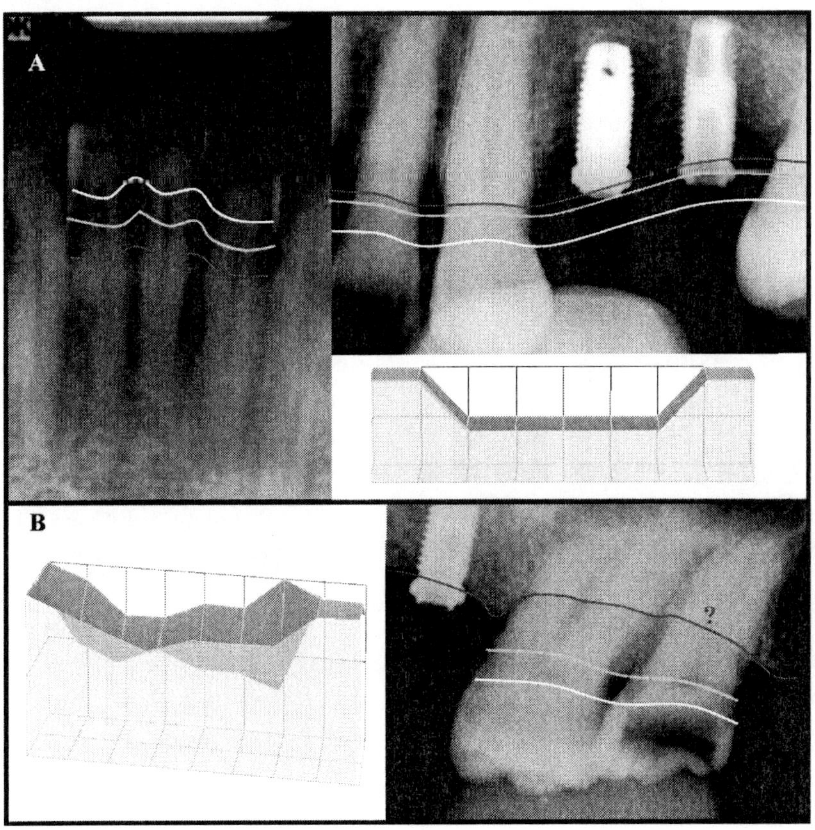

In addition, there is strong evidence that periodontal diseases are associated to certain systemic diseases such as cardiovascular disorders (Khader, 2004). Many studies have shown the importance of early detection of periodontal disease, in relation to the prevention of tooth loss and/or the patient's general health (Oliveira Costa, 2007; Slots, 2003; Seymour, 2007). Diagnostic tools are therefore crucial for accurate assessment of the periodontal status. One problematic issue is the fact that the pattern of attachment loss is extremely variable. The loss of bony support can reveal either a horizontal breakdown (horizontal bone loss) or an angular breakdown (vertical bone loss) (see Figure 1). A normal alveolar crest lies within 1 to 1.5mm distance of the cemento-enamel junction (CEJ).

Especially these angular defects vary tremendously and many different architectural patterns have been described (Hamp 1975; Karn, 1984; Tarnow, 1984). Infrabony defects are a perfect habitat for pathogenic bacteria which may invade the space between roots of multi-rooted teeth to cause furcation problems that are more likely to progress and are associated with poor prognosis (Loos, 1989). Infrabony defects thus vary in severity but -as important- also vary in location and frequency (Jeffcoat, 1991). Furthermore, the disease activity is unpredictable because of these complexities. Examination of the bony architecture is therefore a crucial aspect in periodontal diagnosis and treatment planning. The choice of certain periodontal surgical techniques such as bone regeneration using membranes or bone grafting procedures are highly depending upon the 3-dimensional topography of periodontal breakdown (Muller, 1995). Interestingly, the most commonly used diagnostic tools in this field have barely changed over the years. Traditional screening methods still exist of a thorough clinical examination complemented with panoramic and/or intraoral radiographs. However, recently introduced low dose cone beam computed tomography may bring new potential in the early detection and/ or follow-up of periodontal bone loss.

In this chapter, traditional diagnostic methods for periodontal diagnosis are reviewed showing their limitations and followed by a description of available advanced imaging tools to optimize current methods. Furthermore, this chapter will focus on new three-dimensional computed tomography, discuss current literature and explain the latest three-dimensional analysis tools which may demonstrate the need for new guideline development in the radiographic examination of periodontal breakdown.

CURRENT CONCEPTS IN PERIODONTAL DIAGNOSIS

The management of periodontal patients requires an in depth clinical and radiographic examination (Nyman & Lindhe, 1997). The inflammatory signs associated of gingivitis and periodontitis are easily assessed clinically, but the extent of tissue breakdown should also be investigated. Since clinical measurements of connective tissue loss do not provide information on the relation of alveolar bone loss to the roots, authors agree that both clinical and radiographic tools are complementary (Tugnait, 2000). However, the use of ionizing radiation –how small it may be- should always be justified so that the clinical benefit outweighs the radiation risk. Furthermore, many radiographic techniques exist for dental imaging -each having their own benefits and drawbacks- which can make, together with the various manifestations of periodontal diseases, the choice of examination more complex. Although technology advances and new modalities are being developed, it is always careful to adopt a clinical approach that is supplemented with local imaging where necessary.

Clinical Examination

Methods

Following the medical and dental history collection, both gingival tissues and periodontal ligament space surrounding each tooth, need careful examination. Clinical signs of gingivitis are discoloration and texture change of the marginal soft tissues surrounding the teeth and is associated with the presence of dental plaque and (supra-) gingival calculus. Using a periodontal probe, the bleeding tendency can be assessed which is increased when inflammation is present. The probe is used to measure clinical attachment loss (distance from the CEJ to the alveolar bone) and pocket depths (distance from the gingival margin to the alveolar bone) around each individual tooth. Tooth mobility may indicate a more severe stage of bone loss causing instability in the alveolar socket because of insufficient bony support. Several indices have been proposed for these diagnostic markers and these methods are well established, simple and cost effective. Much information can thus be derived from the clinical examination alone, although this only pertains to establishing disease extent and predicting its progression.

Limitations

Probing attachment levels or pockets depths are aiming to measure a distance from respectively the CEJ or gingival margin until the base of the pocket or in other words the most apical cells of the dentogingival epithelium. The latter measurements can rapidly be recorded and are the most common in dental practice since the CEJ tends to be found more difficult to locate clinically because of poor visualization or local factors like dental restorations. However, these measurements may overestimate the depth when tissues are locally inflamed or underestimate destruction when gingival recession has occurred. In addition, both types of measurements are prone to inter- and intra-observer errors. In a review paper by Hefti (1997) errors due to probing force, angle, positioning, diameter of the tip and read-out are described and research on methods to reduce these are discussed. With correct standardization and protocols, accuracy of clinical measurements using conventional probes has been found to be within approximately 1mm which is similar to using semi-automated electronic probes (Quirynen, 1993). It must be mentioned that in clinical practice these measurement errors are often exceeded. Interestingly, even though much research and progress has been made over the last 30 years, the current clinical protocol has changed little and is often found a painful process by the patient, thus still indicating room for improvement. Furthermore, these clinical tools do not provide any information on current or future disease activity. For instance, at this moment, it does not seem to be possible to know exactly when gingivitis progresses to periodontitis.

Advanced Techniques

The traditional clinical tools seem to be insufficient or lack accuracy for the exact determination of diseases activity and progression. Therefore, many studies are being conducted investigating potential markers of disease activity. Eley & Cox (1998) have published a series of articles describing these advanced research areas and categorize potential biomarkers in bacterial flora and their products, inflammatory and immune products, enzymes released from inflammatory or dead cells and connective tissue degraded products. Although some of these tests to detect disease progression or to detect genetic susceptibility to periodontitis seem very promising, they still need further research and clinical validation and are beyond the scope of this chapter. Furthermore, the exact extent as well as osseous morphology –needed for adequate treatment choice- cannot be determined using these various tests. The use of a radiographic method to assess damage caused to the bony tissues will continue to play a central role in diagnosis (Armitage, 2003; Eley & Cox 1998; Brägger 2005).

Radiographic Examination

Several important additional findings on radiographs will help to determine actual disease extent and treatment plan. Foremost important in the ability to visualize the subgingival periodontal tissues is the evaluation of the alveolar crest and alveolar bone loss. In this way, one can form a visual image of the clinical measurements (gingival soft tissues are not visible on intraoral radiographs) and relate this to the remaining bony support of the dentition for evaluation of the disease extent. Measurements from the CEJ to the alveolar crest are performed after the examination and other important periodontal markers are evaluated, including periodontal ligament (PDL) space, the presence of a lamina dura, trabecular architecture of the alveolar bone, subgingival calculus and overhanging restorations. In addition, the periapical region is imaged which allows not only disease extent estimation, but also visualization of possible apical periodontitis and related endodontic problems. With the current advent of digital intraoral receptors and computer-assisted analysis of digital images, new areas have been explored for follow-up of bony lesions using densitometric analysis. A striking fact is that although it is without a doubt that the radiographic examination is a necessary adjunct to the clinical examinations, traditional clinical charting is rarely complemented with the radiographic measurements. Pocket probing showing changes in the gingival tissues is indeed an easy tool to instruct the patient on their condition, but the above mentioned limitations should make clinicians aware of including radiographic measurements in their analysis of the periodontal condition. Brägger (2005) describes a method where electronic clinical probe and radiographic measurements from the same anatomical fiducial (CEJ) to the alveolar crest are superimposed on panoramic images. Although panoramic images might not be the most optimal imaging method for this purpose, the method does reveal new possible research areas for complete periodontal charting and diagnosis (see Figure 2).

Figure 2. Periodontal measurements in the diagnosis and estimation of disease and extent. (A) Clinical pocket depths (gingival margin) are often the measurement of choice in clinical practice. (B) On intraoral radiographs the distance from CEJ to alveolar crest can be measured. (C) Display of both clinical as well as radiographic measurements on an image –weather intraoral, panoramic or tomographic- may provide easier diagnosis and follow-up (green line= alveolar crest, pink line=gingival margin).

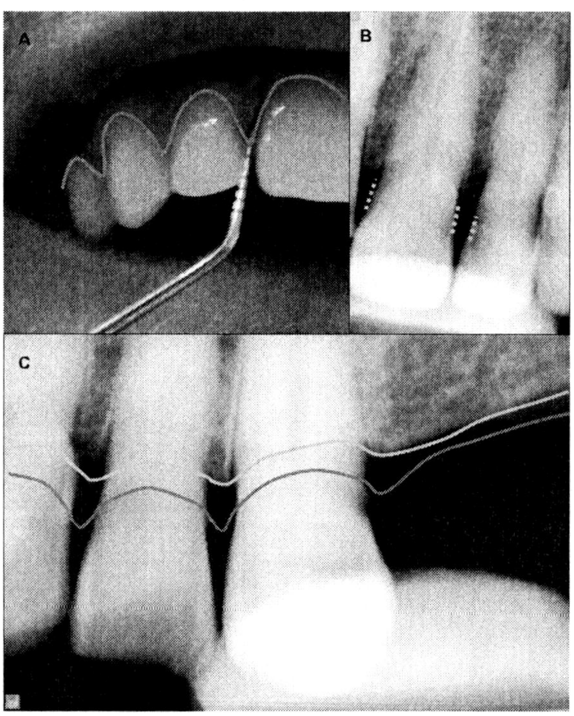

Methods and Limitations

The two main radiographic examinations for periodontal diagnosis are intraoral –periapical as well as bitewing- and panoramic radiographs. Traditionally, the examination consists of a full mouth

Figure 3. (A) When correctly using the paralleling technique, the alveolar crest of the periodontal bone is displayed at true distance from the CEJ (left). Incorrect positioning results in a more apical or coronal projected alveolar crest (right). (B) Buccal plate and oral defect are marked with the two arrows on the dry skull specimen. The two-dimensional radiograph shows projection of the buccal plate on the oral defect.

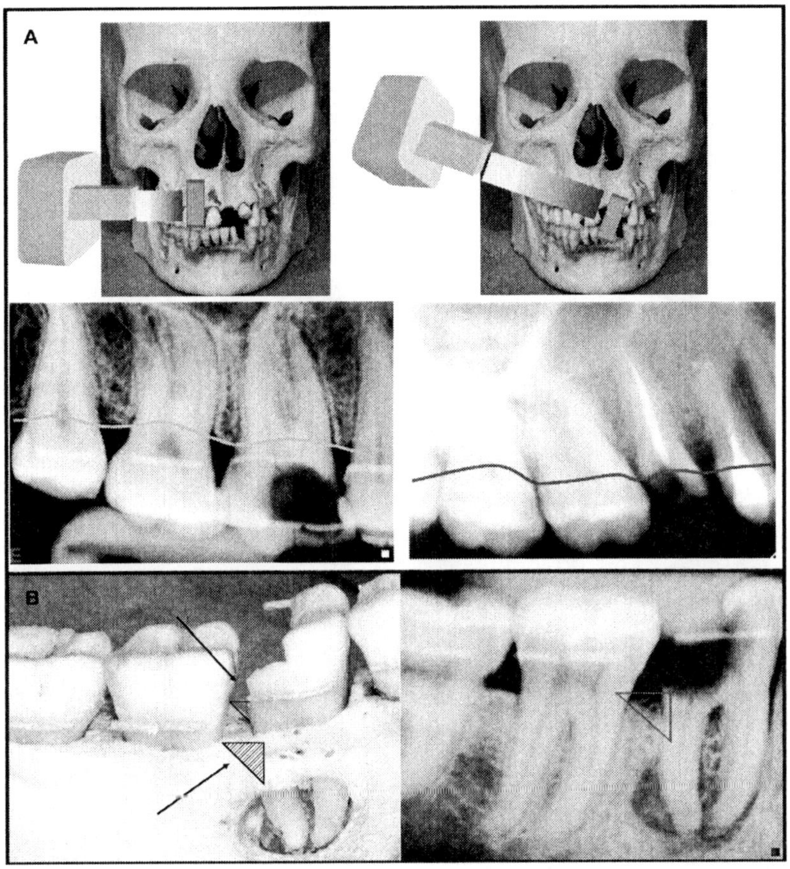

radiographic survey (FMX), which is a series of 18 to 22 periapical and bitewing radiographs. In order to carefully follow the ALARA (As Low As Reasonably Achievable) principle, it has also been suggested to use a panoramic radiograph in combination with a limited number of intraoral radiographs indicated by the severity of the clinical findings. Unfortunately, studies have shown that general recommendations are often not followed in clinical practice and given the limitations of current techniques and the advent of three-dimensional imaging, more evidence-based research needs to be performed using the latest tools and protocols to ensure high standards of radiographic practice (Tugnait, 2004).

Intraoral Radiography

Compared to panoramic radiographs, intraoral radiographs have the advantage of high spatial resolution and, with the optimal exposure settings, a vast amount of contrast information. Using a steady x-ray source and an image receptor (film or digital), the periodontal structures are displayed without any magnification or distortion, but only when properly using the paralleling technique. Unfortunately, even when using aiming devices and correct positioning, the inherent property of intraoral radiographs is a two-dimensional (2D) projection. Buccal and oral structures are superimposed on each other and it is therefore difficult to distinguish buccal from oral alveolar bone (see Figure 3).

Another important factor that may hinder optimal periodontal diagnosis is the exposure condition. Digitalization has drastically changed the face of dentistry and many studies have researched its validity compared to conventional films in the detection of periodontal bone loss (Wolf, 2001; Borg, 1997; Jorgenson, 2007; Li, 2007; Kaeppler, 2000; Pecoraro, 2005). The image quality of digital images is at least equal to conventional image quality at a lower exposure time. This reduction in patient exposure is significant, but also depending on the x-ray generator type (McDavid, 1982) and image receptor used (Berkhout, 2004; Borg, 2000). Photostimulable storage phosphor (PSP) plates are indirect imaging plates that require read-out of the latent image after exposure. Charged couple device (CCD) or complementary metal-oxide semiconductor (CMOS) sensors are direct image receptors that are connected to the computer with a cable. Both PSP and CCD/CMOS technology is different and one of the properties that distinct them is the dynamic range. PSP plates have a wide dynamic range which allows correction for under- or overexposure of the radiograph: the image will appear the same over a wide range of exposures (see Figure 4). For CCD/CMOS sensors, this is not the case. They are more sensitive than PSP plates and produce adequate image quality at very low exposure times, but they only have a small dynamic range: when rising exposure time, the image will therefore darken (see Figure 4). This darkening phenomenon produces so called blooming artefacts when exposure time is too high (Berkhout, 2004). This may give appearance of larger destruction or bone loss of the alveolar crest, infrabony defects and furcation involvements.

Alveolar Bone Loss

Clinically, a precise parallel geometry is necessary to counteract possible projection errors with associated over- or underestimations of the alveolar bone levels (Zulqarnain, 1998). In in-vitro studies, under standardized conditions using proper positioning, accuracy of alveolar bone loss measurements on intraoral radiographs is high with strong inter-observer agreement (deviation within 1mm) (Pecoraro, 2005). Clinically, this standardization may often be more difficult, but studies have for instance reported deviations from the surgical gold standard between 0.4mm and 1.4mm (Borg, 1997) or a mean deviation of 1.41mm (Eickholz, 2000). Pepelassi & Diamanti-Kipioti (1997) report 80% of their measurements within 1mm, 91% within 2mm and 96% within 3mm. Measurement deviations are also depending on the severity of the alveolar destruction and the tooth type. In general, assessments on radiographs tend to underestimate the amount of bone loss, but for severe osseous defects overestimations are more common. Larger measurement deviations are typically seen in the molar regions. This is due to the usually more complex nature of the alveolar loss.

Another aspect within the radiographic examination of periodontal diseases is the need to follow-up periodontal disease progression. Serial radiographs may allow the practitioner to evaluate the disease over time but this requires again careful standardization of the radiographic protocol. An individual occlusal key on the aiming device can be used to warrant reproducibility of the radiographic projection geometry and in addition, the same exposure settings are necessary to obtain identical radiographic contrast. Hausmann & Allen (1997) reported that the measurement error of change in bone height on serial radiographs using a standardized exposure set-up was as small as 0.52mm. Again, more problematic is the follow-up of large infrabony defects since the exact depth estimation is more difficult. Furthermore, when analyzing three-dimensional angular defects, one linear depth measurement does not provide sufficient information on its topography. More advanced techniques have been developed to assess the disease in three dimensions.

Figure 4. PSP (left column) and CCD (right column) radiographs of a dry skull's mandibular molar region at different exposure times. PSP plates are less sensitive than the CCD system and produce artefacts at low exposure times. However, because of their wide dynamic range, the images appear alike when rising exposure time. Using the CCD, the mesial and intra-radicular furcation defects of the 3rd molar are darkening at rising exposure time, simulating larger osseous destruction.

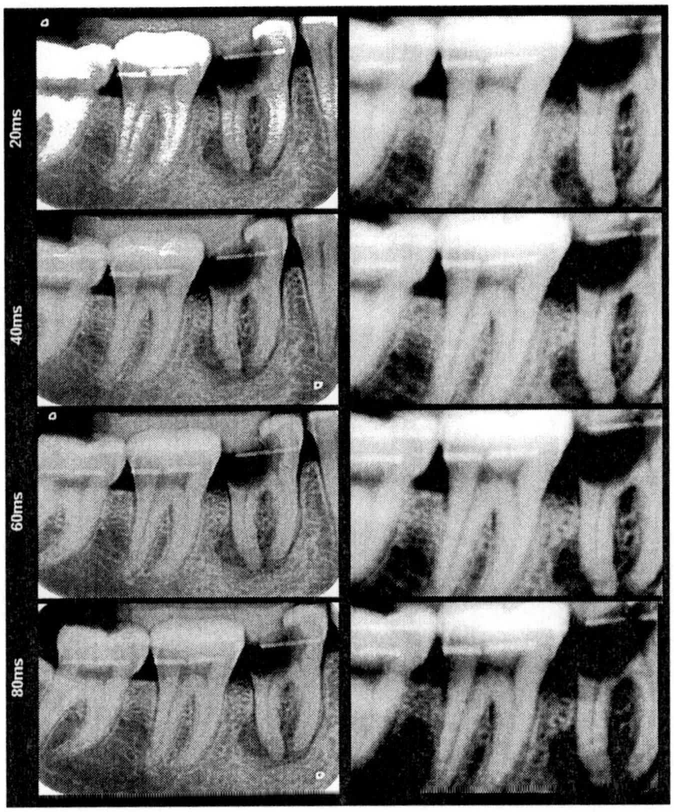

Infrabony Defects: Crater and Furcation Involvements

Besides the ability to measure the extent or depth of an infrabony defect, it is just as important to be able to diagnose them and determine their 3D topography. Already in 1962, Ramadan and Mitchell confirmed that most funnel-shaped defects or lingually located defects cannot be detected. Buccal plate destruction could also not be distinguished from lingual plate destruction. In 1976, Bassiouny & Grant proposed a method where three intraoral radiographs were taken at different angulations to determine the defect topography. This is of course not feasible or justified in modern clinical practice. In the following years, many attempts have been made researching alveolar bone loss on radiographs, but often studies only research linear or horizontal bone loss. With the rise of three-dimensional imaging, Fuhrmann et al (1997) investigated the identification and classification of furcation involvements on intraoral radiographs and using high resolution computed tomography (CT). They found that only 21% of the simulated defects were found on intraoral radiography compared to 100% using CT. These results seem to indicate that three-dimensional imaging may be the method of choice to diagnose complex infrabony defects.

Other Periodontal Landmarks: Subjective Image Quality

The radiographic examination also provides information on the presence of a lamina dura, the periodontal ligament space, the trabecular pattern of periodontal bone and the periapical region. Intraoral radiographs are images with high contrast and spatial resolution and are therefore very suitable for the depiction of these fine structures of the periodontium.

One of the parameters often utilized for evaluation of periodontal stability is the appearance of a lamina dura. Rams et al (1994) studied this phenomenon and found that absence of the lamina dura had a high specificity for predicting attachment loss, although with a low specificity. When the lamina dura was present at baseline, no disease progression was seen for the next two years. Another radiographic parameter is the periodontal ligament space which may reveal disease activity when widening of the space is visible. Few studies have investigated the role or influence of these markers but one of the interesting research areas explored the last few years is the depiction of trabecularization of alveolar bone for bone quality and density assessments. Many of the tools for quantifying or rating bone quality are still being researched and are not yet routinely used in clinical practice. Therefore, these research tools will be discussed in a seperate section (2.2.2.3).

Panoramic Radiography

Orthopantomography is an extraoral imaging technique where x-ray source and image receptor rotate in opposite direction around the patient's head. The movement is in such a way that only anatomical structures in the curvilinear focal trough or image layer are sharply imaged, while the rest of the structures are blurred out. Panoramic radiographs are often used as an initial evaluation tool, e.g. in Orthodontics, Periodontology or for the assessment of 3rd molars. Based on these images, clinicians may decide on the need for further examinations. Despite the lack of evidence to support panoramic radiography as a "screening" tool, this practice is common (Rushton et al 2001). Many studies have found that periapical radiographs are superior to panoramic imaging in detecting and assessing periodontal osseous destruction. Still, Molander et al (1995) suggested using panoramic radiography with restricted intraoral radiographs in the comprehensive oral radiographic diagnosis to minimize radiation dose to the patient.

Amongst the disadvantages of panoramic images is the inability to display fine anatomic detail. The reason for this is not only the 2D projection of 3D structures, but also the magnification and geometrical distortion of the image. Due to the tomographic nature of the technique with a thin image layer, patient positioning is critical to properly visualize both dental arches. Asymmetrical positioning will not only cause certain structures to fall out of the image layer but also asymmetrical geometric distortion (see Figure 5).

Furthermore, the spatial resolution is not as high as intra-oral radiographs. This hampers the detection of minor or nascent lesions. Certainly, panoramic radiography is useful in clinical practice, especially in terms of patient comfort for initial treatment planning and detection of important anatomical structures using only small radiation exposure. However, the actual diagnostic accuracy of panoramic imaging in the assessment of periodontal structures is too low to use it without any supplemental radiographs.

Alveolar Bone Loss and Infrabony Defects

Since one of the major drawbacks of pantomographic imaging is the critical dependence of patient positioning and the local magnification of anatomical structures, it may not be a surprise that linear measurements or detection of complex infrabony defects are often not accurate on panoramic radiographs. Rohlin et al (1989) compared bone level measurements and detectability of bone defects and furcation involvements on panoramic and intraoral radiography in 100 patients. Bone

Figure 5. Panoramic radiograph showing many positioning errors limiting its diagnostic value. Overlap of the right premolar region hinders visibility of the alveolar crest (circle). The right mandibular ramus is wider than the left one (double arrow) which is due to a sideways tilting of the head during acquisition and results in unequal magnification. The spine is projected onto the incisor region (arrow) and the ghost image of the right mandible can be seen projected over the left teeth (line).

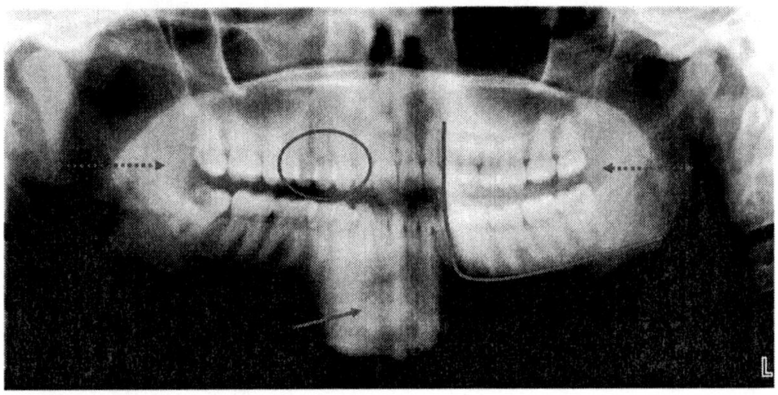

loss measurements on both modalities were only in concordance in sites with small to no bone loss, but varied especially for larger osseous defects. Bone defects were also more easily identified on intraoral radiographs. In a clinical study from Pepelassi et al (1997), 5072 proximal surfaces of 2536 teeth of 100 patients were assessed using intraoral and panoramic images. The results were compared to the intrasurgical gold standard measurements and it was found that intraoral radiography was not only more accurate but also more successful in detecting osseous destruction.

Other Periodontal Landmarks: Subjective Image Quality

Visibility of lamina dura, periodontal ligament space or trabecular pattern is often obscured because of superposition of anatomical structures on the jaws. The same is true for factors related to periodontal disease like overhanging restorations and calculus deposits. These problems are due to positioning errors and are often seen in the lower incisor region (see Figure 5). However, on panoramic screening images the cortical border of the mandible is clearly depicted and this has been one of the research areas in the assessment of jaw bone quality (see 2.2.2.3).

Advanced Techniques

Contrast Enhancement

One of the most important properties of digital imaging is the ability to manipulate the digital image. This advantage makes, together with the greater sensitivity of digital image receptors and the associated dose reduction, modern dental offices rapidly moving towards this technology. Image enhancement can be accomplished by optimizing contrast and/or brightness, or reducing sharpness and noise (see 2.2.2.2).

Contrast resolution indicated the amount of grey values that can be imaged. For digital receptors, contrast resolution is expressed in bit depth, where bits represent the amount of grey values that can be imaged. Computer language is written in a binary language with 0 and 1 bits and therefore 8 bit-language systems can only represent 2^8 or 256 bytes. The pixel from an 8bit image receptor can thus only provide 256 shades of gray. The use of these grey values in an image can easily be seen in the histogram. In this histogram, the number of grey values is represented on the x-axis (for 8bit: 0 to 255) and the number of pixels having a specific grey value is presented on the y-axis. By dynamically choosing the grey values from the

Figure 6. Digital periapical radiograph with histogram of a left upper molar region after image acquisition (top). When choosing different upper and lower limits of the grey values to be displayed, the image is brightened (left) or darkened (right).

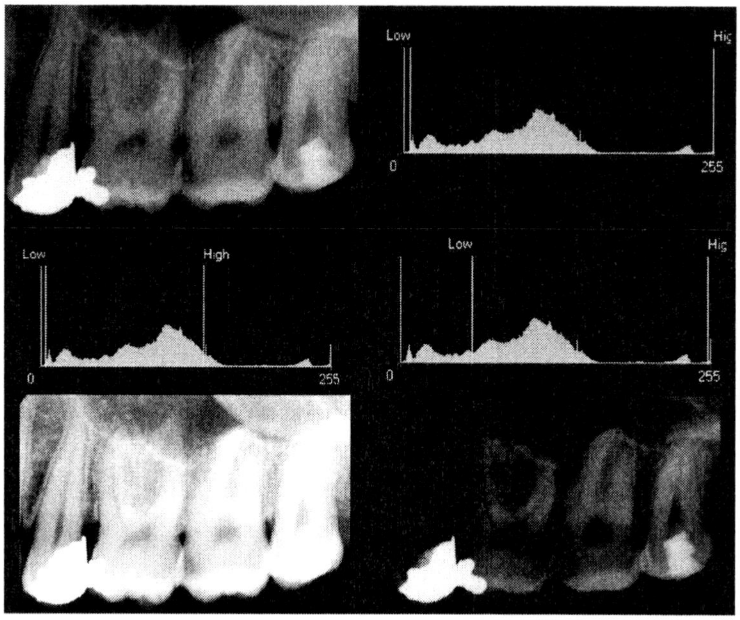

histogram, the image can be darkened or brightened (Analoui, 2001) (see Figure 6).

Although conventional films show excellent contrast since any shade of grey can be displayed, a higher exposure time is required with higher associated patient doses. Furthermore, only illumination and a magnification glass are at hand for analysis. The human eye can namely only distinguish approximately 60 shades of grey at once without any aids (Künzel, 2003). This is of course also true for digital images and in addition, the resolution of the display screen can limit the display of many grey values at once. On the other hand, digital enhancement may thus help in visualizing the whole dynamic range and even adjust for small over- or underexposures.

Much research has been done to compare conventional films with digital systems for periodontal diagnosis and no difference in accuracy is perceived. This is especially due to improving resolution of digital sensors. Newer systems have now reached higher bit depths (12bit= 2^{12} or 4096 gray shades, 16bit= 2^{16} or 65.536 gray shades) which may influence the diagnostic image quality of intraoral radiographs (Heo, 2009; Wenzel, 2007). For periodontal diagnosis, the ability of newer systems to depict more grey values may thus cause a better visualization of the alveolar crest, especially when keeping in mind that this crest can be deteriorated by blooming artefacts at high exposure times (see Figure 4). Nevertheless, image enhancement is the ability to change an image in order to make it more visually appealing. In other words, this does not mean that this manipulation will lead to a better diagnosis. Therefore, given the limited literature on the use of these high contrast resolutions for periodontal diagnosis, more research needs to be conducted to demonstrate its influence on diagnosis.

Image Filtering

Another form of image enhancement is the use of image filters. Filters are simple mathematical operations that are applied to the image pixels with as result a visually more appealing image (see Figure 7).

Figure 7. (A) Original image with filter window, a filter matrix and mask width can be chosen for the mathematical operation to be applied on the image (B) sharpened image (C) edge enhancement (D) inverse function

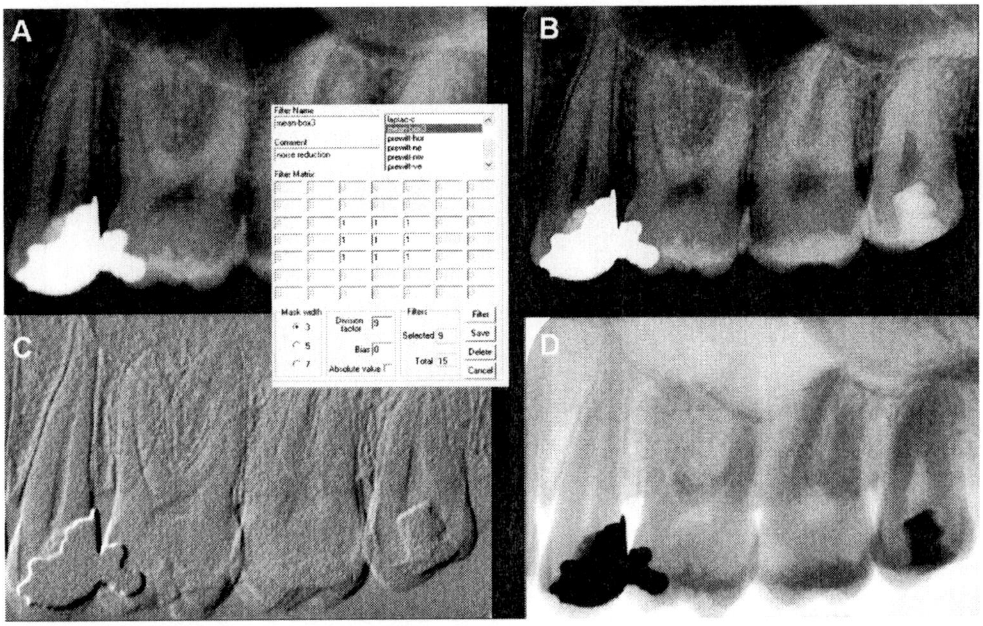

The description of these operators is beyond the scope of this chapter, but it is important to note that much research is ongoing to demonstrate the value of these operations. When assessing caries lesions, filters like image sharpening and noise reduction may indeed prove to influence diagnosis. The same seems applicable for endodontic imaging of small file sizes. Although literature seems to indicate additional benefits, some researchers have found no differences between enhanced and unenhanced digital images. This may be due to several factors like the use of older image receptors with lower contrast and/or spatial resolution, the use of different computer displays or viewing conditions. Because of the many variables in the image process, it is important to fully standardize the research protocol for adequate assessments and demonstration of filter influence.

For periodontal diagnosis, research is limited. Eickholz et al (1999) and Wolf et al (2001) did not find any significant differences when using digital enhancement, although digitized conventional films with a 10bit flatbed scanner were used. Li et al (2007) also did not find any differences for bone level measurements using enhanced images but no information is provided on the exposure protocol. More research in this field is needed, not only for the value of filters when assessing bone loss, but also for detection and measurements of craters depths and furcation involvements.

Qualitative and Quantitative Analysis: Jaw Bone Quality Assessment

The assessment of jaw bone quality is an important but often forgotten parameter in the clinical diagnosis of periodontal disease. Jaw bone quality assessments are important in the preoperative planning of implant placement and the follow-up of bone changes as a result of disease progress or therapy. Bone healing can be hampered in poor bone quality which may be prone to rapid bone loss and even tooth loss (Lerner, 2006). Successful oral implant placement and osseointegration are to a large extent determined by the quantity (width and height) but also by the quality of the available jaw bone (Herrmann, 2005). Therefore, the

Figure 8. Mandibular Cortical Index (MCI) and panoramic radiograph detail for each category (Klemetti, 1993)

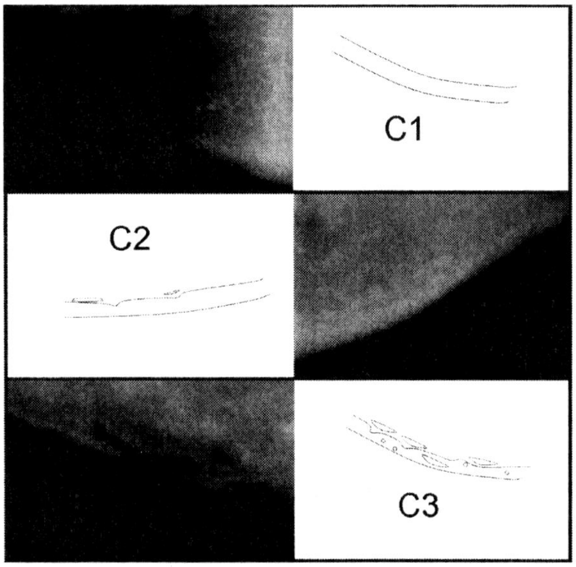

availability of bone quality data prior to surgery should be considered a prerequisite as such to adapt surgical procedures, alter implant sites and types to avoid surgical complications and/or to enhance implant outcome. Furthermore, radiographic jaw bone quality assessments are gaining importance in oral pathology to detect systemic diseases like osteoporosis. In addition, there is evidence that periodontal disease is increasing in the presence of osteoporosis (Swoboda, 2008) which makes this screening quite important.

The assessment methods vary from subjective ordinal classifications to mathematical processing of the radiographic material. A recurrent obstacle in studying these techniques is the acquisition of standardised images. More than in other skeletal sites, this standardisation is hard to achieve considering the complex jaw bone anatomy. Follow-up studies that require exact repositioning are hampered by this lack of standardisation as well as by potential changes that may occur intra-orally (tooth migration, attrition, extraction, bone loss …).

Clinical tools for objective *quantification* of jaw bone quality are sparse. Studies on this often use image registration methods that are not easily accessible in most patient care facilities or are not validated (Ribeiro-Rotta, 2007). For *qualitative evaluation* of jaw bone, no readily available and clinically reliable tools are present for routine use. Indeed, radiology is still to a large extent based on visual interpretation of radiographs, but the reliability of this interpretation has often been questioned (Ribeiro-Rotta, 2007). Therefore, assessment of bone quality and its importance in therapeutic planning and monitoring the progress of local or systemic bone disease will require more sophisticated methods.

Ordinal Classification

Several classifications based on oral radiographs are used in research and clinical practice. These classifications enable quantification, albeit simple, of otherwise subjective observation of the radiographic characteristics of the jaw bones.

On panoramic images, the Mandibular Cortical Index (MCI) subdivides the mandibular inferior cortex distally from the mental foramen into 3 classes: normal cortex (C1), mildly to moderately eroded cortex (C2) and severely eroded cortex (C3) (Klemetti, 1993) (see Figure 8). The MCI is often used in research on osteoporosis screening (Taguchi 2008).

The Bone Quality Index (BQI) is often used in implant planning. Lekholm & Zarb (1985) developed the index as a predictive tool for implant success. Although it was intended for use in tomographic images, the BQI is nowadays mostly based on panoramic radiographs. There are 4 classes: homogeneous cortical bone (1), thick cortical bone with marrow cavity (2), thin cortical bone with dense trabecular bone of good strength (3) and very thin cortical bone with low density trabecular bone of poor strength (4) (see Figure 9).

Figure 9. Bone Quality Index (BQI) by Lekholm & Zarb, 1985 (modified from Brånemark P. I. et al. (1985). Tissue-integrated prostheses: osseointegration in clinical dentistry, Chicago: Quintessence Publishing)

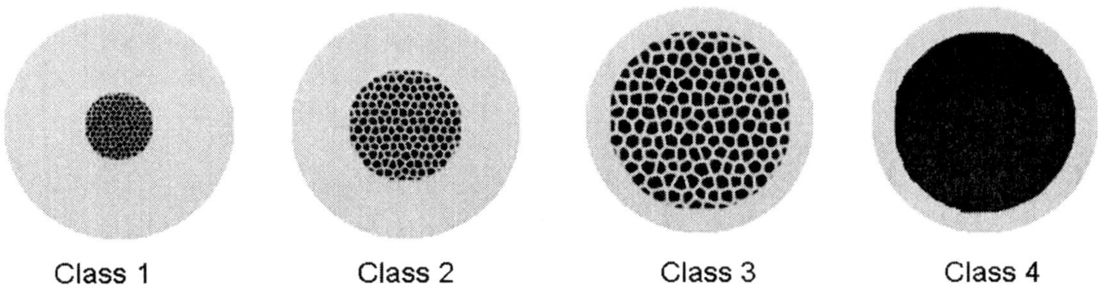

Lindh et al (1996) developed a classification of the trabecular pattern in intra-oral radiographs, classifying the pattern into: dense and homogeneous (1), heterogeneous (2) and sparse homogeneous (3). When performing the classification, reference radiographs are used to enhance inter-rater agreement (Figure 10). The Lindh classification is used in the assessment of bone quality before endosseous implant treatment and in research on osteoporosis screening.

In these ordinal classifications, good inter- and intra-rater agreement seems to be tricky, so whenever they are used in research, several observers should be included, as well as a training session to calibrate the observers. Moreover, it is not evident to find studies assessing the diagnostic accuracy of such classifications that fulfil the methodological criteria for diagnostic accuracy studies. Examples of problem issues in this context are the presentation of results that do not allow the actual assessment of diagnostic accuracy or biased interpretation of test results (Ribeiro-Rotta et al 2007). Although truly interesting from a clinical point of view, validation studies are needed to determine the true relevance in clinical practice of these classifications.

Radiographic Density

The degree of darkening of an image receptor exposed by X-rays is referred to as radiographic density. The radiographic density is influenced by

Figure 10. Reference radiographs showing the trabecular pattern on intraoral radiographs described by Lindh et al (1996) (modified from Lindh, C. et al, 2008). The use of visual assessment of dental radiographs for identifying women at risk of having osteoporosis, the OSTEODENT project.

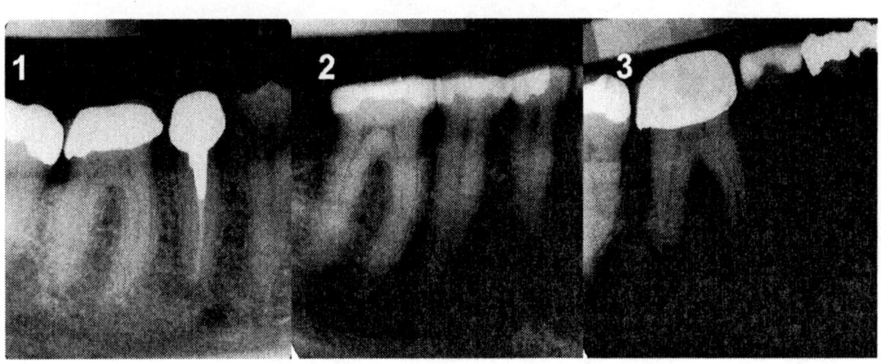

exposure time, thickness and density of a subject. In the assessment of bone quality, the mean and standard deviation of grey values in the region of interest can be used. However, grey values have limited use, as they can be influenced by many other factors, apart from actual bone changes or characteristics.

To obtain a more meaningful result, many researchers have used subtraction radiography for bone density changes on follow up radiographs. Digital subtraction radiography has been used for many years as a visual aid in the progression of bony lesions. It involves the acquisition of periapical radiographs at various time points, using reproducible angulation and exposure methods. Software is available to subtract the radiographs and underscore changes. Although a promising technique if applied with high precision (Jeffcoat, 1992; Du Tré, 2006), digital subtraction radiography is hardly feasible in clinical studies. The accurate interpretation of subtraction images demands pairs of radiographs of close to identical x-ray beam projection geometry, film position and contrast (Brägger, 2005). Digital image subtraction may yield quantitative, albeit relative, results, expressed as 'number of changed pixels x mean grey level change', when using computer assisted densitometric image analysis (CADIA). Although this is a step forward towards quantification of bone densitometric analysis, the comparison of change at different regions of interest requires a mineral or aluminium stepwedge for internal references. An aluminium stepwedge has similar absorption and scatter properties of bone and is therefore suitable for densitometric analysis and follow-up (see Figure 11).

Figure 11. (A) Aluminum step wedge integrated in the aiming device for radiographic acquisition. (B) Pre- and post- radiographs of the molar region of a dog. An artificial defect was created in the post radiograph. By subtracting both images, quantification of bone loss is possible.

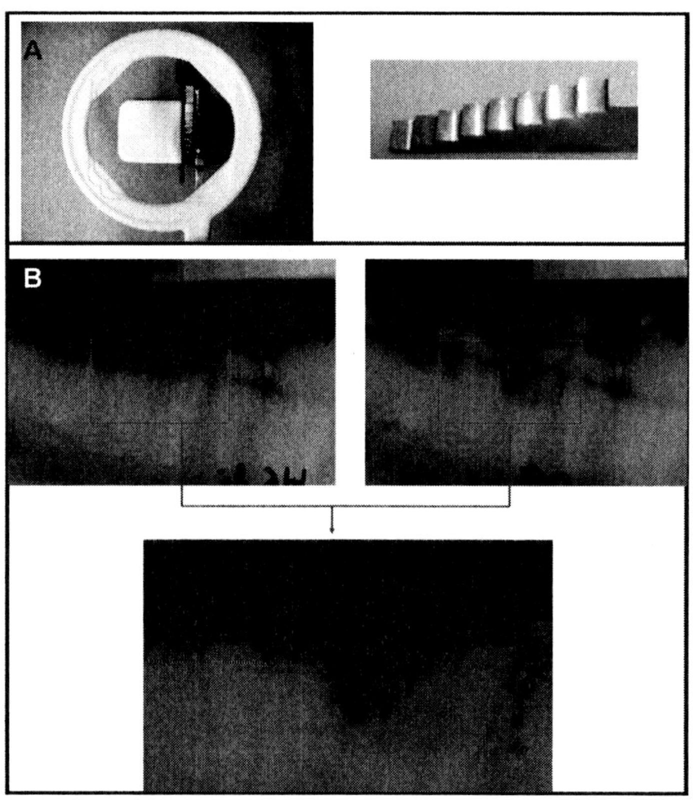

Radiomorphometry

Radiomorphometry is the application of anthropologic indices of bone morphology to radiographs. Mostly, these indices are based on measurements of cortical bone because it is more distinct on radiographs than trabecular bone.

Panoramic Mandibular Index (PMI)

The PMI was initially developed as a tool for osteoporosis screening by dentists, using a relative measure for cortical thickness (Benson et al, 1991). First, the shortest distance between the inferior border of the mandible and the superior and inferior margins of the mental foramen on panoramic radiographs is determined. On this line, the cortical width is measured and PMI is calculated as:

PMI (superior) = Thickness of cortex/Distance from superior margin of mental foramen to inferior border of mandible

PMI (inferior) = Thickness of cortex/Distance from inferior margin of mental foramen to inferior border of mandible.

Mandibular Cortical Thickness

In several studies, the PMI showed poor interobserver agreement, which is not surprising since the location of the mental foramen on a panoramic radiograph is not always unequivocal, let alone the definition of the upper and lower border. Furthermore, the index is based on two linear measurements, which introduces a cumulative error in the measurement. At present, the mandibular cortical thickness is more often used as a morphometric jaw bone index on panoramic radiographs. To determine the width, first a tangent to the lower mandibular border is drawn. Through the mental foramen, a perpendicular line to the first is created. On this perpendicular line, the cortical width is measured. If the cortex shows erosion, the thinnest compact cortical width should be considered.

Residual Ridge Height

Besides absolute and relative measures of local alveolar bone height in the evaluation of periodontal bone loss, residual ridge height is used to assess generalised ridge resorption (Xie, 1997). It is usually measured at the mental foramen site. It is also based on the tangent to the inferior mandibular border. The perpendicular to this tangent intersecting the inferior border of the mental foramen is the line used for measuring the ridge height; it is measured from the lower border of the mandible to the top of the alveolar crest.

Texture Analysis

Texture analysis of trabecular bone requires digital manipulation of the images. Due to the application of mathematical operations on the image, the results often depend on the applied parameters, but the analysing methods are more robust in quantifying the images than all previously mentioned methods (Apostol, 2006). This often makes textural analysis the method of choice in imaging research. A vast number of texture parameters exist; the ones described below do not form an exhaustive list, but are a selection of frequently used parameters in describing jaw bone structural properties.

The processing of 2D radiographs for texture analysis of bone starts with a binarisation of the image or the region of interest (see Figure 12). The bone is segmented as the foreground signal, often following an initial filtering to remove noise from the image. The segmentation is usually done with a thresholding technique. A binarised image can be seen in Figure 12, B. Based on the binary image, the bone area can be calculated, as well as the background area. The number of black and/or white regions can be counted, to have an idea of connectivity of the bone. By further skeletonising the binary image (see Figure 12, C), a number of measurements can be done on the wire version of the image. These are for instance the total frame length, the number of endpoints and the number

Figure 12. (A) Region of interest from original radiograph, (B) binarised region of interest, (C) skeletonised region of interest

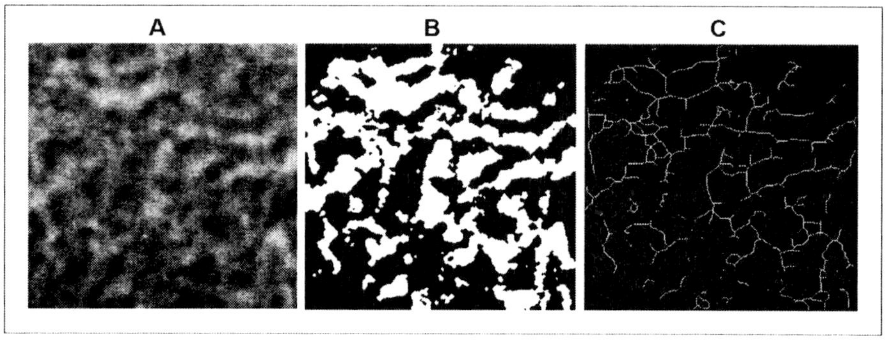

of nodes. This can be done for the white skeleton as well as the black.

Another form of textural analysis that is now widely used in all areas of science is fractal analysis. It can thus also be used for the characterisation of bone. Fractal analysis divides objects into fractals which are complex geometric shapes that have properties like self-similarity. Trabecular bone has a branching pattern which also exhibits this property. Research in this field using traditional dental imaging modalities is still sparse and with the rise of 3D modalities a new exciting approach to 3D texture analysis may arise.

NEW DEVELOPMENTS: PERIODONTAL DIAGNOSIS IN THREE DIMENSIONS

Two-dimensional radiographs are still the most commonly used modalities for periodontal diagnosis. Nevertheless, the process of bone remodeling is a dynamic process of osteoblastic and osteoclastic activity in three dimensions. Alveolar bone loss often presents infrabony defects with complex architecture which are difficult to image using these 2D techniques. The reason for their widespread recommendation is the ease of use, the low dose and the easy access of these technologies in clinical practice. Modern tomographic technologies have brought the third dimension into play, but it is only with the recent introduction of low dose cone beam CT, that a drastic change in periodontal diagnosis may occur.

Tuned Aperture and Traditional (Computed) Tomography

Conventional tomography produces a 2-dimensional cross-section by moving x-ray source and detector in opposite direction and in such a way that only the objects in a line of interest are imaged and the rest is blurred because of movement (cfr pantomography, but here a linear line of interest or a cross-section). Unfortunately, this technique causes magnification of the cross-section and is of poor diagnostic quality due to the inherent blur of the method (Kassebaum, 1990). In addition, multiple slices have to be obtained successively for adequate diagnosis and treatment planning of the region of interest which makes the process time-consuming and is associated with a relatively high radiation dose.

To further address the need of three dimensional imaging, tuned aperture computed tomography (TACT™) was introduced. It is based on principles of tomosynthesis but uses traditional projection radiography. By shifting the x-ray tube, projections can be obtained from multiple angles and cross-sections can be reconstructed using the TACT

Figure 13. (A) Principle of spiral CT, multiple convolutions are needed to scan the entire dental region (B) cone beam computed tomography utilizes a conical beam which makes one rotation sufficient for imaging the whole dento-alveolar area

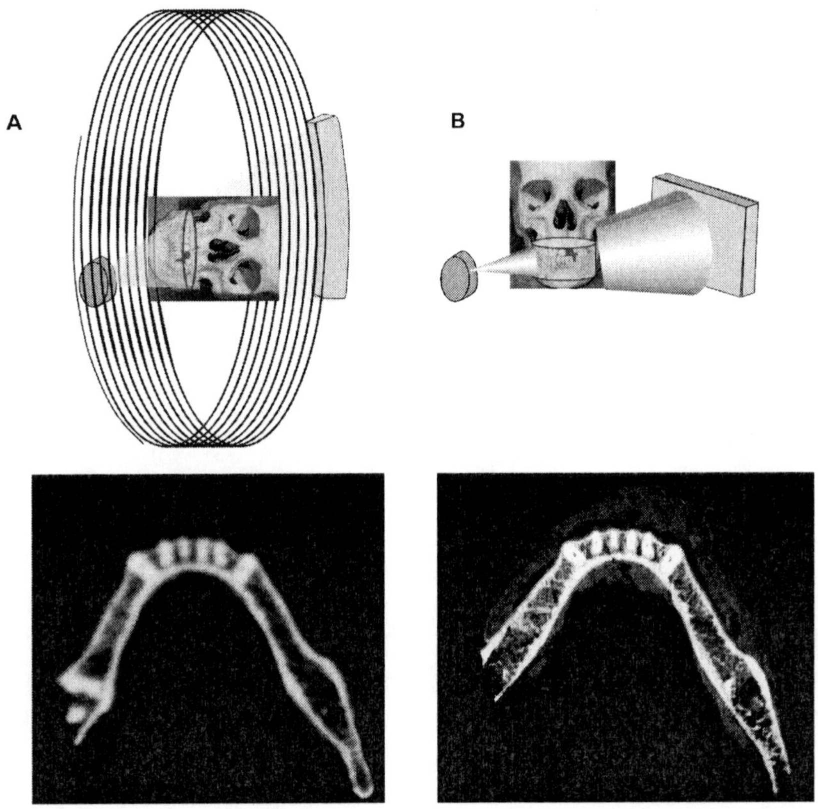

algorithm, which eliminates blur and sharpens the view of sections through defects. Many studies have shown the potential of this technique for detection of osseous defects and the advantage over traditional radiography (Webber, 1997). However, the method –just like for DSR- requires a complex multiradiographic method with precise and similar projection geometry, making this approach appropriate for research but unpractical for clinical practice.

A more promising technique for 3D imaging was the development of axial computed tomography (CT) which uses a narrow fan beam that rotates around the patient to generate an axial slice without distortion or magnification. A sequential scanning for multiple slices was still needed but spiral CT quickly filled in this need. By moving the patient (table) into the gantry of the unit and using a continuous rotation of the x-ray beam, a helical or spiral path is described which generates multiple slices that can be stacked into a volume (see Figure 13, A). This stack of slices can be reformatted into the sagittal or coronal direction which is called multiplanar reformatting (MPR). Primarily, CT is being used in medicine for imaging the whole body, but because of these excellent 3D capabilities, its use in dentistry has been researched and validated for many years. The third dimension namely allows locating important anatomical structures like the inferior alveolar canal and maxillary sinusses, or allows assessing the width and height of the alveolar process, thus aiding in precise planning of implant surgery (Preda, 1997). For the detection of periodontal defects causing furcation problems, Fuhrmann et al (1997) performed a comparison between intraoral radiographs and CT scanning and found that only 21% of the furcation defects were visible using radiography compared to 100% for CT.

Despite its excellent contrast resolution, the major drawbacks of this technology are high cost, limited spatial resolution and a high radiation dose. Further improvements have already been made for the latter two and modern multi-slice spiral CT units have reached sub-millimeter accuracy at lower radiation doses.

Cone Beam Computed Tomography

In contrary to medical computed tomography, cone beam computed tomography (CBCT) distinguishes itself by a different scan procedure. In stead of obtaining the region of interest (ROI) or volume slice-by-slice using a fan-shaped beam, it utilizes a conical beam which only makes one convolution around the patient's head: the dentomaxillofacial complex is scanned entirely in one rotation (see Figure 13, B).

The detector row used in spiral CT is replaced by a plat panel detector which allows acquiring radiographic projections of the jaws from all angles in a 360° rotation. From the scanned volume, axial slices are reconstructed and MPR is made possible. The different method to obtain these axial cross-sections makes that both CT and CBCT have some different intrinsic properties. Since only one rotation is needed, the associated high radiation dose of medical CT has greatly been decreased. Furthermore, the CBCT detectors have an excellent spatial resolution and reach sizes as small as 75micron (compared to 0.5-1mm for medical CT). This allows for an excellent and detailed visualization of the bony structures in the maxillofacial complex (see Figure 13). Furthermore, CBCT units are compact-sized and the cost is drastically less than medical CT. Disadvantage of CBCT is the lower contrast resolution which limits imaging of low contrast structures like soft tissue imaging. Also, the conical shape of the beam makes reconstruction more difficult since the algorithm has to take account for this beam angle. In contrary, with spiral CT, slices are generated horizontally. The advantage of CT over CBCT is the high contrast resolution which allows distinguishing tissues with very small differences in physical density like for instance different soft tissues.

A drastic change has occurred in dental imaging since the introduction of modern CBCT technology. When making the cost-benefit analysis for decision making of a patient's examination type, the clinician should always justify the use of ionization radiation and follow the ALARA (as low as reasonably achievable) principle and this for each patient individually. When the added value of 3D information is required -for instance in the planning of dental implants- CBCT is thus the imaging modality of choice given the small radiation dose. The latter has been found to be within the range of an intraoral FMX or of only a couple of panoramic radiographs. When using the latest imaging protocols for adequate dose reductions with fast films or digital systems, the dose of an FMX using a PSP system may be around 34.5 μSv, but this may run up to 100 μSv when following incorrect or outdated guidelines (Ludlow, 2008, Gibbs, 2000). This range is also found for CBCT examinations although it depends on the specific type of CBCT unit and its settings like the field-of-view (FOV), kV and mAs (Palomo, 2008).

For periodontal diagnosis, the discussion on CBCT examinations has only recently started and it seems to be a controversial topic considering the limited research published in the field and the already controversial discussion around the usefulness of a radiographic examination in Periodontology (Tugnait, 2000). Much information can be derived from the clinical examination alone, but for more complex patterns of bone destruction and the multitude of modern regenerative treatment techniques, the 3-dimensional examination seems inevitable.

Figure 14. (A) Axial slice through the dry skull at the level of the furcation of the right mandibular first molar. A disto-lingual defect of the first right molar is already visible (Note that this is a view from below). The orange line is the sagittal slice in the multiplanar view of the skull (B). When moving the slice from buccal to oral (green arrow), the clinician can scroll through the region of interest (C).

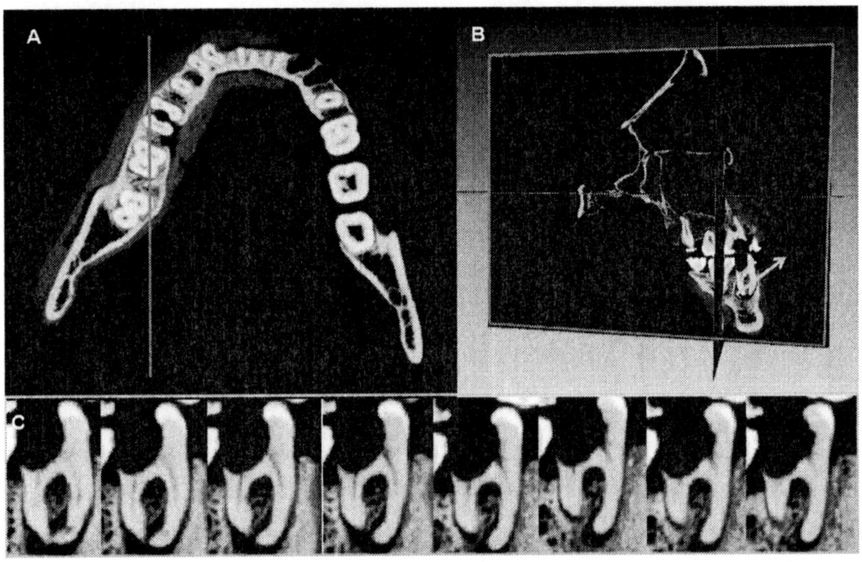

3D Periodontal Assessments

Adding a third dimension to the radiographic image of the periodontium, requires a thorough understanding of periodontal anatomy in 3D. While only two interproximal mesial and distal measurements on intraoral radiographs are used to estimate alveolar bone loss, many more measurements are possible in 3D. Furthermore, not only buccal and oral measurements are possible, but the exact topography of infrabony craters can be derived by scrolling through the data. In Figure 14, the same molar region of the dry skull in Figure 3B is imaged using CBCT.

On the standardized projection radiograph in Figure 3B, an infrabony defect distally of the first molar and possibly a furcation involvement are suspected, but no information can be derived on the exact interproximal, buccal or palatal bone topography. The CBCT data in Figure 14 allows orthogonal reconstructions of axial, sagittal and coronal slices (Figure 14B). By scrolling through the sagittal slice (Figure 14C, from left to right= buccal to lingual) it can be noticed that the distal bone of the first molar is present buccally, but is slowly breaking down towards the lingual side. This confirms the lingual position of the infrabony crater which was suspected in the radiograph. When inspecting the furcation when scrolling, bone loss can be seen when moving lingually, which allows correct classification of the involvement.

Besides orthogonal reslicing or MPR of the axial data, oblique reslicing in all directions is also possible. One useful example of this is the simulation of a panoramic overview. By drawing an oblique line that follows the jaw's arch, an overview of the periodontal bone is possible at sub-millimeter slice thickness (see Figure 15A). By raising the slice thickness -or in other words stacking several slices on top of each other- a high resolution panoramic reconstruction is simulated without the several image artefacts of the pantomographic technique (see Figure 15B).

Furthermore, true 3-dimensional evaluation is made possible by software which allows render-

Figure 15. (A) The oblique line drawn onto the axial slice through the mandible is reconstructed as an oblique reformatting of the CBCT data. (B) By raising the slice thickness, the oblique reformat is widened to include more structures and simulate a high resolution panoramic overview.

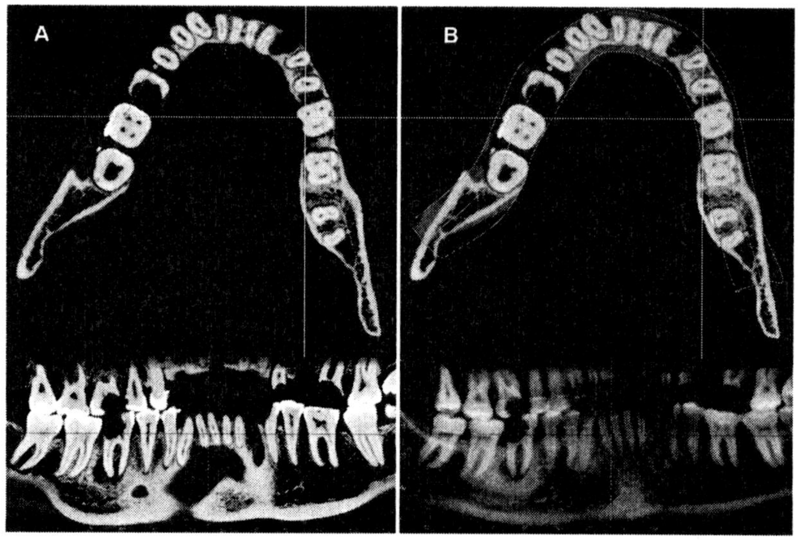

ing of the CBCT data into a volume (see Figure 16). Just like any digital image, CBCT data has a histogram showing the grey values attributed to each pixel or voxel. By choosing a threshold value, all grey values below or above this threshold are included in the rendered volume. This allows for 3-dimensional display of different structures, like the bony contours with or without the overlying soft tissues. A careful interpretation of the CBCT data is thus a prerequisite, and a diagnosis should never only be based on such display tools. For instance, bony particles can have many dif-

Figure 16. (A) Rendered volume showing the dry bony skull from Figure 15 and 3. A soft tissue simulating material was modelled over the upper and lower jaw. (B) Rendered volume without the soft tissues revealing the alveolar bone (Note that CBCT images do not properly allow to discern the gingival tissues from the surrounding lips and cheeks). (C) The right mandibular sided cropped out of the volume and seen from lingual to inspect the lingual bone loss of the first mandibular molar.

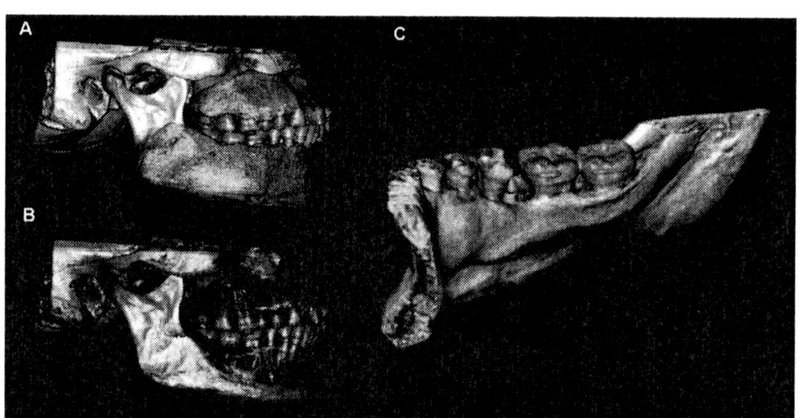

Figure 17. (A) CBCT scanning was done by aiming the horizontal positioning line parallel to the mandibular border. Since the molar teeth are inclined, the coronal slice -standard reformatted orthogonally onto the axial- is not parallel to the longitudinal axes of the teeth. (B) By adjusting the coronal slice (oblique reformat), correct measurements, parallel to the teeth's axes, can be done.

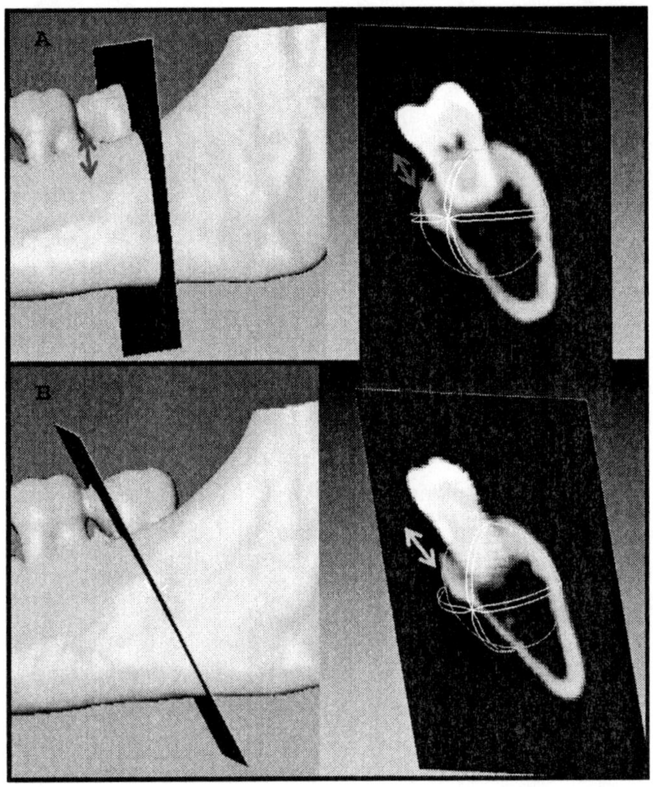

ferent grey values depending on their density (calcification degree). Thus, a certain threshold may exclude some bony particles in the rendered volume. Therefore, the histogram should be used to see which structures are displayed in 3D.

Alveolar Bone Loss: Measurement Accuracy

When making measurements on CBCT data -weather it is for alveolar bone loss or for implant site assessment- it is foremost important to mention that patient positioning is crucial when investigating alveolar bone. When scanning a patient along the occlusal plane, axial slices are obtained parallel this plane, while the reformatted orthogonal cross-sections will be perpendicular to the axial one. Assuming a normal occlusal pattern with normal dental alignment, the sagittal and coronal slice should then be approximately parallel to the central axes of the teeth. This will allow for correct measurements. However, when tilting the scan plane or when certain teeth are abnormally tilted in the dentition, alveolar bone level measurement deviations will increase or decrease because orthogonal reslices are not parallel to the teeth's axes. Figure 17 is an example of this phenomenon when a jaw is scanned along the border of the mandibular body.

For this reason, it is important to scan along the occlusal plane, or in inevitable or incorrect cases, to adjust the orthogonal slices and create oblique ones.

Many recent in-vitro studies have compared the accuracy of alveolar bone loss measurements on intraoral radiographs and CBCT cross-sections.

Some of them use in-vitro standardization methods which cannot be used in clinical practice but find that CBCT reaches an excellent sub-millimeter measurement accuracy which indicates that no magnification of the images is present (Mengel, 2005). Other studies with cadaver jaws use occlusal alignment of the specimens and still found that measurement accuracy of alveolar bone loss assessed on 1mm CBCT cross-sections is at least as reliable as intraoral radiography and as good as direct measurements using a probe (Misch, 2007). Vandenberghe et al (2008) compared alveolar bone loss assessment on 5.2mm oblique reformatted slices (panoramic overview) and found these measurements as reliable as intraoral radiographic measurements (0.03-1.69mm deviation error for CBCT compared to 0.01-1.65mm for intraoral radiography). When measuring on orthogonal slices of 0.4mm thickness, CBCT was found more accurate than intraoral radiography (deviation errors of 0.04-0.9mm for CBCT 0.4mm cross-sections.

These studies thus point out that accuracy is at least equal or higher using CBCT and that it is not only important to use a correct scanning protocol, but also to use an adequate voxel-size or slice thickness for the assessments. However, clinical studies have to be conducted to see if these results are similar in a clinical environment.

Infrabony Defects and Furcation Involvement Diagnosis

Since many modern periodontal treatment techniques are dependent of the topography of infrabony craters or on the degree of furcation involvement, these may be the periodontal manifestations that need standard 3D assessment. Therefore, laboratory studies have compared the diagnostic accuracy of CBCT compared to 2D radiographs in the detection of these defects. All these studies point out that CBCT is a superior imaging technique (Mengel, 2005; Misch, 2006; Vandenberghe, 2007; Vandenberghe, 2008). One clinical study from Walter et al confirmed these results. They conclude that CBCT may be a suitable imaging modality to make adequate treatment decisions of periodontally affected maxillary molars. These are encouraging results and preliminary guidelines for CBCT use have already included that CBCT may be a desirable method in selected cases where complex periodontal defects cannot be adequately assessed clinically and radiographically.

Other Periodontal Landmarks: Subjective Image Quality

The visualization of periodontal landmarks like lamina dura, periodontal ligament (PDL) space and trabecularization of alveolar bone is also possible using CBCT. However, in general, these landmarks seem to be better perceived on intraoral radiography (Vandenberghe, 2008). This is due to the limited contrast resolution of CBCT and the many artefacts present. However, more research needs to be performed since modern CBCT units are showing improved contrast and spatial resolution while new metal artifact reduction (MAR) algorithms are being developed.

Liang et al compared the subjective image quality of five different CBCT units to multi-slice computed tomography (MSCT) and found that image quality was comparable or even superior to MSCT. Still, lamina dura delineation, PDL space and trabecular pattern of bone scored the least and ratings vary depending on the CBCT unit.

Bone Density Assessments

Because of the nature of the CBCT technique, Hounsfield units, the standard in bone density evaluation on CT images, are not applicable. The CT numbers derived from CBCT deviate depending on CBCT unit and even on patient positioning. However, since high resolution images of the jaw bone can be produced, without the need for biopsies as would be the case for μ-CT or histology, it is worthwhile investigating methods for objectively quantifying bone quality on CBCT images. One study from Hua et al (2009) using mandibular bone samples seems to point out

Figure 18. (A) Optical scan alignment with the CBCT reconstruction of the dentition. (B) Registered optical scan on the CBCT slices or volume. (Courtesy of Sirona Dental Systems GmbH, Bensheim, Germany).

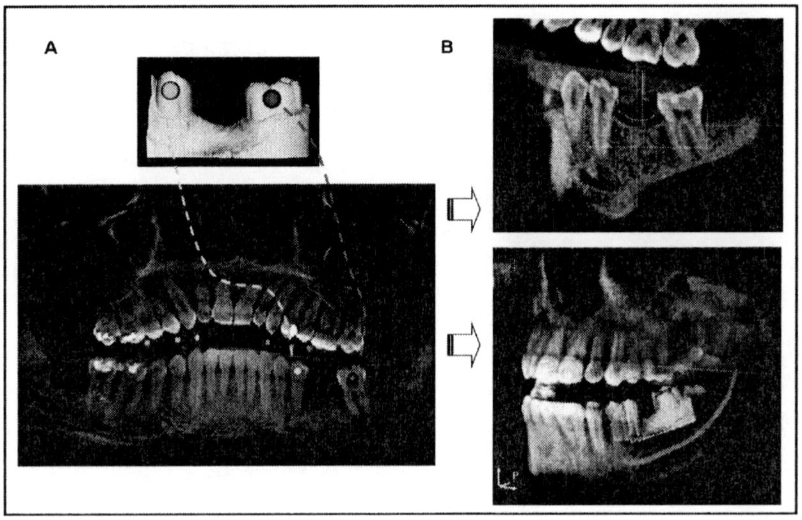

that methods like fractal analysis and bone area measurements may have potential in assessment of bone quality on CBCT images but that density measurements do not seem to be valid.

To analyse the bone structure, 3D characteristics as in μ-CT can be applied. After segmentation, morphological measures like trabecular number, trabecular separation, trabecular thickness and bone volume relative to the total volume can be calculated.

Future and Advanced Applications

Although low dose 3D CBCT has opened the door for exploration of many research areas and applications in clinical and computerized dentistry, only two important aspect will briefly be covered in the future expectations of CBCT related to periodontal diagnosis.

Soft Tissue Imaging

One of the standard clinical assessments in periodontal diagnosis is the clinical probing of the pockets around each tooth. This process is quite painful for the patient, is time-consuming and is observer-dependent. Unfortunately, CBCT does not allow visualizing the gingival tissues around the teeth which makes computerized assessments of these measurements not possible. Researchers are starting to investigate this area and several paths towards this goal are being followed.

A modification of the CBCT scanning protocol has been proposed by Januario et al (2008). Using a lip retractor during scanning, the cheeks and lips are being separated from the gingival tissues and the tongue is pressed down in the oral cavity. This soft tissue CBCT or ST-CBCT protocol allowed the researchers to measure the relation of soft and hard tissues with measurements of the CEJ to the gingival margin, of the bony crest to the gingival margin and of the gingival thickness.

Recently, CBCT images have been combined or fused with optical scanning of the dentition in the planning of implants. This would allow for a more precise design of the implant prosthesis and planning of proper occlusal relations (see Figure 18). CBCT has namely often many artefacts at the level of the enamel, especially when the patient is in occlusion during scanning. Perfect occlusal pattern segmentation is therefore almost not feasible and accuracy should be doubted upon.

Optical scans of the dentition are able to visualize the gingival tissues (see Figure 18) and more research should be conducted in its accuracy for registration with CBCT images. This fusion of images from different modalities may thus bring many more possibilities in the near future.

3D Follow-Up

An interesting and very promising area is the follow-up of bone in three dimensions. This would allow for accurate assessment of periodontal regenerative therapy or even implant evaluation. Grimard et al (Grimard, 2009) compared clinical, periapical radiograph and CBCT measurement techniques for assessing bone level changes after periodontal regenerative surgery and found that CBCT measurements correlated strongly with surgical ones. Still, only two dimensions are actually used since assessments were done on 2D slices of CBCT. Furthermore, the question arises if one or two (width and/or height) measurements are actually enough for assessment of 3D treatment outcomes. Better would be to use a volumetric (in mm^3) analysis which may be one of the powerful tools of the future.

No published studies have been conducted using CBCT volumes for periodontal bone follow-up. Feichtinger et al (2007) used medical CT to assess bone resorption after secondary bone grafting. A manual segmentation method was used in this study: by drawing the borders of the region of interest (ROI), namely the bony grafting site at start, on each slice using specific software, a small volume is segmented that can be compared to a follow-up scan at a later time. These volumetric assessments were found a very useful method. Nevertheless, CT was used in this study with a slice thickness or spatial resolution of 1mm. In addition, this method also may be quite labor intensive.

Therefore, researchers are investigating new image analysis tools for volumetric follow-up using CBCT. In a recent ongoing study from Vandenberghe et al (abstract presented at IADMFR

Figure 19. (A) CBCT scan volume of a dry skull prior to defect creation (blue) and CBCT scan volume after defect creation (red) in the buccal plate of the incisor region, with respective sagittal slices. (B) Both PRE and POST scan are displayed on top of each other for final registration (bottom).

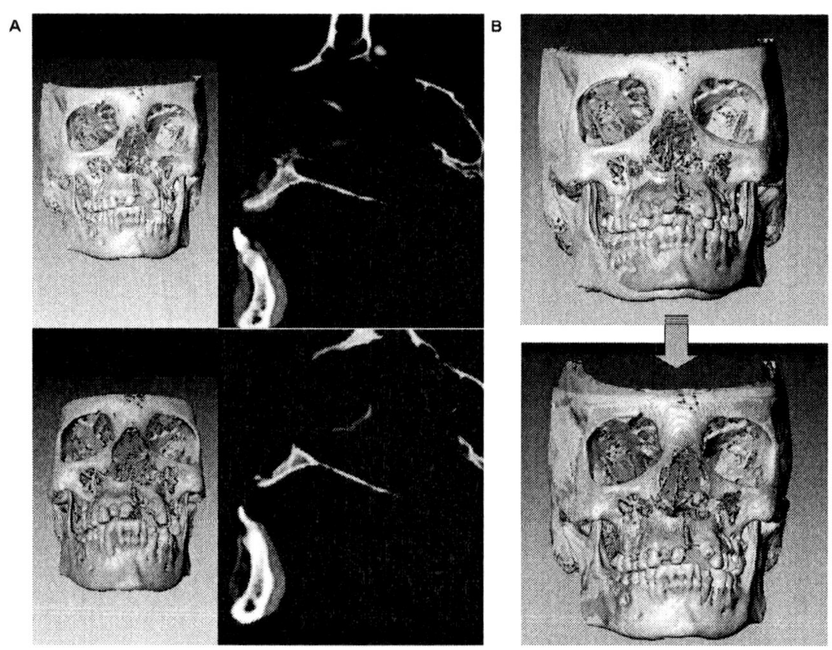

2009), several specimens (dry skulls and cadaver jaws) were scanned using CBCT before and after defect creation. The small defects were created at the level of the buccal plate of the incisor region. This defect type was chosen, in order to simulate buccal bone loss after buccal grafting or site preservation, which is an often encountered problem in clinical practice (see Figure 19).

Bone loss was estimated using different segmentation tools and compared to the gold standard, being the negative of the defect volume (imprint using hard wax and scanned with μ-CT). Preliminary results indicate that the typical manual slice-by-slice segmentation results in the largest volumetric measurement deviations. Other segmentation strategies like simple thresholding or region growing are more promising methods, especially when combining them with image registration. This registration is the translation and rotation of the CBCT scans in order to obtain identical spatial coordinates. Still, only future studies will point out which method may be desirable, not only as a research tool, but also as a tool for clinical use.

REFERENCES

Analoui, M. (2001). Radiographic image enhancement. Part I: spatial domain techniques. *Dento Maxillo Facial Radiology*, *30*(1), 1–9. doi:10.1038/sj.dmfr.4600562

Apostol, L., Boudousq, V., Basset, O., Odet, V., Yot, S., & Tabary, J. (2006). Relevance of 2D radiographic texture analysis for the assessment of 3D bone micro-architecture. *Medical Physics*, *33*(9), 3546–3556. doi:10.1118/1.2211727

Armitage, G. C., Research, Science and Therapy Committee of the American Academy of Periodontology. (2003). Diagnosis of periodontal diseases. *Journal of Periodontology*, *74*(8), 1237–1247. doi:10.1902/jop.2003.74.8.1237

Bassiouny, M. A., & Grant, A. A. (1976). Radiographic assessment of infrabony pocket topography. *Journal of Periodontology*, *47*(8), 440–443.

Berkhout, W. E., Beuger, D. A., Sanderink, G. C., & van der Stelt, P. F. (2004). The dynamic range of digital radiographic systems: dose reduction or risk of overexposure? *Dento Maxillo Facial Radiology*, *33*(1), 1–5. doi:10.1259/dmfr/40677472

Borg, E., Attaelmanan, A., & Gröndahl, H. G. (2000). Subjective image quality of solid-state and photostimulable storage phosphor systems for digital intra-oral radiography. *Dento Maxillo Facial Radiology*, *29*(2), 70–75. doi:10.1038/sj.dmfr.4600501

Borg, E., Gröndahl, K., & Gröndahl, H. G. (1997). Marginal bone level buccal to mandibular molars in digital radiographs from charge-coupled device and storage phosphor systems. An in vitro study. *Journal of Clinical Periodontology*, *24*(5), 306–312. doi:10.1111/j.1600-051X.1997.tb00762.x

Brägger, U. (2005). Radiographic parameters: biological significance and clinical use. *Periodontology 2000*, *39*, 73–90. doi:10.1111/j.1600-0757.2005.00128.x

Du Tré, F., Jacobs, R., Styven, S., & van Steenberghe, D. (2006). Development of a novel digital subtraction technique for detecting subtle changes in jawbone density. *Clinical Oral Investigations*, *10*(3), 235–248. doi:10.1007/s00784-006-0055-2

Eickholz, P., & Hausmann, E. (2000). Accuracy of radiographic assessment of interproximal bone loss in intrabony defects using linear measurements. *European Journal of Oral Sciences*, *108*(1), 70–73. doi:10.1034/j.1600-0722.2000.00729.x

Eickholz, P., Riess, T., Lenhard, M., Hassfeld, S., & Staehle, H. J. (1999). Digital radiography of interproximal bone loss: validity of different filters. *Journal of Clinical Periodontology*, *26*(5), 294–300. doi:10.1034/j.1600-051X.1999.260506.x

Eley, B. M., & Cox, S. W. (1998). Advances in periodontal diagnosis. 3. Assessing potential biomarkers of periodontal disease activity. *British Dental Journal*, *184*(3), 109–113. doi:10.1038/sj.bdj.4809556

Feichtinger, M., Mossbock, R., & Karcher, H. (2007). Assessments of bone resorption after secondary alveolar bone grafting using three-dimensional computed tomography: a three-year study. *The Cleft Palate-Craniofacial Journal*, *44*(2), 142–148. doi:10.1597/06-047.1

Fuhrmann, R. A., Bücker, A., & Diedrich, P. R. (1997). Furcation involvement: comparison of dental radiographs and HR-CT slices in human specimens. *Journal of Periodontal Research*, *32*(5), 409–418. doi:10.1111/j.1600-0765.1997.tb00553.x

Gibbs, S. J. (2000). Effective dose equivalent and effective dose: comparison for common projections in oral and maxillofacial radiology. *Oral Surgery, Oral Medicine, Oral Pathology, Oral Radiology, and Endodontics*, *90*(4), 538–545. doi:10.1067/moe.2000.109189

Grimard, B. A., Hoidal, M. J., Mills, M. P., Mellonig, J. T., Nummikoski, P. V., & Mealy, B. L. (2009). Comparison of clinical, periapical radiograph, and cone-beam volume tomography measurement techniques for assessing bone level changes following regenerative periodontal therapy. *Journal of Periodontology*, *80*(1), 48–55. doi:10.1902/jop.2009.080289

Hamp, S. E., Nyman, S., & Lindhe, J. (1975). Periodontal treatment of multirooted teeth. Results after 5 years. *Journal of Clinical Periodontology*, *2*(3), 126–135. doi:10.1111/j.1600-051X.1975.tb01734.x

Hausmann, E., & Allen, K. (1997). Reproducibility of bone height measurements made on serial radiographs. *Journal of Periodontology*, *68*(9), 839–841.

Hefti, A. F. (1997). Periodontal probing. *Critical Reviews in Oral Biology and Medicine*, *8*(3), 336–356. doi:10.1177/10454411970080030601

Heo, M. S., Choi, D. H., Benavides, E., Huh, K. H., Yi, W. J., Lee, S. S., & Choi, S. C. (2009). Effect of bit depth and kVp of digital radiography for detection of subtle differences. *Oral Surgery, Oral Medicine, Oral Pathology, Oral Radiology, and Endodontics*, *108*(2), 278–283. doi:10.1016/j.tripleo.2008.12.053

Herrmann, I., Lekholm, U., Holm, S., & Kultje, C. (2005). Evaluation of patient and implant characteristics as potential prognostic factors for oral implant failures. *The International Journal of Oral & Maxillofacial Implants*, *20*(2), 220–230.

Hua, Y., Nackaerts, O., Duyck, J., Maes, F., & Jacobs, R. (2009). Bone quality assessment based on cone beam computed tomography imaging. *Clinical Oral Implants Research*, *20*(8), 767–771. doi:10.1111/j.1600-0501.2008.01677.x

Januario, A. L., Barriviera, M., & Duarte, W. R. (2008). Soft tissue cone-beam computed tomography: a novel method for the measurement of gingival tissue and the dimensions of the dentogingival unit. *Journal of Esthetic and Restorative Dentistry*, *20*(6), 366–373. doi:10.1111/j.1708-8240.2008.00210.x

Jeffcoat, M. K., & Reddy, M. S. (1991). Progression of probing attachment loss in adult periodontitis. *Journal of Periodontology*, *62*(3), 185–189.

Jeffcoat, M. K., Reddy, M. S., van den Berg, H. R., & Bertens, E. (1992). Quantitative digital subtraction radiography for the assessment of peri-implant bone change. *Clinical Oral Implants Research*, *3*(1), 22–27. doi:10.1034/j.1600-0501.1992.030104.x

Jorgenson, T., Masood, F., Beckerley, J. M., Burqin, C., & Parker, D. E. (2007). Comparison of two imaging modalities: F-speed film and digital images for detection of osseous defects in patients with interdental vertical bone loss. *Dento Maxillo Facial Radiology*, *36*(8), 500–505. doi:10.1259/dmfr/29704550

Kaepller, G., Vogel, A., & Axmann-Krcmar, D. (2000). Intra-oral storage phosphor and conventional radiography in the assessment of alveolar bone structures. *Dento Maxillo Facial Radiology*, *29*(6), 362–367. doi:10.1038/sj.dmfr.4600556

Karn, K. W., Shockett, H. P., Moffitt, W. C., & Gray, J. L. (1984). Topographic classification of deformities of the alveolar process. *Journal of Periodontology*, *55*(6), 336–340.

Kassebaum, D. K., Nummikoski, P. V., Triplett, R. G., & Langlais, R. P. (1990). Cross-sectional radiography for implant site assessment. *Oral Surgery, Oral Medicine, and Oral Pathology*, *70*(5), 674–678. doi:10.1016/0030-4220(90)90421-N

Khader, Y. S., Albashaireh, Z. S., & Alomari, M. A. (2004). Periodontal diseases and the risk of coronary heart and cerebrovascular diseases: a meta-analysis. *Journal of Periodontology*, *75*(8), 1046–1053. doi:10.1902/jop.2004.75.8.1046

Klemetti, E., Kolmakov, S., Heiskanen, P., Vainio, P., & Lasilla, V. (1993). Panoramic mandibular index and bone mineral densities in postmenopausal women. *Oral Surgery, Oral Medicine, and Oral Pathology*, *75*(6), 774–779. doi:10.1016/0030-4220(93)90438-A

Künzel, A., Scherkowski, D., Willers, R., & Becker, J. (2003). Visually detectable resolution of intraoral dental films. *Dento Maxillo Facial Radiology*, *32*(6), 385–389. doi:10.1259/dmfr/22478778

Lekholm, U., & Zarb, G. A. (1985). Patient selection and preparation. In P. I. Brånemark, G.A. Zarb, T. Albrekttson, (Ed.), *Tissue-integrated prostheses: osseointegration in clinical dentistry*, (pp. 1-356). Chicago: Quintessence Publishing.

Lerner, U. H. (2006). Inflammation-induced bone remodelling in periodontal disease and the influence of post-menopausal osteoporosis. *Journal of Dental Research*, *85*(7), 596–607. doi:10.1177/154405910608500704

Li, G., Engström, P. E., Nasström, K., Lü, Z. Y., Sanderink, G., & Welander, U. (2007). Marginal bone levels measured in film and digital radiographs corrected for attenuation and visual response: an in-vitro study. *Dento Maxillo Facial Radiology*, *36*(1), 7–11. doi:10.1259/dmfr/28315324

Liang, X., Jacobs, R., Hassan, B., Li, L., Pauwels, R., Corpas, L., Souza, P. C., Martens, W., et al. (2009). A comparative evaluation of Cone Beam Computed Tomography (CBCT) and Multi-Slice CT (MSCT) Part I. On subjective image quality. *Eur J Radiol,* (e-pub ahead of print).

Lindh, C., Horner, K., Jonasson, G., Olsson, P., Rohlin, M., & Jacobs, R. (2008). The use of visual assessment of dental radiographs for identifying women at risk of having osteoporosis: the OSTEODENT project. *Oral Surgery, Oral Medicine, Oral Pathology, Oral Radiology, and Endodontics*, *106*(2), 285–293. doi:10.1016/j.tripleo.2007.09.008

Lindh, C., Petersson, A., & Rohlin, M. (1996). Assessment of the trabecular pattern before endosseous implant treatment: diagnostic outcome of periapical radiography in the mandible. *Oral Surgery, Oral Medicine, Oral Pathology, Oral Radiology, and Endodontics*, *82*(3), 335–343. doi:10.1016/S1079-2104(96)80363-5

Loos, B., Nylund, K., Claffey, N., & Egelberg, J. (1989). Clinical effects of root debridement in molar and non-molar teeth. A 2-year follow-up. *Journal of Clinical Periodontology, 16*(8), 498–504. doi:10.1111/j.1600-051X.1989.tb02326.x

Ludlow, J. B., Davies-Ludlow, L. E., & White, S. C. (2008). Patient risk related to common dental radiographic examinations: the impact of 2007 International Commission on Radiological Protection recommendations regarding dose calculation. *The Journal of the American Dental Association, 139*(9), 1237–1243.

McDavid, W. D., Welander, U., Pillai, B. K., & Morris, C. R. (1982). The Intrex—a constant-potential x-ray unit for periapical dental radiography. *Oral Surgery, Oral Medicine, and Oral Pathology, 53*(4), 433–436. doi:10.1016/0030-4220(82)90448-0

Mengel, R., Candir, M., Shiratori, K., & Flores-de-Jacoby, L. (2005). Digital volume tomography in the diagnosis of periodontal defects: an in vitro study on native pig and human mandibles. *Journal of Periodontology, 76*(5), 665–673. doi:10.1902/jop.2005.76.5.665

Misch, K. A., Yi, E. S., & Sarment, D. P. (2006). Accuracy of cone beam computed tomography for periodontal defect measurements. *J Peridontol, 77*(7), 1261–1266. doi:10.1902/jop.2006.050367

Molander, B., Ahlqwist, M., & Gröndhal, A. G. (1995). Panoramic and restrictive intraoral radiography in comprehensive oral radiographic diagnosis. *European Journal of Oral Sciences, 103*(4), 191–198. doi:10.1111/j.1600-0722.1995.tb00159.x

Nyman, S., & Lindhe, J. (1997). Examination of patients with periodontal disease. In J. Lindhe, T. Karring, N. P. Lang (Ed.), *Clinical periodontology and implant dentistry, 3* (pp. 383-395). Copenhagen: Munksgard.

Oliveira Costa, F., Cota, L. O., Costa, J. E., & Pordeus, I. A. (2007). Periodontal disease progression among young subjects with no preventive dental care: a 52-month follow-up study. *Journal of Periodontology, 78*(2), 198–203. doi:10.1902/jop.2007.060150

Palomo, J. M., Rao, P. S., & Hans, M. G. (2008). Influence of exposure conditions on radiation dose. *Oral Surgery, Oral Medicine, Oral Pathology, Oral Radiology, and Endodontics, 105*(6), 773–782. doi:10.1016/j.tripleo.2007.12.019

Pecoraro, M., Azadivatan-le, N., Janal, M., & Khocht, A. (2005). Comparison of observer reliability in assessing alveolar bone height on direct digital and conventional radiographs. *Dento Maxillo Facial Radiology, 34*(5), 279–284. doi:10.1259/dmfr/13900561

Pepelassi, E. A., & Diamanti-Kipioti, A. (1997). Selection of the most accurate method of conventional radiography for the assessment of periodontal osseous destruction. *Journal of Clinical Periodontology, 24*(8), 557–567. doi:10.1111/j.1600-051X.1997.tb00229.x

Preda, L., Di Maggio, E. M., Dore, R., La Fianza, A., Solcia, M., & Schifino, M. R. (1997). Use of spiral computed tomography for multiplanar dental reconstruction. *Dento Maxillo Facial Radiology, 26*(6), 327–331. doi:10.1038/sj.dmfr.4600290

Quirynen, M., Callens, A., van Steenberghe, D., & Nys, M. (1993). Clinical evaluation of a constant force electronic probe. *Journal of Periodontology, 64*(1), 35–39.

Ramadan, A. B., & Mitchell, D. F. (1962). A roentgenographic study of experimental bone desctruction. *Oral Surgery, Oral Medicine, and Oral Pathology, 15*, 934–943. doi:10.1016/0030-4220(62)90087-7

Rams, T. E., Listgarten, M. A., & Slots, J. (1994). Utility of the radiographic crestal lamina dura for predictiong periodontitis disease-activity. *Journal of Clinical Periodontology*, *21*(9), 571–576. doi:10.1111/j.1600-051X.1994.tb00745.x

Ribeiro-Rotta, R. F., Lindh, C., & Rohlin, M. (2007). Efficacy of clinical methods to assess jaw bone tissue prior to and during endosseus dental implant placement: a systematic literature review. *The International Journal of Oral & Maxillofacial Implants*, *22*(2), 289–300.

Rohlin, M., Akesson, L., Hakansson, J., Hakansson, H., & Nasstrom, K. (1989). Comparison between panoramic and periapical radiography in the diagnosis of periodontal bone loss. *Dento Maxillo Facial Radiology*, *18*(2), 72–76.

Rushton, V. E., Horner, K., & Worthington, H. V. (2001). Screening panoramic radiology of adults in general dental practice: radiological findings. *British Dental Journal*, *190*(9), 495–501. doi:10.1038/sj.bdj.4801014a

Seymour, G. J., Ford, P. J., Cullinan, M. P., Leishman, S., & Yamazaki, K. (2007). Relationship between periodontal infections and systemic disease. *Clinical Microbiology and Infection*, *13*(Suppl 4), 3–10. doi:10.1111/j.1469-0691.2007.01798.x

Slots, J. (2003). Update on general health risk of periodontal disease. *International Dental Journal*, *53*(Suppl 3), 200–207.

Swoboda, J. R., Kiyak, H. A., Darveau, R., & Persson, G. R. (2008). Correlates of periodontal decline and biological markers in older adults. *Journal of Periodontology*, *79*(10), 1920–1926. doi:10.1902/jop.2008.080005

Taguchi, A., Asano, A., Ohtsuka, M., Nakamoto, T., Suei, Y., & Tsuda, M. (2008). Observer performance in diagnosing osteoporosis by dental panoramic radiographs: results from the osteoporosis screening project in dentistry (OSPD). *Bone*, *43*(1), 209–213. doi:10.1016/j.bone.2008.03.014

Tarnow, D., & Fletcher, P. (1984). Classification of the vertical component of furcation involvement. *Journal of Periodontology*, *55*(5), 283–284.

Tugnait, A., Clerehugh, V., & Hirschmann, P. N. (2000). The usefulness of radiographs in diagnosis and management of periodontal diseases: a review. *Journal of Dentistry*, *28*(4), 219–226. doi:10.1016/S0300-5712(99)00062-7

Tugnait, A., Clerehugh, V., & Hirschmann, P. N. (2004). Use of the basic periodontal examination and radiographs in the assessment of periodontal diseases in general dental practice. *Journal of Dentistry*, *32*(1), 17–25. doi:10.1016/S0300-5712(03)00126-X

Vandenberghe, B., Hassan, B., Armellini, D., Maes, F., & Jacobs, R. (2009, July). Volumetric quantification of bone loss for determination of bone grafting accuracy: a pilot study. *Programme and abstract book of the 17th International Congress of Dentomaxillofacial Radiology 2009*, (p. 59).

Vandenberghe, B., Jacobs, R., & Yang, J. (2007). Diagnostic validity (or acuity) of 2D CCD versus 3D CBCT-images for assessing periodontal breakdown. *Oral Surgery, Oral Medicine, Oral Pathology, Oral Radiology, and Endodontics*, *104*(3), 395–401. doi:10.1016/j.tripleo.2007.03.012

Vandenberghe, B., Jacobs, R., & Yang, J. (2007). Topographic assessment of periodontal craters and furcation involvements by using 2D digital images versus 3D cone beam CT: an in-vitro study. *The Chinese Journal of Dental Research*, *10*(1), 21–29.

Vandenberghe, B., Jacobs, R., & Yang, J. (2008). Detection of periodontal bone loss using digital intra-oral and CBCT images: an in-vitro assessment of bony and/or infrabony defects. *Dento Maxillo Facial Radiology*, *37*(5), 252–260. doi:10.1259/dmfr/57711133

Walter, C., Kaner, D., Berndt, D. C., Weiger, R., & Zitzmann, N. U. (2009). Three-dimensional imaging as a pre-operative tool in decision making for furcation surgery. *Journal of Clinical Periodontology*, *36*(3), 250–257. doi:10.1111/j.1600-051X.2008.01367.x

Webber, R. L., Horton, R. A., Tyndall, D. A., & Ludlow, J. B. (1997). Tuned-aperture computed tomography (TACT). Theory and application for three-dimensional dento-alveolar imaging. *Dento Maxillo Facial Radiology*, *26*(1), 53–62. doi:10.1038/sj.dmfr.4600201

Wenzel, A., Haiter-Neto, F., & Gotfredsen, E. (2007). Influence of spatial resolution and bit depth on detection of small caries lesions with digital receptors. *Oral Surgery, Oral Medicine, Oral Pathology, Oral Radiology, and Endodontics*, *103*(3), 418–422. doi:10.1016/j.tripleo.2006.05.016

Wolf, B., von Bethlenfalvy, E., Hassfeld, S., Staehle, H. J., & Eickholz, P. (2001). Reliability of assessing interproximal bone loss by digital radiography: infrabony defects. *Journal of Clinical Periodontology*, *28*(9), 869–878. doi:10.1034/j.1600-051x.2001.028009869.x

Xie, Q., Ainamo, A., & Tilvis, R. (1997). Association of residual ridge resorption with systemic factors in home-living elderly subjects. *Acta Odontologica Scandinavica*, *55*(5), 299–305. doi:10.3109/00016359709114968

Zulqarnain, B. J., & Almas, K. (1998). Effect of x-ray beam vertical angulation on radiographic assessment of alveolar crest level. *Indian Journal of Dental Research*, *9*(4), 132–138.

KEY TERMS AND DEFINITIONS

Alveolar Crest: The most coronal portion of the alveolar bone.

Angular or Vertical Bone Loss: Local manifestation of periodontal disease showing more severe or aggressive bone loss localized around a tooth's proximal surface. It is often associated with an irregular pattern and creates craters and furcation involvements.

Clinical Attachment Loss: Distance between the cemento-enamel junction and the base of the gingival sulcus or periodontal pocket.

Computed Tomography: Extraoral radiographic technique using a fan-shaped x-ray beam and a detector row (which rotate around the subject) to scan sections of the body layer by layer until the desired volume is scanned. The computer then calculates axial cross-sections of the body which can be reformatted in all planes.

Cone Beam Computed Tomography: Computed tomography using a cone-shaped x-ray beam projected on a two-dimensional x-ray sensor. The conical beam makes one convolution around the subject, capturing all the image data. This is followed by axial and multiplanar reformatted slice reconstruction by the computer.

Contrast Enhancement: Image enhancement technique to improve visibility by increasing or decreasing contrast.

Contrast Resolution: The ability of an imaging modality to display differences between structures having different densities.

Crater: Irregular depression or infrabony defect in alveolar bone due to vertical bone loss.

Furcation Involvement or Defect: Vertical bone loss spread out in the furcation area of a tooth, where the root divides into 2, 3 or more segments.

Gingivitis: Inflammation of the gingival tissues or gums caused by bacterial plaque.

Histogram: Graphical representation of the grey values in a digital radiograph.

Horizontal Bone Loss: Manifestation of periodontal disease where bone loss is more generalized and involves the four walls surrounding the tooth roots. This results in equal flattening of the alveolar crest.

Image Filtering: Mathematical operations applied onto image pixels to make it visually more appealing or to enhance the image.

Image Registration: Process transforming two data sets into one coordinate system.

Image Segmentation: Process of dividing a digital image into segments.

Intraoral Radiography: Radiographic technique based on projection radiography. A film or digital receptor is placed in the oral cavity and the extraoral x-ray source is pointed towards the sensor using aiming devices for radiographic visualization of teeth and supporting tissues.

Lamina Dura: Radiographic term used for the radiopaque dense or compact bony plate adjacent to the periodontal ligament space.

Multiplanar Reformatting: Viewing of the captured image volume into axial, coronal and sagittal cross-sections.

Panoramic Radiography: Extraoral radiographic technique based on tomography, where x-ray source and sensor rotate in opposite direction around the subject and image objects within the focal plane, being a curvilinear plane centered on the dental arches. Objects outside this field are blurred out.

Periodontal Ligament Space: Space adjacent to the tooth root containing the connective tissue fibers that attach the teeth to the alveolus.

Periodontitis: Alterations in the periodontium or tooth supporting tissues after inflammations. Also commonly used to denote the next stage after gingivitis where inflammation spreads to the alveolar bone and bone loss is present.

Pocket Depths: Distance between the gingival margin and the base of the pocket.

Radiographic Density: The degree of darkening of an exposed film or digital radiograph.

Radiomorphometry: Application of anthropologic indices of bone morphology to radiographs.

Spatial Resolution: Resolving power of an imaging modality referring to the ability to display small details.

Subtraction Radiography: Process of subtracting two geometrically standardized radiographs taken at two time points from one another. It enhances the visualization of mineral changes over time and also allows for quantification of density measurements over time.

Texture Analysis: The characterization of regions in an image by their texture content.

Tomography: Extraoral radiographic technique where x-ray source and receptor rotate in opposite direction and sharply image objects in a line of interest creating cross-sections.

Tuned Aperture Computed Tomography: Radiographic technique based on the principle of tomosynthesis but using traditional radiographic projections from different angles to reconstruct cross-sections.

Volume Rendering: Method to display the 2D projection of a 3D data set and to extract a surface from a volumetric data.

Section 4
Bioinformatic Applications in Bacterial Identification

Chapter 14
Meta-Analysis Approach for the Identification of Molecular Networks Related to Infections of the Oral Cavity

Andriani Daskalaki
Max-Planck-Institute for Molecular Genetics, Germany

Axel Rasche
Max-Planck-Institute for Molecular Genetics, Germany

ABSTRACT

Chronic periodontitis is the most common infection of the oral cavity. Understanding how and why bacteria enter host cells, and how barrier cells respond to limit their impact, provides a biological basis of infection in the mixed bacterial-human ecosystem of the oral cavity. In addition, elucidation of the underlying shared pathogenic mechanisms of complex diseases like diabetes and oral infections can lead to new insight into the involvement of genes in increased susceptibility of patients with oral infections to complex systemic diseases and vice versa. Transcriptional profiling, statistical and ontology tools are used to uncover and dissect genes and pathways of human gingival epithelial cells that are modulated upon interaction with the periodontal pathogens. Affymetrix microarrays are applied to search the gene expression underlying infection with oral bacteria and identify distinct classes of up- and down-regulated genes during this process. The developed meta-analysis approach can help to extract sets of genes related to oral infection and interaction networks by integrating and combining quantitative gene expression data using statistical approaches. By means of overrepresentation analysis, the authors discovered molecular networks related to immune systems responses.

BACKGROUND

Humans are hosts of a complex population of microorganisms that colonize the oral mucosal membranes. More than 700 species of bacteria can inhabit the oral cavity (Aas et al., 2005).

A subset of oral microorganisms, including *F. nucleatum*, *Aggregatibacter* (*Actinobacillus*) *actinomycetemcomitans*, and *P. gingivalis*, can invade host cells (Han et al., 2000;Handfield et

DOI: 10.4018/978-1-60566-733-1.ch014

al., 2005; Lamont & Jenkinson 1998; Tribble et al., 2006).

Although it is well established that the bacterial inhabitants of the subgingival crevice are direct precursors of periodontal disease, the oral microorganisms form a spectrum ranging from commensals, such as *Streptococcus gordonii*, to aggressive pathogens, such as *P. gingivalis*. Other species like *F. nucleatum*, are frequently found in individuals with good oral health but are also able to contribute to disease (Avila-Campos et al., 1999; Dzink et al. 1988, Feng & Weinberg 2006).

Periodontitis is a common chronic inflammatory disease which may lead to tooth loss.

Inflammation involves production of reactive oxygen species (Chapple & Matthews 2007), raised levels of proinflammatory cytokines (Graves 2008), and elevated concentrations of matrix metalloproteinases (Sorsa et al., 2006) within periodontal tissues and fluid. Some of the genes that encode the molecular components involved in the inflammatory process might confer susceptibility to both periodontitis and rheumatoide arthritis (De Pablo et al., 2009; Nilsson & Kopp, 2008), resulting in an association between the two diseases. Furthermore, periodontal infections have been associated with systemic inflammation and risk for atherosclerosis and vascular disease (Desvarieux et al., 2004).

The goal of periodontal therapy is complete regeneration of the tissues lost as a result of periodontitis. Clinical and radiographic measurements are applied for the diagnosis of periodontitis but offer little information regarding the pathogenesis of the disease. Therefore, the comparison of diseased to healthy gingival tissue transcriptomes provide a valuable scientific tool that may reveal insights of the pathobiology of periodontitis (Demmer et al., 2008). The interdependency between host and pathogen in an infectious disease involves changes in gene expression. Clinical studies have investigated the similarities in cytokine profiles and gene expression profiles in blood cells between patients with and those without periodontitis.

MICROARRAY ANALYSIS TO STUDY ORAL INFECTION

Microarray analysis allows the simultaneous investigation of thousands of genes. The use of microarrays has become the method of choice for gene expression analysis of host-pathogen interaction (McGuire & Glass, 2005).Transcriptional profiling using microarrays provided a way to monitor host cell responses to microorganisms on a global scale (Cummings & Relman 2000; Mans 2006) and revealed differentially expressed up-regulated and down-regulated genes in oral infection.

Innate immune factors, have been found to be differentially regulated in host cells infected with pathogenic organisms compared to the regulation in uninfected controls (Handfield et al., 2005; Jenner, & Young 2005; Mans et al., 2006). Transcriptional profiling has been used to uncover and dissect genes and pathways of human gingival epithelial cells that are modulated upon interaction with periodontal pathogens like *Actinobacillus actinomycetemcomitans* and *Porphyromonas gingivalis*. Demmer et al. (2008) examined gene expression signatures in healthy and diseased human gingival tissues by using the Affymetrix platform (AffymetrixU133Plus2.0 arrays). Handfield et al. (2005) analyzed the gene expression of human immortalized gingival keratinocytes (HIGK) cells with transcriptional profiling by using Affymetrix microarrays to define the biological pathways of HIGK cells modulated by the oral pathogenic *Porphyromonas gingivalis* and *Aggregatibacter* (formerly actinobacillus) *actinomycetemcomitans*. The authors analyzed the gene expression underlying infection and identified up- and down-regulated genes between infected with either the oral pathogenic P. gingivalis (Pg) or A. actinomycetemcomitans (Aa). and non infected HIGK cells. In another study (E-GEOD-10526) HIGK cells were infected with either the oral pathogen *P. gingivalis* (Pg) or an isogenic mutant for SerB (Hasegawa et al.,

2008). Classes of up- and down-regulated genes have been identified by using transcriptional profiling of oral keratinocytes to analyse the gene expression underlying infection with a P. gingivalis mutant (P. gingivalis SerB). Papapanou et al. (2007) investigated the effects of periodontal therapy on gene expression of peripheral blood monocytes by using Affymetrix U133 Plus 2.0 chips Approximately 1/3 of the patients showed changes in gene expression relevant to pathways related to innate immunity, apoptosis, and cell signaling. The authors concluded that periodontal therapy may alter monocytic gene expression of peripheral blood monocytes creating a systemic anti-inflammatory effect.

Lichanska et al. (2005) used microarrays (Hu133A Affymetrix array) to identify differentially expressed genes and pathways that were characteristic of ligament, gingiva and regenerating cells. Proteases/Protease inhibitors were differentially expressed between the ligament and gingiva highlighting high ECM remodeling activity by gingival cells. On the other hand, ligament cells were shown to have increased protein synthesis by increasing their nucleolar and ribosomal gene complement. Lichanska et al identified signaling pathways which are consistent with clinical observations of the regenerative properties of gingival and periodontal ligament cells. These pathways provide candidate targets that can be manipulated in order to achieve a superior regenerative clinical outcome.

ANALYSIS WORKFLOW

The concept of the analysis workflow and applied pipeline for data processing is presented in Figure 2. The meta-analysis approach has been implemented in the software platform R (R-2.7.0) using the BioConductor package collection (BioC 2.2, Gentleman 2004). The process include the standard steps for processing microarrays. The first step of the workflow is the determination of test cases based on the published experimental data. The input in the pipeline (Figure 2) are microarray data cel files related to the phenotypic information of its experiment. Each test case represents a grouping of microarray cel files according to the phenotype. The one group include samples treated under a specific condition like cells infected with a pathogen, and the other group is considered as control and include the healthy or non treated samples. After manual determination of the test cases the data is processed automatically.

For the processing of every test case specific steps are as follows.

A preprocessing part includes three steps: a. intrachip normalisation, which corrects for the GC content of the probes, b. interchip normalisation, which reduces non-biological differences between chips, and c. summarisation, a step which combines the probe intensities into single gene expression values.

The second step would be the analysis of differential expression (DE).

The whole processing script is based on Ensembl genes (www.ensembl.org). The gene sets have different gene or protein identifers and are mapped to Ensembl genes before evaluation.

The output of the genewise evaluation is amended with HUGO identifiers and gene descriptions. The gene set level was evaluated through enrichment and group testing. Output are several evaluation tables and images (Figures 3, 6, 8). The evaluation tables comprise hybridisation and expression values, genewise evaluation of the normalised expression of all genes on the chip and the therefrom filtered differentially expressed genes as well as lists for the gene set level analysis.

Microarray data sets are generated with a specific research question in mind. One of the main current challenges in microarray research is the comparison between different data sets. A meta-analysis helps to identify general disease markers exceeding results possible with specific data sets.

Figure 1. Overview of the datasets used for the meta-analysis approach. Streptococcus pyogenes: St Streptococcus gordonii, Aa: Actinobacillus actinomycetemcomitans, Pg Porphyromonas gingivalis, Sg: S. gordonii, Fn: F. nucleatum, Oral: oral bacteria

Organism	Publication	PMID	Tissue	Pathogen	GEO ID	ArrayExpress ID
Homo sapiens	Handfield M et al. 2005	15888084	Gingival epithelial HIGK cells	*Pg /Aa*	GSE9723	E-GEOD-9723
Homo sapiens	Hasegawa Y et al. 2007	17307939	Gingival epithelial HIGK cells	*Sg/Fn*	GSE6927	E-GEOD-6927
Homo sapiens	Demmer RT et al. 2008	18980520	Healthy and diseased gingival tissues	Oral	GSE10334	E-GEOD-10334
Homo sapiens	_	18391005	Diseased gingival tissues	Oral	GSE10526	E-GEOD-10526
Mus musculus	Goldmann et al. 2007	17526748	Macrophages	*St*	GSE7769	E-GEOD-7769
Homo sapiens	_	_	Periodontium	Oral	GSE2525	E-GEOD-2525
Homo sapiens	_	_	Inflamed periodontal ligament cells	Oral	GSE7321	E-GEOD-7321
Homo sapiens	Papapanou et al. 2007	17716309	Diseased gingival tissues	Oral	GSE6751	E-GEOD-6751

We present a meta-analysis pipeline including methods that allow study of gene up- and down-regulation using statistical methodologies. We applied these to understand the signaling pathways affected by inflammatory factors. This approach combined individual studies related to healthy versus diseased oral conditions by extracting consistent information. We have retrieved publicly available microarray data. We have analysed the data from a total of 8 studies. These studies were carried out with homogeneous technical platforms, on similar model systems (human tissues, human cell lines, mouse tissues). We included a total of 6 manucripts and 8 experiments from the ArrayExpress repository and related to Affymetrix microarray expression data. The experiments were split into studies in function of pathogen infection and tissue regeneration. The studies were only included when the raw information (CEL files) were available.

Figure 1 contains seven columns related to the studied species (Organism), the reference (Publication), the cells of tissue (Tissue), the oral environmental specified conditions (Pathogen), and the experimental ID's derived from the GEO and ArrayExpress public databases for transcriptomics data (GEO ID, ArrayExpress ID).

The concept of the analysis workflow and applied pipeline for data processing is presented in Figure 2. The meta-analysis approach has been implemented in the software platform R (R-2.7.0) using the BioConductor package collection (BioC 2.2, Gentleman 2004).

MICROARRAY DATA SET PROCESSING

The process follows the standard guidelines for processing microarrays. The first step is the determination of test cases based on the published experimental data. The input in the pipeline (Figure 2) are microarray data files related to the phenotypic information of its experiment. In order to reduce technical bias of transcriptome measurements we restrict to experiments performed on the Affymetrix GeneChip platform and start with CEL files. Each test case represents a grouping of microarray cel files according to the phenotype. The one group includes samples treated under a specific condition like cells infected with a pathogen, and the other group is considered as control and include the healthy or non treated samples.

Arrays from the same test case are preprocessed in three steps: (a) intrachip normalisation, which corrects for the GC content of the probes; (b) interchip normalisation, which reduces non-biological differences between chips and (c) summarisation, a step which combines the probe intensities into single gene expression values.

After preprocessing we assess differential expression between samples taking into account the strength of the change and its significance. Values are averaged within conditions over the arrays. Three statistical values are stored for every test case and gene: (1) The fold change between samples, (2) the standard error of the fold change as well

Figure 2. Illustration of the workflow design for the meta-analysis pipeline. This workflow describes the steps from data processing to pathway annotation.

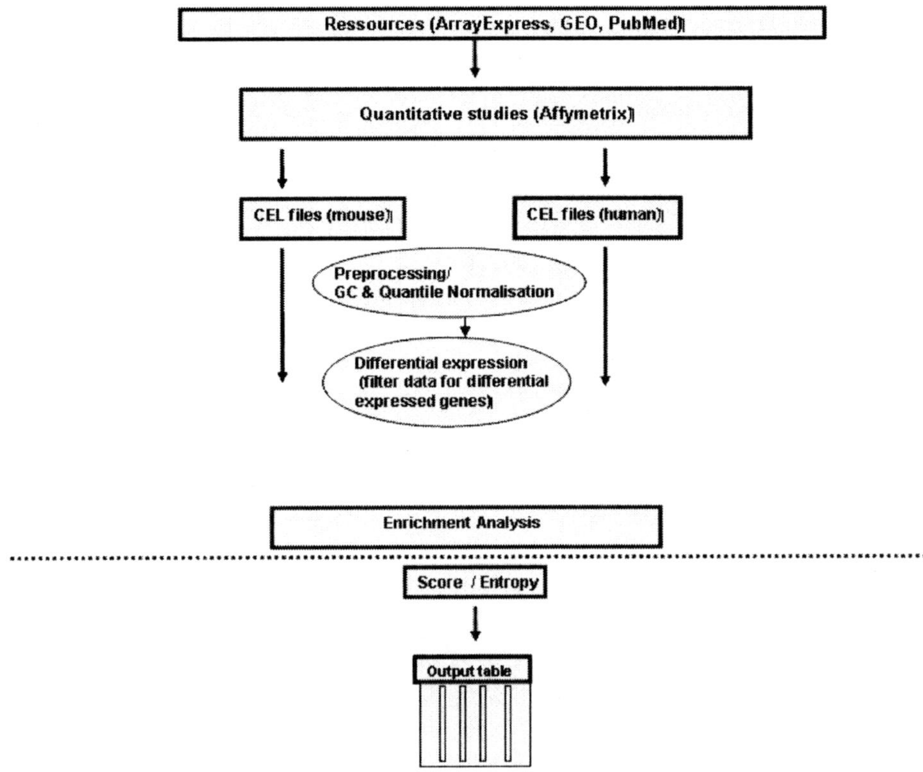

as (3) a presence p-value indicating if the gene is expressed within at least one of the samples.

The whole processing script is based on Ensembl genes (www.ensembl.org). Ressources with different gene or protein identifiers are mapped to Ensembl genes before evaluation.

SCORING GENES WITH RELEVANCE TO ORAL INFECTION BY META-ANALYSIS

In order to rate the contribution of single genes in specific experiments, we calculated scores of the individual studies, from quantitative gene expression values.

The score of the i-th gene in the j-th study, was computed as follows:

$$s_{ij} = \begin{cases} \left|\log 2\left(r_{ij}\right)\right|\left(1 - \frac{e_{ij}}{r_{ij}}\right)\left(1 - p_{ij}\right), & p_{ij} < 0.1 \text{ and } e_{ij} / r_{ij} \leq 1 \\ 0, & else \end{cases}$$

Here, r_{ij} is the fold change, p_{ij} is the average detection p-value and e_{ij} is the standard error of the ratio derived from the experimental replicates of the study. Thus, the fold change is weighted with its reproducibility across the experimental replicates and with the likelihood of the gene being expressed in the study's target samples. A similar formula applies for correlation studies:

$$s_{ij} = \begin{cases} \left|c_{ij}\right|\left(1 - v_{ij}\right)\left(1 - p_{ij}\right), & p_{ij} \leq 0.1 \text{ and } v_{ij} \leq 1 \\ 0, & else \end{cases}$$

In the formula above, c_{ij} is the correlation to a certain phenotypic parameter, p_{ij} the average detection p-value and v_{ij} the coefficient of variation

Figure 3. To compare the different experimental gene expression data a correlation heatmap is provided. **AavsPg** *(treatment = Aa, control = Pg),* **AavsnoInfection** *(treatment = Aa, control = no infection),* **StvsFuso** *(treatment = St, control = Fuso),* **PgvsnoInfection** *(treatment = Pg, control = no infection),* **FusovsnoInfection** *(treatment = Fuso, control = no infection), StvsnoInfection (treatment = St, control = no infection),* **HealthvsDiseased** *(treatment = infected gingival tissues, control = healthy gingival tissues),* **PgvsPg_mut** *(treatment = Pg mutated, control = Pg).* **InfvsnonInf** *related to [E-GEOD-7321], treatment = chronic periodontal lesions, control = healthy periodontium),* **Orligvsreg** *(treatment =ligament, control =reg cells),* **Orregvsging** *(treatment =regenerating cells, control = gingiva),* **Orligvsging** *(treatment =ligament, control = gingiva).* **Aa** *= Actinobacillus actinomycetemcomitans,* **Pg.** *= Porphyromonas gingivalis,* **St** *= Streptococcus gordonii,* **Fuso***= Fusobacterium nucleatum.*

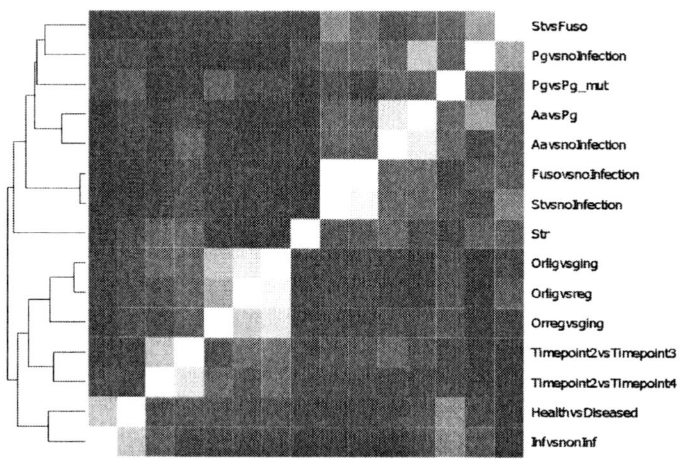

of the gene's signal across experimental replicas. The formula is applied on the data of Papapanou et al. (2007).

To assess the similarity of the data sets we computed a distance matrix between studies based in two correlation indices (Pearson) and a good correlation between studies indicates that the results are consistent. In Figure 3 the correlations are visualised with a heatmap.

IDENTIFICATION OF CELL RESPONSE CANDIDATE GENES: GENERALITY VERSUS SPECIFICITY

The total score for each gene was computed as the sum across all scores from the individual experiments. In order to assess the significance of the overall gene scores we generated random gene scores. Using a Bootstrap (Bradley 1979) scoring approach we computed a core set of genes that show significant relevance related to oral infection in the gene expression data sets under study. We have drawn a random score from each experiment and using a random background distribution as sample we assigned as "significant" the genes that are above the 99.9 percentile of the background distribution (Figure 4). Based on this analysis we identified 131 genes (Score >7.27).

Since we have analysed data from human and mouse exposed to different pathogenetic conditions, it is likely that for some cases an individual experiment is dominating the score, for example if the gene is active only in mouse or after the host-pathogen interaction with a specific pathogen. In order to identify those genes we have computed an entropy-based numerical criterion. Entropy is low if a single study has a major contribution

Figure 4. In this figure is illustrated the histogram of the gene score distribution based on experimental data (black line) and of the background distribution of scores derived from bootstrap sampling (blue line). The dashed vertical red line indicates the cut-off for the candidate gene list.

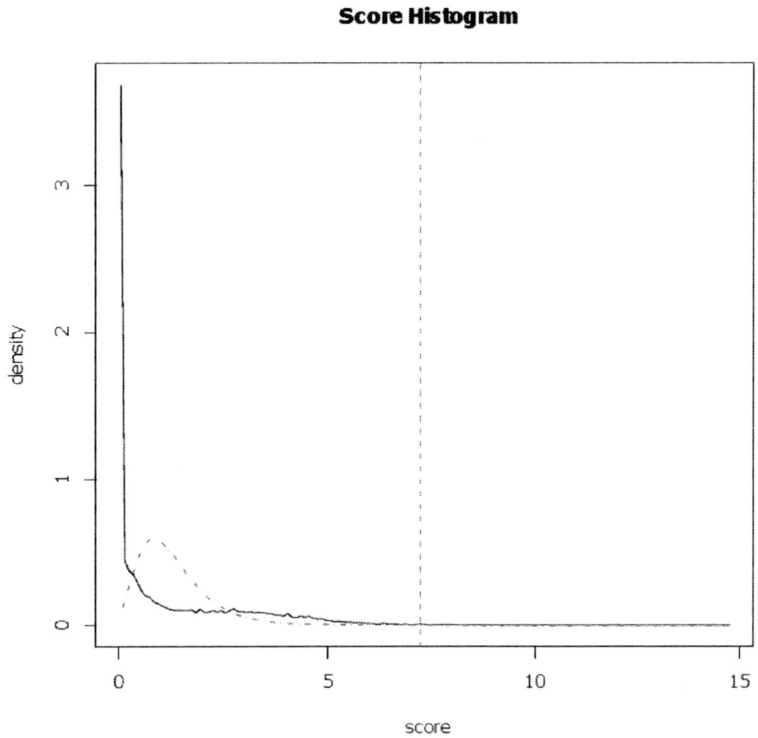

on the overall score. On the other hand, entropy is high if most of the studies account equally for the score.

Entropy express a measure for the uniformity of the score distribution over the individual experiments. The computation of Entropy E_i is based on the following formula, where s_i the score of the i-th gene in the j-th study.

$$E_i = -\sum_j \frac{s_{ij}}{\sum_k s_{ik}} \log_2 \left(\frac{s_{ij}}{\sum_k s_{ik}} \right)$$

The gene PFKFB3 (Figure 5) presents a relative high score (9.046, rank 46/131 significant genes) in our meta-analysis, and showed consistent alterations across many different studies indicated by high entropy (3.422, rank 220/9314). This gene is known to be activated by inflammatory and hypoxic stimuli (Chesney, 2006).

CHROMOSOME DISTRIBUTION OF DISEASE MARKERS

The superset of disease genes already facilitates a first genomic analysis of the disease looking at the chromosomal distribution, markers highlighted in red. The distribution of disease markers showed a preference for human chromosome 1, 9, 11, 19, 20 (Figure 6), 10 weeks after treatment which resulted in substantial improvement in clinical periodontal status and reduction in levels of several periodontal pathogens. (based on Papapanou et al. 2007).

Figure 5. Distribution of experimental gene expression values for PFKFB3

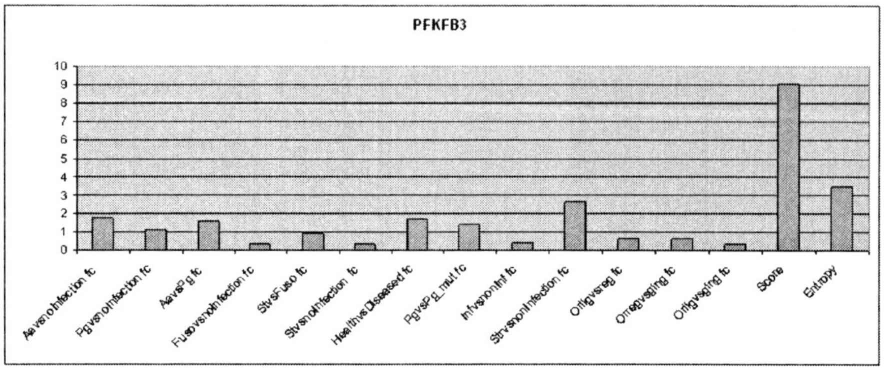

Figure 6. Distribution of marker genes across human chromosome at baseline/time point 2 (right) vs 10 weeks after treatment/time point 4 (left) periodontal status was recorded)

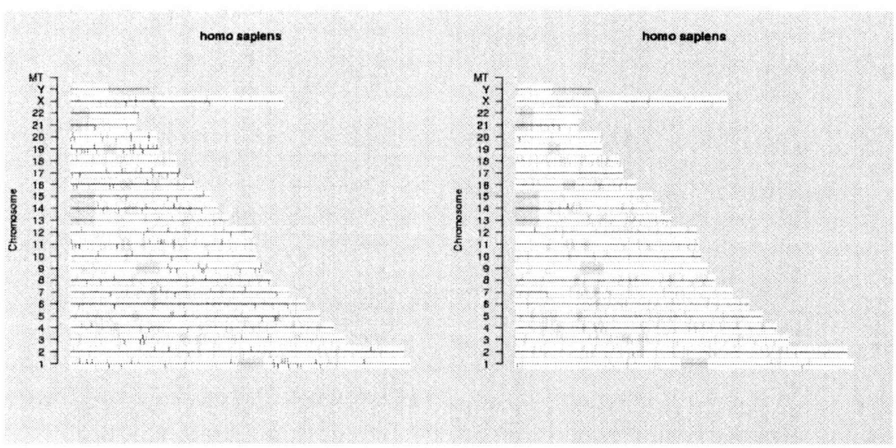

IDENTIFICATION OF DISEASE RELATED NETWORKS WITH ENRICHMENT ANALYSIS

Gene ontology (GO) analysis identified differentially expressed groups of genes related to the biological pathways of apoptosis, antimicrobial humoral response, antigen presentation, regulation of metabolic processes, signal transduction, and angiogenesis. Disease related networks can be analyzed with four different types of networks – biological pathways, protein-protein interaction networks, gene regulatory networks, and functional annotation using GO annotations (Ashburner et al., 2000). These networks define subsets of associated genes. The goal of this analysis is to identify genes or gene sets associated with particular phenotypes. One such method of analysis is the Gene Set Enrichment Analysis (GSEA). GSEA uses a Kolmogorov-Smirnov-style statistic to identify groups of genes that are regulated together (Subramanian et al., 2005).

Enrichment analyses were carried out in order to assess whether the selected set of genes is overrepresented with respect to a certain functional category.

Enriched sets are searched among two categories of predefined gene sets: neighborhood-based sets and pathway-based sets. A pathway-based set contains all the proteins and genes that are involved in some biochemical pathway. pathway-based sets are used for over-representation and/or gene set enrichment analysis.

Using overrepresentation based on hypergeometric distribution we were able to assign each pathway a p-value reflecting the occurrence of candidate genes selected by our meta-analysis approach (Figure 7). The hypergeometric distribution (Klipp et al. 2005) compares the overlap between our gene set and the gene group assigned to a specific annotation object (pathway, GO term) to the overlap of a random selection of two gene sets equal in size.

Two pathways (Figure 7), that were significantly impacted by oral infection (p=0.00046 and p=0.0036) involve Glucose transport and metabolism.

The interaction networks are illustrated in ConsensusPathDB (Figure 8) by graphs. The ConsensusPathDB (http://cpdb.molgen.mpg.de/) web interface supports functional annotation of gene lists that are significantly over- or underexpressed in a gene expression study. Based on the results of the meta-analysis we have generated molecular networks which can

Figure 7. Top 15 over-represented pathways

Pathways	P-value	SigSet	Set
Dissolution of Fibrin Clot	3.67E-05	3	8
glutathione biosynthesis	0.000231	2	3
Glutathione synthesis	0.000231	2	3
Glucose is carried across the plasma membrane by a glucose transport protein (GLUT)	0.00046	2	4
Cellular roles of Anthrax toxin	0.00268	2	9
Glucose metabolism	0.0036	4	71
il-10 anti-inflammatory signaling pathway	0.00405	2	11
fibrinolysis pathway	0.00658	2	14
Glutathione conjugation	0.00755	2	15
cadmium induces dna synthesis and proliferation in macrophages	0.00858	2	16
COX reactions	0.00884	1	1
Metabolism of small molecules	0.00933	4	93
Metabolism of carbohydrates	0.00933	4	93
Canonical NF kappa B Pathway	0.0108	2	18
Wnt Signaling-Canonical Pathway	0.016	2	22

Figure 8. In this figure is illustrated the pathway COX reactions in the database ConsensusPathwayDB. PGHS exhibits a catalytic activity, as a cyclooxygenase and a peroxidase. Here is illustrated the oxidation of Arachidonic acid to PGG2 catalyzed by the cyclooxygenase PGHS and the PGHS – peroxidase mediated reduction of PGG2 to PGH2.

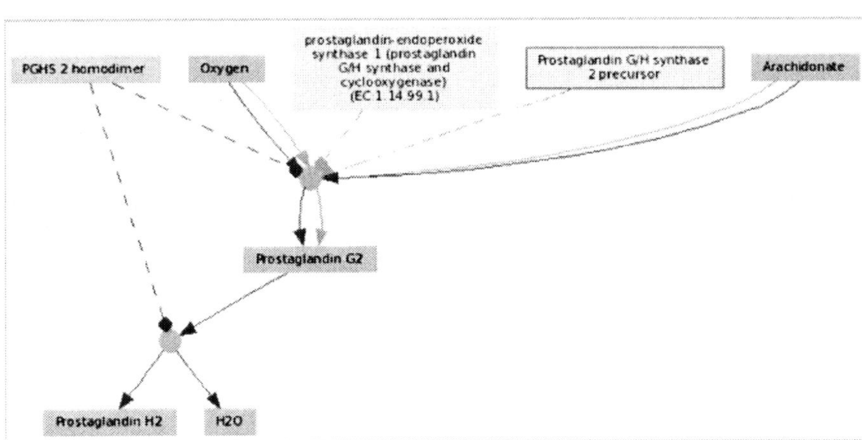

be visualized by graphs in the ConsensusPathDB (Figure 8).

The network in Figure 8 contains three biochemical reactions indicated by green circles representing functional interaction nodes. PGH2 (Figure 8) plays a critical role in immune function regulation, it exists in two isoforms, 1 and 2. Isoform 1 is involved in performing normal physiological functions. Isoform 2, in contrast, is involved in critical steps of inflammation.

DISCUSSION

The oral cavity is characterized by complex and dynamic interactions between host epithelial cells and endogenous bacteria that can cause opportunistic infections.

Periodontitis is an oral infection disease related to diabetes mellitus, obesity, and gender (Saremi et al., 2005; Desvarieux et al., 2004]. Periodontitis is a leading cause of tooth loss in adults, which can impair nutritional status. Results from clinical studies point towards a potential association between chronic periodontitis and systemic inflammatory diseases — in particular, rheumatoid arthritis (Lee et al., 2008; Lee et al., 2009).

Studies also demonstrated similarities in the spectrum of bacteria in the oral cavity and in coronary plaques [Desvarieux et al., 2005; Ott et al., 2006], and both diseases are characterized by an imbalanced immune reaction and a chronic inflammatory process [Assuma et al., 1998; Kaplan et al., 2001]. Periodontitis is also associated with elevated C-reactive protein levels [Hettne et al., 2007], a phenotype for which common genetic risk factors for periodontitis and atherosclerosis have been discussed [Paraskevas et al., 2008]. Polymorphisms in genes implicated in chronic periodontitis, such as interleukin-1 and Fcγ receptor, have also been implicated as susceptibility factors for rheumatoid arthritis. (Lee et al. 2008). These findings indicate a possible mutual genetic basis underlying this oral infection and systemic diseases.

The aim of the meta-analysis presented in this chapter was to investigate the molecular mechanisms that are involved in oral tissue response against infection and regeneration. The applied meta-analysis approach is generic and can be used as a template for studies in different disease domains like diabetes (Rasche et al. 2008). This is a meta-analysis approach to characterize the gene expression profile of periodontal cells and allowed to gain valuable insights into the cellular and molecular mechanisms that occur during the infectious as well as regenerative process in case of periodontitis.

The goal of the application of our meta-analysis pipeline in the analysis of quantitive genomic data related to periodontal tissues was to identify genes causative of this oral infection disease. Therefore we combined individual studies and used data sources from the Affymetrix platform which was compatible to our pipeline .

Linkage of specific bacterial components to host pathways and networks provide an insight into the pathogenic process of oral periodontitis. A targeted therapy based on these molecular networks could contribute to the therapeutic success in case of inflammatory diseases of the oral cavity like periodontitis.

Furthermore, by integrating data related to the periodontium regeneration studies we were focused to the interaction of oral tissues with the oral cavity environment during the regenerative process.

In the first part of this work, genes were scored in each individual study according to their oral infection relevance, showing high scores in many different experiments as well as genes that have a specific relevance to oral infection expressing high scores in only few experiments. Data sets were selected from infected and non infected oral tissue/cells treated with oral pathogens. For each gene and each source we computed a numerical value that expressed its likelihood for being oral infection relevant.

In a second part, the significant gene set based on statistical significance was used to identify biological networks related to signaling pathways.

Enrichment analyses based on the hypergeometric distribution were carried out in order to assess whether our periodontal candidate list is over-represented with respect to a certain biological pathway.

The molecular networks that have been identified included pathways known to be involved in signal transduction and previously examined in the context of diabetes (Nadler et al., 2000).

Nevertheless, for a better analysis of the common transcriptional response of epithelial cells to different bacteria, more data need to be integrated to the meta -analysis to better analyze predominant results based on organism-specific responses.

ACKNOWLEDGMENT

This work was supported by the EU FP6 grant SysCo (LSHG-CT-2006-37231), SysPro (LSHG-CT-2006-37457) and the Max Planck Society.

REFERENCES

Aas, J. A., Paster, B. J., Stokes, L. N., Olsen, I., & Dewhirst, F. E. (2005). Defining the normal bacterial flora of the oral cavity. *Journal of Clinical Microbiology*, *43*, 5721–5732. doi:10.1128/JCM.43.11.5721-5732.2005

Ashburner, M., Ball, C. A., Blake, J. A., Botstein, D., Butler, H., & Cherry, J. M. (2000). Gene Ontology: tool for the unification of biology. *Nature Genetics*, *25*, 25–29. doi:10.1038/75556

Assuma, R., Oates, T., Cochran, D., Amar, S., & Graves, D. T. (1998). IL-1 and TNF antagonists inhibit the inflammatory response and bone loss in experimental periodontitis. *Journal of Immunology (Baltimore, MD.: 1950)*, *160*, 403–409.

Avila-Campos, M. J., Sacchi, C. T., Whitney, A. M., Steigerwalt, A. G., & Mayer, L. W. (1999). Arbitrarily primed-polymerase chain reaction for identification and epidemiologic subtyping of oral isolates of *Fusobacterium nucleatum*. *Journal of Periodontology*, *70*, 1202–1208. doi:10.1902/jop.1999.70.10.1202

Bradley, E. (1979). Bootstrap Methods . *Another Look at the Jackknife.*, *7*, 1–27.

Chapple, I. L., & Matthews, J. B. (2007). The role of reactive oxygen and antioxidant species in periodontal tissue destruction. *Periodontology 2000*, *43*, 160–232. doi:10.1111/j.1600-0757.2006.00178.x

Chesney, J. (2006). 6-phosphofructo-2-kinase/fructose-2,6-bisphosphatase and tumor cell glycolysis. *Current Opinion in Clinical Nutrition and Metabolic Care*, *9*(5), 535–539. doi:10.1097/01.mco.0000241661.15514.fb

Cummings, C. A., & Relman, D. A. (2000). Using DNA microarrays to study host-microbe interactions. *Emerging Infectious Diseases*, *6*, 513–525. doi:10.3201/eid0605.000511

De Pablo, P., Chapple, I. L. C., Buckley, C. D., & Dietrich, T. (2009). Periodontitis in systemic rheumatic diseases. *Nature Reviews Rheumatology, 5*, 218 – 224. Retrieved from doi: 10.1038/nrrheum.2009.28

Demmer, R. T., Behle, J. H., Wolf, D. L., Handfield, M., Kebschull, M., & Celenti, R. (2008). Transcriptomes in healthy and diseased gingival tissues. *Journal of Periodontology*, *79*, 2112–2124. doi:10.1902/jop.2008.080139

Desvarieux, M., Demmer, R. T., Rundek, T., Boden-Albala, B., & Jacobs, D. R. Jr (2005). Periodontal microbiota and carotid intima-media thickness: the Oral Infections and Vascular Disease Epidemiology Study (INVEST). *Circulation*, *111*, 576–582. doi:10.1161/01.CIR.0000154582.37101.15

Desvarieux, M., Schwahn, C., Volzke, H., Demmer, R. T., & Ludemann, J. (2004). Gender differences in the relationship between periodontal disease, tooth loss, and atherosclerosis. *Stroke*, *35*, 2029–2035. doi:10.1161/01.STR.0000136767.71518.36

Dzink, J. L., Socransky, S. S., & Haffajee, A. D. (1988). The predominant cultivable microbiota of active and inactive lesions of destructive periodontal diseases. *Journal of Clinical Periodontology*, *15*, 316–323. doi:10.1111/j.1600-051X.1988.tb01590.x

Feng, Z., & Weinberg, A. (2006). Role of bacteria in health and disease of periodontal tissues. *Periodontology 2000*, *40*, 50–76. doi:10.1111/j.1600-0757.2005.00148.x

Gentleman, R. C., Carey, V. J., Bates, D. M., Bolstad, B., Dettling, M., & Dudoit, S. (2004). Bioconductor: Open software development for computational biology and bioinformatics. *Genome Biology*, *5*, R80. doi:10.1186/gb-2004-5-10-r80

Graves, D. (2008). Cytokines that promote periodontal tissue destruction. *Journal of Periodontology*, *79*, 1585–1591. doi:10.1902/jop.2008.080183

Han, Y. W., Shi, W., Huang, G. T., Kinder, S., Haake, N. H., & Park, H. (2000). Interactions between periodontal bacteria and human oral epithelial cells: *Fusobacterium nucleatum* adheres to and invades epithelial cells. *Infection and Immunity*, *68*, 3140–3146. doi:10.1128/IAI.68.6.3140-3146.2000

Handfield, M., Mans, J. J., Zheng, G., Lopez, M. C., Mao, S., & Progulske-Fox, A. (2005). Distinct transcriptional profiles characterize oral epithelium-microbiota interactions. *Cellular Microbiology*, *7*(6), 811–823. doi:10.1111/j.1462-5822.2005.00513.x

Hasegawa, Y., Mans, J. J., Song, M., Lopez, M. C., Baker, H. V., Handfield, M., & Lamont, R. J. (2007). Gingival epithelial cell transcriptional responses to commensal and opportunistic oral microbial specie. *Infection and Immunity*, *75*(5), 2540–2547. doi:10.1128/IAI.01957-06

Hasegawa, Y., Tribble, G. D., Baker, H. V., & Mans, J. J. (2008). Role of Porphyromonas gingivalis SerB in gingival epithelial cell cytoskeletal remodeling and cytokine production. *Infection and Immunity*, *76*(6), 2420–2427. doi:10.1128/IAI.00156-08

Hettne, K. M., Weeber, M., Laine, M. L., Cate, H., & Boyer, S. (2007). Automatic mining of the literature to generate new hypotheses for the possible link between periodontitis and atherosclerosis: lipopolysaccharide as a case study. *Journal of Clinical Periodontology*, *34*, 1016–1024. doi:10.1111/j.1600-051X.2007.01152.x

Jenner, R. G., & Young, R. A. (2005). Insights into host responses against pathogens from transcriptional profiling. *Nature Reviews Microbiology*, *3*, 281–294. doi:10.1038/nrmicro1126

Kaplan, R. C., & Frishman, W. H. (2001). Systemic inflammation as a cardiovascular disease risk factor and as a potential target for drug therapy. *Heart Disease*, *3*, 326–332. doi:10.1097/00132580-200109000-00009

Klipp, E., Herwig, R., Kowald, A., Wierling, C., & Lehrach, H. (2005). *Biology in Practice*. Hoboken, NJ: Wiley-VCH.

Lamont, R. J., & Jenkinson, H. F. (1998). Life below the gum line: pathogenic mechanisms of *Porphyromonas gingivalis*. *Microbiology and Molecular Biology Reviews*, *62*, 1244–1263.

Lee, Y. H. (2008). Associations between FCGr3A polymorphisms and rheumatoid arthritis susceptibility: a metaanalysis. *The Journal of Rheumatology*, *35*, 2129–2135. doi:10.3899/jrheum.080186

Lee, Y. H. (2009). Association between interleukin 1 polymorphisms and rheumatoid arthritis susceptibility: a metaanalysis. *The Journal of Rheumatology*, *36*(1), 12–15.

Lichanska., et al. (2005). Retrieved from http://www.ebi.ac.uk/microarray-as/ae/ (E-GEOD-2525)

Mans, J. J., Baker, H. V., Oda, D., Lamont, R. J., & Handfield, M. (2006). Distinctive characteristics of transcriptional profiles from two epithelial cell lines upon interaction with *Actinobacillus actinomycetemcomitans*. *Oral Microbiology and Immunology*, *21*, 261–267. doi:10.1111/j.1399-302X.2006.00281.x

Mans, J. J., Lamont, R. J., & Handfield, M. (2006). Microarray analysis of human epithelial cell responses to bacterial interaction. *Infectious Disorders Drug Targets*, *6*, 299–309. doi:10.2174/187152606778249926

McGuire, K., & Glass, E. J. (2005). The expanding role of microarrays in the investigation of macrophage responses to pathogens. *Veterinary Immunology and Immunopathology*, *105*, 259–275. doi:10.1016/j.vetimm.2005.02.001

Nadler, S. T., Stoehr, J. P., Schueler, K. L., Tanimoto, G., Yandell, B. S., & Attie, A. D. (2000). The expression of adipogenic genes is decreased in obesity and diabetes mellitus. *Proceedings of the National Academy of Sciences of the United States of America*, *97*(21), 11371–11376. doi:10.1073/pnas.97.21.11371

Nilsson, M., & Kopp, S. (2008). Gingivitis and periodontitis are related to repeated high levels of circulating tumor necrosis factor-alpha in patients with rheumatoid arthritis. *Journal of Periodontology*, *79*, 1689–1696. doi:10.1902/jop.2008.070599

Ott, S. J., El Mokhtari, N. E., Musfeldt, M., Hellmig, S., & Freitag, S. (2006). Detection of diverse bacterial signatures in atherosclerotic lesions of patients with coronary heart disease. *Circulation*, *113*, 929–937. doi:10.1161/CIRCULATIONAHA.105.579979

Papapanou, P. N., Sedaghatfar, M. H., Demmer, R. T., Wolf, D. L., Yang, J., & Roth, G. A. (2007). Periodontal therapy alters gene expression of peripheral blood monocytes. *Journal of Clinical Periodontology*, *34*(9), 736–747. doi:10.1111/j.1600-051X.2007.01113.x

Paraskevas, S., Huizinga, J. D., & Loos, B. G. (2008). A systematic review and meta-analyses on C-reactive protein in relation to periodontitis. *Journal of Clinical Periodontology*, *35*, 277–290. doi:10.1111/j.1600-051X.2007.01173.x

R Development Core Team. (2005). *R: A Language and Environment for Statistical Computing*. Vienna, Austria: R Foundation for Statistical Computing.

Rasche, A., Al-Hasani, H., & Herwig, R. (2008). Meta-Analysis Approach identifies Candidate Genes and associated Molecular Networks for Type-2 Diabetes Mellitus. *BMC Genomics*, *9*, 310. doi:. doi:10.1186/1471-2164-9-310

Saremi, A., Nelson, R. G., Tulloch-Reid, M., Hanson, R. L., & Sievers, M. L. (2005). Periodontal disease and mortality in type 2 diabetes. *Diabetes Care*, *28*, 27–32. doi:10.2337/diacare.28.1.27

Sorsa, T. (2006). Matrix metalloproteinases: contribution to pathogenesis, diagnosis and treatment of periodontal inflammation. *Annals of Medicine*, *38*, 306–321. doi:10.1080/07853890600800103

Subramanian, A., Tamayo, P., & Mootha, V. K. (2005). Gene set enrichment analysis: a knowledge-based approach for interpreting genome-wide expression profiles . *Proceedings of the National Academy of Sciences of the United States of America*, *102*(43), 15545–15550. doi:10.1073/pnas.0506580102

Tribble, G. D., Mao, S., James, C. E., & Lamont, R. J. (2006). A *Porphyromonas gingivalis* haloacid dehalogenase family phosphatase interacts with human phosphoproteins and is important for invasion. *Proceedings of the National Academy of Sciences of the United States of America, 103*, 11027–11032. doi:10.1073/pnas.0509813103

KEY TERMS AND DEFINITIONS

Actinobacillus Actinomycetemcomitans: Aggregatibacter actinomycetemcomitans is a gram-negative facultatively aerobic bacterium occurring as pathogen in mammals. The presence of this bacterium serve as an indicator for aggressive periodontitis.

Array-Express Repository: ArrayExpress (http://www.ebi.ac.uk/microarray-as/ae/) is a public archive for expression data from a subset of experiments.

Differential Expression: Process to filter data for differentially expressed genes between treatment and control groups.

Down-Regulated Genes: Genes with decreased expression within a cell.

Enrichment Analysis: Analysis to recognize genes overrepresented in gene sets.

Gene Expression: The process by which information from a gene is used in the synthesis of a functional gene product which could be a protein, or functional RNA in case of non-protein coding genes such as rRNA genes or tRNA genes.

Gene Expression Omnibus: Gene Expression Omnibus (http://www.ncbi.nlm.nih.gov/projects/geo/) is a public archive for expression data from a subset of experiments.

Gene Expression Signatures: Functionally relevant gene sets characterizing each individual. These gene sets indicate intra-individual or between-groups tissue differences.

Microarray: A microarray is a collection of microscopic spots, commonly representing sequence extracts of single genes, arrayed on a solid surface by covalent attachment to a chemical matrix. DNA microarrays are commonly used for monitoring expression levels of thousands of genes simultaneously.

Periodontium: The tissues that surround and support the teeth. It is comprised from gingival epithelium: gingival connective tissue, periodontal ligament, aveolar bone and cementum.

Periodontitis: An inflammatory disease affecting the periodontium. Periodontitis is caused by bacteria that adhere to and grow on the tooth's surfaces, along with an overly aggressive immune response against these bacteria.

Porphyromonas Gingivalis: A gram-negative, anaerobic bacterium, considered to be an important pathogen in periodontal disease.

Transcriptional Profiling: The measurement of the activity (the expression) of thousands of genes at once, to provide insight to cellular function.

Up-Regulated Genes: Genes with increased expression which occurs within a cell triggered by a signal.

Chapter 15
A Comprehensive Evaluation of the Virulence of Oral Flora

Yoshihisa Yamashita
Kyushu University, Japan

Toru Takeshita
Kyushu University, Japan

ABSTRACT

The oral cavity is inhabited by more than 700 species of commensal bacteria. Several have been identified as pathogens of oral diseases, dental caries, and periodontal diseases. However, the lack of information concerning the interaction between pathogens and the remaining commensal bacteria has made it difficult to understand the precise etiologies of oral diseases. We need to identify the comprehensive species found in individual oral flora and compare these results with corresponding oral health conditions. In this chapter, the authors delineate the previous attempts to identify oral commensal bacterial flora and discuss the potential capability of modern molecular genetic technologies such as terminal restriction fragment length polymorphism, DNA microarray and pyrosequencing analyses utilizing bioinformatics.

INTRODUCTION

Oral Diseases and Microbes

Two major oral diseases, dental caries and periodontitis, occur at different rates among countries (Petersen, 2003). Dental caries is most widespread in several Asian and Latin American countries but is less common in most African countries. Although developed countries have shown a marked decrease in the prevalence of dental caries in children over the past decades, dental caries is still a major oral health problem in most industrialized countries, affecting 60–90% of schoolchildren and most adults. It is rare to find a person from a developed country who has not experienced dental caries. It is the most common chronic disease affecting children, including those in the United States, and is five times more common than the second most prevalent chronic disease, asthma (American Academy of Pediatrics, 2009). Periodontal diseases are also highly prevalent and affect up to 90% of the world's population. Most

DOI: 10.4018/978-1-60566-733-1.ch015

children exhibit signs of gingivitis (the mildest form of periodontal disease), redness, or swelling of gum tissue and bleeding from the gingival sulcus. Persons generally experience the initial stages of periodontal diseases as adults, and the likelihood of moderate or severe periodontitis, which has been reported in 13% of the United States population, increases with age (Albandar et al., 1997). Periodontitis may also be a main cause of tooth loss. Juvenile or early-onset aggressive periodontitis, which affects about 2% of youth, can lead to premature tooth loss (Albandar et al., 1997).

The etiologies of both oral diseases have been extensively pursued for more than 100 years. These diseases are believed to be infectious diseases caused by several specific oral bacterial species, although some features show signs of a multifactorial disease. W. D. Miller, an American dentist, visited Koch's laboratory to seek the specific pathogens of oral diseases. However, he concluded in his publication "The Micro-organisms of the Human Mouth" (1890) that no single species of microorganism caused dental caries, but rather that the process (a chemo-parasitic process) was mediated by a microorganism capable of producing acid and digesting protein. His concept conformed to the modern interpretation of the dental caries etiology based on the mutual interaction of multi-bacterial species. However, many successors continued to chase the actual culprits among the acid-producing candidates in accordance with Koch's postulate and Miller's chemo-parasitic theory. *Streptococcus mutans*, which is presently being reclassified into seven detailed species (*mutans*, *sobrinus*, *cricetus*, *rattus*, *ferus*, *macacae*, and *downei*) known as the "mutans streptococci" group (Bratthall, 1970; Ota et al., 2006), was the favored candidate during the mid-1900s. Animal experiments clearly demonstrated the dental caries etiology of *S. mutans* (Loesche, 1986). Much epidemiological research confirmed the etiology based on the *S. mutans* story; however, the subjects in these studies were biased to infants with deciduous teeth or young subjects with permanent teeth immediately after tooth eruption. As far as we know, few epidemiological studies support that *S. mutans* causes dental caries in adults. Of interest is that a recent study with restricted adult subjects reported contrasting results to the *S. mutans* theory (Nishikawara et al., 2006). Hence, bacteriological etiology has not yet been established.

The bacteriological etiology of periodontal diseases is much more complicated than that of dental caries because of the complex modification of the former by multiple host immune-inflammatory responses. The host's response should be protective, but hypo- and hyper-responsiveness can lead to the destruction of periodontal tissues. Studies have been dedicated to understanding the relationship between periodontal diseases and microflora using conventional modern molecular techniques. The putative anaerobic pathogens, such as *Porphyromonas gingivalis*, *Tannerella forsythia*, and *Treponema denticola*, were frequently detected in the subgingival sites with periodontitis. These bacterial species release proteolytic enzymes that can damage host tissue and produce various putative virulence factors. However, it is difficult to declare these particular bacterial species as the causative species or as being able to adapt to the anaerobic conditions of the deep pocket in the periodontal lesion. One of the reasons that it is difficult to ascertain the exact periodontal pathogen is because the field lacks an appropriate animal model that can establish the relationship between bacterial infection and periodontitis.

Problems in Oral Microbiology

Should we pursue the pathogen directly responsible for oral diseases without considering the more than 700 bacterial species inhabiting the oral cavity? There must be an interaction among or between pathogens, and possibly the surrounding non-virulent bacterial species, that can regulate the expression of virulence factors from pathogens. We may also have to consider the virulence of oral microflora in perspective rather than in particulars of each species within the flora.

In dental plaque formation, streptococci and actinomyces are the early dominant colonizers that attach between the bacterial adhesin and its specific salivary receptor on tooth surfaces. Fusobacteria, veillonellae, propionibacteria, rothiae, capnocytophagae, and prevotellae subsequently bind to the streptococci and/or actinomyces by specific molecular interactions between the adhesins and receptors on their cell surfaces. Bacterial interactions between *F. nucleatum* and other oral bacteria are especially important for late colonizers (Figure 1; Kolenbrander et al., 2006). Although these molecular interactions have been demonstrated in a number of studies using different model systems, it is still unclear which interaction is critical for virulent biofilm formation.

Catabolic competence among oral bacteria has also been reported. *Streptococcus sanguinis* or *S. oligofermentans* compete against *S. mutans* by producing ammonium or hydrogen peroxide and subsequently suppress the expression of cariogenicity in *S. mutans* or its growth (Kreth et al., 2005; Tong et al., 2007). Alternatively, alkali production through the arginine deiminase system or urease activity in microflora was recently found to modify cariogenicity of comprehensive oral microflora, suggesting that the proportion of acid- or alkali-producing microorganisms is important when evaluating the cariogenicity of oral microflora (Nascimento et al., 2009). However, the co-culture of a combination of well-known periodontopathic bacteria, such as *P. gingivalis*, *T. denticola*, *T. forsythia*, and *Fusobacterium necleatum*, resulted in synergistic biofilm formation (Kuramitsu et al., 2005). Quorum-sensing via AI-2 between *P. gingivalis* and *S. gordonii* is imperative for their biofilm formation (McNab et al., 2003). Hence, identifying the existence of several specific pathogens is not sufficient for evaluating the virulence of oral microflora. Conversely, most of the information available was derived from *in vitro* experiments, which

Figure 1. Proposed molecular interactions within dental biofilm, from Kolenbrander (2006)

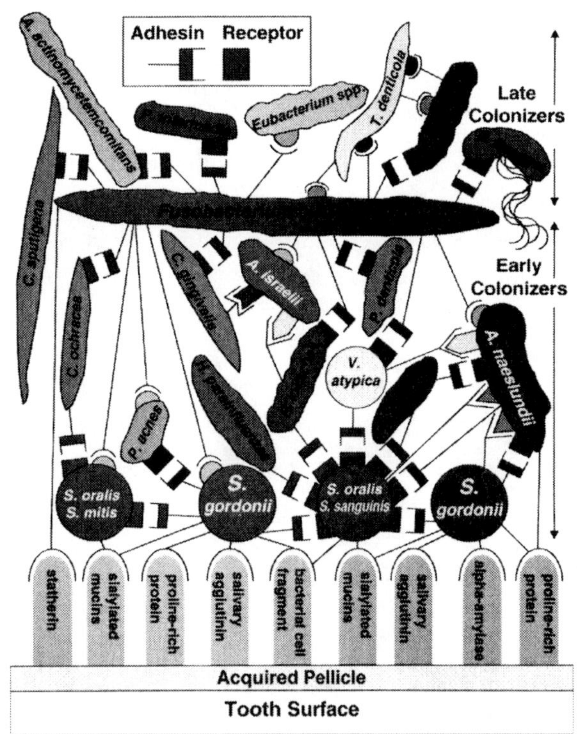

provided definitive data. However, experimental data obtained *in vitro* may not necessarily represent a genuine, complex biological system. We need to face the complexity of the microflora community and overcome the difficulties encountered while studying the etiology of oral diseases surrounded by these microflora.

It is commonly thought that special science laws, especially those in the biological sciences, are not as easily established as in physics and chemistry (Elgin, 2006). Difficulties in the biological sciences consist of the following: (1) organisms are very complex and behave differently under the same circumstances; and (2) biological objects, such as genes, groups, and species, are constantly fluctuating and are subject to the forces of evolution. As described previously, biology may have an inherent complexity that is not easily revealed in a single cell. Furthermore, in the case of multicellular organisms, many exceptions arise because of the different kinds of cell types. Oral microflora, which are composed of numerous bacterial species, may mimic the interaction of cells seen in multicellular organisms. It is important to identify the biological and physiological properties of purified cultures of living cells to better understand the biological system of multicellular organisms. However, isolated cells do not necessarily behave as do those found in multicellular organisms. Mutual interactions between similar or different types of cells are important for performing proper biological functions. This is also true for oral microflora. Which interactions between bacteria are critical for oral health or diseases? What balance, in terms of plaque bacteria, is conducive to oral health or disease?

What Methods Are Needed for Microfloral Analysis in Dentistry?

We would like to explore the methods needed to identify the comprehensive species that make up the oral flora and compare these results with corresponding oral health conditions. In this chapter, we delineate previous attempts to identify oral commensal bacterial flora and discuss the potential capability of modern molecular genetic technologies such as terminal restriction fragment length polymorphism (T-RFLP), DNA microarray and pyrosequencing analyses utilizing bioinformatics. These techniques generate large data sets, but challenges remain in terms of significant scientific meaning.

Finally, we introduce here a recent approach that is applicable for analyzing microflora related to oral health conditions with a large number of subjects and that is able to specify the organisms or plaque composition associated with the health condition. Because the analytical methods used remain incomplete and complex, we also discuss the difficulties associated with analyzing these data and our search for the next approach based on a new paradigm.

In the near future of dentistry, the drill-and-fill approach will be replaced with oral health care based on the proper diagnosis and risk assessment of oral diseases. Oral health is closely connected with a systemic health condition. Much attention has been focused on the association of periodontal health with cardiovascular disease, stroke, diabetes, and pulmonary disease, which are serious problems in the elderly population. Japan is the leading country in terms of population aging: The proportion of Japanese adults aged 65 years or older was 17.4% in 2000 and is estimated to be more than 35% by 2050 (Health and Welfare Statistics Association, 2003). Maintaining healthy conditions for the elderly must be one of the most important and contemporary policies addressed by the governments of most developed countries. The development of floral analyses contributes to the diagnosis of oral flora associated with the risk of oral and systemic diseases, which gives a suitable guideline for maintaining proper oral health conditions.

TECHNIQUES FOR ASSESSING THE COMPOSITION OF THE COMPLEX MICROBIAL COMMUNITY

There is little doubt that the oral microbial community is one of the most complex of microbial floras in the human body. Previous studies using traditional cultivation-based methods and culture-independent molecular techniques have identified more than 700 bacterial species in the human oral cavity. Each person is thought to have 100–200 species, and the composition greatly varies among individuals (Paster et al., 2006). In addition, these bacteria construct distinct microbial communities as biofilms on the saliva-bathed surfaces of various oral structures, such as the dorsum of the tongue, the periodontal pocket, the hard palate, the soft palate, the teeth, and the buccal mucosa.

Cultivation Techniques to DNA Molecular Techniques

The population structure of the oral microbial community has been classically investigated using cultivation-dependent methods that provided substantial evidence of the relationship between commensal microbes and the host. For example, Gram-positive bacteria, such as streptococci and lactobacilli, are predominant in supragingival plaque, whereas subgingival plaque is more dominated by Gram-negative anaerobic bacteria, including *Tannerella forthythensis*, *Prevotella intermedia*, *P. gingivalis*, *T. denticola*, and *F. nucleatum*. Alternation of the bacterial community in the succession of dental plaque was also demonstrated using a cultivation-based method (Ritz, 1967). However, limitations of the cultivation technique have prevented an accurate understanding of the oral microbial community. One drawback of this method is the risk of not identifying bacteria that are difficult to culture or that are non-culturable. Staley and Konopka indicated that only 1% of organisms are able to be grown *in vitro* (Staley & Konopka, 1985). Although the proportion of cultivable oral bacterial species is higher than that of species in other environments, such as soil and sediments, about 50% of bacterial species detected in the oral cavity remain uncultivated. The cultivation method is also very labor intensive and time consuming. A comparative study of bacterial communities using a sufficient sample size was considered to be unrealistic.

The molecular approach, using DNA extracted directly from microbial communities, helps to overcome the limitations of the traditional cultivation technique. The use of the 16S ribosomal ribonucleic acid (rRNA) gene in combination with the polymerase chain reaction (PCR) method has become the most common approach for community analysis. The 16S rRNA gene is thought to be present in all organisms and is approximately 1,500 bp in length. Although its nucleic acid sequence has remained relatively conserved throughout evolution because of its conserved function, it contains nine variable regions that can be used for the classification of bacteria almost to the species level (Pace, 1997). The PCR amplification method uses primers designed from the conservative regions, which allows for the ready collection of the gene from nearly all members of the bacterial community, including non-cultivated species. The population structure of the bacterial community can be characterized based on the amplicon sequence.

Clone Library Analysis

The cloning and sequencing approach is currently regarded as the gold-standard method for analyzing 16S rRNA gene amplicons to identify the composition of microbial consortia, in spite of the fact that the PCR procedure cannot amplify equivalent amounts of different DNA sequences. In general, amplicons are cloned into a plasmid vector, and the resultant plasmids are transformed into *Escherichia coli*. After the construction of the clone library, the inserts are sequenced individually. These sequences are then compared to a large number of sequences deposited in a public database known as the Ribosomal Database Project (http://rdp.cme.msu.edu) to determine their origins or the closest species for identification. More than 800,000 sequences of 16S rRNA gene are presently registered in the database, which is frequently updated.

Since microbial populations in the subgingival plaque were discovered using cloning and sequencing methods (Kroes et al., 1999; Paster et al., 2001), the compositions of different oral bacterial communities from subjects with various symptoms have been continuously investigated using this comprehensive approach. The results of these studies revealed more than 700 members of oral microflora, including more than 300 non-cultivated species (Aas et al., 2005).

It is clear that among the several analytical methods of the 16S rRNA gene, the cloning and sequencing approach provides the most detailed phylogenetic information. However, one disadvantage is that this approach is labor intensive, time consuming, and expensive. It is not well suited for comparing a large number of bacterial communities and monitoring the shift in bacterial compositions. Indeed, Kumar et al. (Kumar et al., 2006) demonstrated by using this method that a change in periodontal status is accompanied by shifts within the subgingival microflora, but more a high-throughput approach of analyzing the population structure is required to create a link between the host's health and the presence or abundance of specific bacterial complexes as well as bacterial species. Nonetheless, nucleic acid sequences play a fundamental role in microbial community analysis.

Denaturing Gradient Gel Electrophoresis (DGGE)

DGGE is the so-called fingerprinting analysis of the 16S rRNA gene amplicons together with T-RFLP analysis. This approach offers a compromise between sample throughput and phylogenetic resolution. DGGE provides a pattern of the community diversity based on the physical separation of unique nucleic acid species (Muyzer et al., 1993). In this approach, internal regions of the 16S rRNA genes (around 200–700 bp) are amplified by PCR, and the products are run on a denaturing gel. Because amplicons with different sequence compositions (GC content) denature at different concentrations, they are separated into distinct bands on the gel. The bacterial community composition can be displayed as a pattern of bands. Theoretically, each band represents a different bacterial population present in a community.

The advantages of this method are its affordability for laboratories and the relative ease in interpreting the results. In particular, it is very useful for assessing the similarity of or variation in different bacterial communities. For example, the similarity in the bacterial populations in saliva between mother and child (Li et al., 2007) and the temporal stability of the bacterial composition in saliva (Rasiah et al., 2005) were clearly revealed by this method. However, it is undeniable that there is a limitation in its phylogenetic resolution. Specific bands of interest can be excised from the gels and identified via sequencing. Direct sequencing of the PCR product occasionally fails because of the mixing of different phylotypes, and cloning of the excised band is more labor intensive. Even if the sequence is determined, the fragment might not contain sufficient information for a precise taxonomic classification. Despite this disadvantage, this method has provided novel evidence of the difference in community structure associated with oral diseases, *e.g.*, severe early childhood caries (Li et al., 2007). DGGE in combination with sequencing is currently one of the most powerful tools used in the comparative analysis of microbial communities.

Terminal Restriction Fragment Length Polymorphism (T-RFLP) Analysis

T-RFLP analysis is another fingerprinting technique that focuses on the size variation of the 5′-end restriction fragments due to restriction enzyme site polymorphisms in the 16S rRNA gene amplicons (Liu et al., 1997). With this method, 16S rRNA genes are PCR-amplified using 5′-end fluorescently labeled primers. The amplicons are digested with a restriction enzyme, and the fragments are separated by capillary electrophoresis. Because only labeled terminal fragments are detected using a laser, the profile is less complex than that of a general RFLP analysis. The sizes and relative abundances of the 5′-terminal fragments reflect the types and abundance of species present in the bacterial community and can be viewed as a peak pattern.

Like DGGE, this method is suitable for making quick comparisons and has been applied to the analysis of various oral bacterial communities, *e.g.*, subgingival plaque (Sakamoto, 2004). The great advantage of T-RFLP over DGGE is its potential to generate a direct phylogenetic assignment to each peak. The mobility of the terminal restriction fragments (T-RFs) is roughly based on fragment size. Therefore, the restriction fragment size of each bacterial species can be predicted from the sequence deposited in the database. T-RFLP analysis can be an analytical method that combines high sample throughput and high phylogenetic resolution.

However, in reality, the interpretation of T-RFLP profiles remains a difficult process. One major reason for this is the presence of similar terminal restriction fragment sizes for multiple species of bacteria. Although the combination of multiple T-RFLP profiles using different restriction enzymes or labeling both ends with different fluorescent dyes can increase specificity, the interpretation of these results is complicated. Furthermore, interpretation can become hampered by discrepancies in fragment size between experimental and theoretical values. Although the combined use of clone libraries of some selected samples may serve for large-scale clinical studies, the enhancement of informatics tools is required to achieve its full potential. We introduce the details of our previous attempts in the next section.

Checkerboard Hybridization and Microarray Analysis

The checkerboard hybridization assay of oral microbial communities was first described in 1994 (Socransky et al., 1994). This methodology enables simultaneous DNA hybridization assays of multiple or selected species present in the microbial community, which helps determine their presence and abundance. The advantage of this method is its high sample throughput. Socransky et al. (1998) investigated 13,261 subgingival plaque samples from 185 subjects using this method and discovered five distinct bacterial complexes related to periodontal health.

In initial reports, whole genomic probes were utilized. Hence, closely related species were occasionally indistinguishable, and identifiable bacterial species were limited to the cultivable species. To overcome these limitations, PCR-based reverse-capture checkerboard hybridization was introduced by Paster et al. (1998). In this modified version of the checkerboard hybridization assay, the 16S rRNA gene amplicons are analyzed in the same manner as the aforementioned approaches. The partial region of the 16S rRNA gene, which is the sequence that is unique to the target bacterial species (about 20 bases), is adapted from the genetic sequence database as a reverse-capture probe. The synthesized oligonucleotide probes (up to 40 probes) are deposited on a nylon membrane in separate horizontal lanes, and the digoxigenin-labeled 16S rRNA gene amplicons derived from the microbial community (up to 45 samples) are hybridized in vertical channels in a Miniblotter apparatus (Paster et al., 1998).

The greatest disadvantage of this method is the limited number of selected species. However, the number of simultaneously analyzable bacterial species increases by more than 300 when one uses the microarray hybridization on glass slides known as the Human Oral Microbe Identification Microarray (http://mim.forsyth.org; Paster et al., 2006). Although quantitative comparison of signal intensities among different bacterial species is not easy to interpreted, it may be the most commonly used approach for characterizing the total bacterial community in the oral cavity.

Pyrosequencing Analysis

Pyrosequencing, which is considered the next-generation sequencing technique, was recently applied to the analysis of oral bacterial communities (Keijser et al., 2008). This method offers numerous sequence data at a much lower cost than the conventional sequencing technique. In this study, almost 200,000 sequences representing 22 taxonomic phyla were determined from bacterial populations in saliva and dental plaque. The addition of a tag sequence to a primer enables the simultaneous analysis of multiple distinct microbial community samples.

The tradeoff for the high processivity of this method is the short length of the individual read. The length restriction of the sequences obtained was about 100 bases for the Genome Sequencer 20 system (Roche, Basel, Switzerland) at 454 Life Sciences (Branford, CT). Nonetheless, the use of the only hypervariable region of the 16S rRNA gene, such as the V6 region, provides a phylogenetic resolution almost to the genus level. In the current GS FLX Titanium series, the readable length has increased up to 400 bases, and more accurate assignments of bacterial taxonomic groups are expected.

The major difficulty associated with using this method is the immense amount of data processing. The procedures, such as classifying based on tag sequence, trimming sequences by removing an adaptor sequence, eliminating low-quality sequences, and searching the corresponding bacterial species from a genetic sequence database, are too labor intensive to perform manually. A suitable support for informatics is indispensable for the future development of this method.

FUTURE TECHNOLOGIES FOR BACTERIAL COMMUNITY ANALYSIS

Our Recent Progress in T-RFLP Analysis

As described previously, targeting the 16S rRNA gene using T-RFLP is a very effective tool for analyzing bacterial communities. In the conventional method, the fragment lengths are calculated as bases, but the order of the fragment lengths does not consistently agree with the order based on molecular weight (Kaplan & Kitts, 2003). A few online databases make archived sequences available, assuming the same or similar sizes for T-RFs from a given endonuclease digestion (Kent et al., 2003; Marsh et al., 2000). However, the discrepancy in molecular sizes resulting from the different composition of nucleic bases may prevent species identification in samples (Kaplan & Kitts, 2003). A ±7-bp range error has been resigned in the conventional T-RFLP, and such a broad range results in too many candidate species to make an accurate identification (Marsh, 2005). Therefore, we developed a Web-based tool, TRFMA, for identifying bacterial species by calculating the molecular weights of the T-RFs (Nakano et al., 2006). TRFMA includes a small and large 16S rRNA genetic database. The small database is composed of sequences from 650 species of oral bacteria and includes the names of species, strains, and Ribosomal Database Project accession numbers. The nucleotide sequences start with the forward primer D88 (5'-GAGAGTTTGATYMTGGCTCAG-3'; Paster et al., 2001)). The large database comprises 50,000 sequences selected from Ribosomal Database Project version 9.35 data by removing those containing more than 10 unidentified nucleotides or lacking primer sequences. The molecular weights of the T-RFs were predicted from 16S rRNA sequences using the forward primer D88 and a set of tetrameric restriction enzymes. This tool in combination with the development of a new size marker successfully reduced the variability to an average discrepancy and displayed accurate candidates for the sample bacterial species.

Limitations in the precise and accurate sizing of DNA fragments based on their mobility during electrophoresis are well described (Luckey & Smith, 1993). When capillary electrophoresis is performed, the observed mobility of an oligonucleotide varies primarily on its molecular mass, but other factors can also strongly affect mobility. To minimize the sizing error and obtain reproducibility, an internal standard can be included in the same lane, and the T-RF size can be estimated from the relative mobility compared to internal standard fragments. However, additional sizing er-

Figure 2. Scheme for the new size definition of the commercially available internal standard GeneScan-1000 ROX. GS# are the fragments in GeneScan-1000 ROX and St# are the self-produced FAM-labeled fragments amplified from the 16S rRNA gene of P. gingivalis. f (x) is the formula of the regression line calculated from the association between the molecular weight (MW) of the FAM-labeled fragments and corresponding their RUM (tSt#). GS# were given the virtual MW of f (t#) according to their own RMU (t#), and the new size definition of GeneScan-1000 ROX was determined. Cited from the reference (Kolenbrander et. al. 2002).

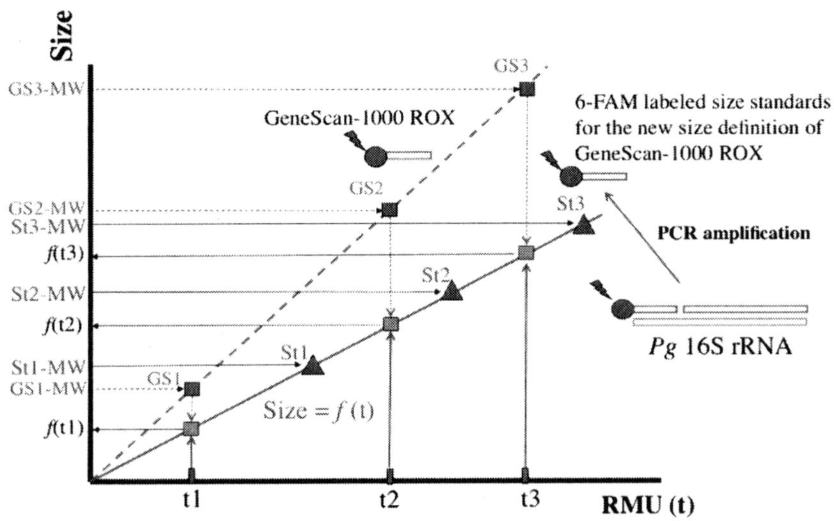

rors can be reproduced even when using an internal standard. Differences in the fluorescent dyes used for labeling can also cause differential mobility (Marsh, 2005), and the diverse 3D-structure derived from sequence variations might cause differential electrophoretic mobility (Kaplan & Kitts, 2003). Therefore, we assumed that sizing errors could be reduced by preparing size markers with structures similar to those of the samples and by using the same fluorescent dye as the standard for the T-RFs (Takeshita et al., 2007). We then prepared a size marker composed of T-RFs that were labeled with 6-carboxyfluorescein (6-FAM) and derived from a 16S rRNA gene of *P. gingivalis*, an oral bacterium (Figure 2). A commercially available internal standard, GeneScan-1000 ROX, was applied to the capillary electrophoresis simultaneously with the FAM-labeled T-RFs derived from the 16S rRNA gene. Based on the result, a new size definition was established for GeneScan-1000 ROX by re-calculating molecular weight sizes of ROX-labeled fragments in regard to the relative mobility of the FAM-labeled T-RFs as shown in Figure 2. Using this definition, the average sizing errors among eight oral bacteria from six phyla were estimated and compared with those obtained using the conventional method. The average sizing error of 2.42 bases for 40 T-RFs was drastically reduced to 0.62 bases, and sizing errors that were more than 2 bases were eliminated, as shown in Figure 3.

Based on these results, the matching window was set to a molecular weight of ±600. Furthermore microbial communities isolated from saliva were analyzed using the new size definition. Bacterial species were assigned to peaks using TRFMA and compared with those identified using the cloning method. More than 90% of the total bacterial clones were detected using the clone library and were assigned by T-RFLP, confirming the accuracy of our method by determining the T-RF sizes derived from various species.

We also modified the T-RFLP method to analyze oral microflora as follows. To analyze the T-RFs for full-length fragments lacking a re-

Figure 3. Sizing error for various bacteria after digestion with HaeIII, HhaI, AluI, BstUI and MspI

Organism[1]	Digestion	Predict size (base)	ROX-base definition (base)	FAM-base definition (base)	FAM-MW definition count as base[2]	MW
Pg	*Alu*I	77	**−3.98**	−0.08	−0.13	−39.26
	*Msp*I	98	0.39	0.03	−0.06	−18.83
	*Hha*I	103	−0.30	−0.17	−0.29	−88.42
	*Bsf*UI	118	**−1.57**	−0.20	−0.37	−114.91
	*Hae*III	922	**1.99**	**1.38**	**1.13**	347.63
Pe	*Alu*I	77	**−3.86**	0.24	0.17	51.69
	*Msp*I	98	0.25	−0.20	−0.22	−69.14
	*Hha*I	103	−0.44	−0.63	−0.53	−162.81
	*Bsf*UI	118	**−1.71**	−0.36	−0.47	−144.47
	*Hae*III	921	**3.42**	**3.85**	**2.98**	921.84
Nm	*Alu*I	76	**−4.11**	−0.19	−0.19	−59.95
	*Msp*I	497	**1.10**	0.51	−0.34	−103.60
	*Hha*I	214	**1.02**	0.82	0.38	116.32
	*Bsf*UI	396	**3.38**	0.43	−0.03	−9.73
	*Hae*III	207	**1.31**	**1.56**	0.80	246.97
Sm	*Alu*I	169	0.06	0.23	−0.13	−41.57
	*Msp*I	564	−4.74	0.64	0.52	161.27
	*Hha*I	223	**1.04**	0.48	0.54	167.39
	*Bsf*UI	105	**−1.05**	−0.55	−0.24	−74.90
	*Hae*III	318	**1.03**	**1.09**	0.66	205.10
Vp	*Alu*I	76	**−4.10**	−0.05	−0.36	−112.34
	*Msp*I	303	0.31	0.30	0.32	97.41
	*Hha*I	591	**−8.49**	0.36	−0.08	−24.87
	*Bsf*UI	116	**−1.53**	−0.10	−0.16	−50.43
	*Hae*III	213	**1.09**	0.95	0.78	239.92
Rd	*Alu*I	73	**−4.65**	**−1.02**	**−1.02**	−314.61
	*Msp*I	164	−0.93	−0.74	−0.93	−286.36
	*Hha*I	375	**4.06**	0.70	−0.17	−52.39
	*Bsf*UI	397	**3.32**	0.04	−0.65	−200.26
	*Hae*III	234	**1.21**	0.58	−0.05	−14.00
Fn	*Alu*I	190	**1.44**	**1.02**	0.99	306.52
	*Msp*I	269	**1.14**	**1.37**	**1.22**	376.54
	*Hha*I	199	**1.39**	0.82	0.85	263.65
	*Bsf*UI	97	0.88	0.43	0.34	104.91
	*Hae*III	272	1.00	**1.44**	**1.26**	390.18
Td	*Alu*I	73	**−3.86**	−0.23	−0.22	−68.31
	*Msp*I	285	**−1.39**	−0.94	**−1.28**	−396.28
	*Hha*I	38	**−9.47**	**−1.48**	**−1.50**	−464.24
	*Bsf*UI	38	**−9.47**	**−1.85**	**−1.70**	−524.84
	*Hae*III	227	−0.25	−0.96	−0.55	−170.54
	Average[3] ± SD		2.42 ± 2.39	0.72 ± 0.70	0.62 ± 0.58	

[1]*Pg, Porphyromonas gingivalis; Pe, Porphyromonas endodontalis; Nm, Neisseria mucosa*
Sm, Streptococcus mutans; Vp, Veillonella parvula;
Rd, Rothia dentocariosa', Fn, Fusobacterium nucleatum; Td, Treponema denticola.
[2]Using the FAM-MW definition, 308.95 (MW) equals 1 base.
[3]Average indicates the average of absolute errors in sizing. The sizing error represents the difference between estimated size after capillary electrophoresis and the size predicted from the sequence. Sizing errors greater than one base are shown in bold.

striction site, we selected a primer set to produce small PCR amplicons. Both forward and reverse primers were labeled with different fluorescence dyes to obtain the information from either side of the T-RFs in a single run. Using the universal forward primer 8F (5'-AGAGTTTGATYMTG-GCTCAG-3'; slightly modified from D88; Paster et al., 2001) labeled at the 5' end with 6-FAM and the universal reverse primer 806R (5'-GGAC-TACCRGGGTATCTAA-3'; slightly modified from F16; Paster et al., 2001) labeled at the 5' end with hexachlorofluorescein, we amplified internal regions of 16S rRNA genes of about 800 bp. Based on the substitution of a primer set, TRFMA was modified to fit a new primer set. The number of deposited sequences in the small database of TRFMAW increased from 650 to 866 derived from 655 species or phylotypes with insufficient sequence information.

A commercially available GeneScan-500 ROX plus 6 additional ROX-labeled self-synthesized DNA fragments derived from a bacterial 16S rRNA gene were used as an internal standard. The new size definition for FAM-labeled primer F8 and primer 806R was performed under the same conditions as described previously. In addition, PCR was performed using KOD DNA polymerase instead of ExTaq DNA polymerase to produce a blunt-ended fragment. *Taq* DNA polymerase possesses terminal transferase activity, resulting in the addition of an adenosine residue at the 3' end of an amplicon. However, none of the amplicons had two peaks derived from a single amplicon (Figure 4 A). KOD DNA polymerase does not exhibit terminal transferase activity, unlike *Taq* DNA polymerase, and generates a single peak from a single amplicon as shown in Figure 4 B. Utilizing these advanced T-RFLP methods, we were able to characterize the microbial community in saliva associated with periodontal diseases (Takeshita et al., 2009).

One approach to solving the problem of identifying the origin of each fragment in the T-RFLP by improving the accuracy of the peak identification has been introduced previously. We propose another method for precisely identifying each fragment with its origin in a calculated sequence database using a correlation matrix of retention times and peak areas of the fragments (Nakano et al., 2008). This strategy was based on the probability that the proportions of two T-RFs from one amplicon should be nearly equal in each analysis. We hypothesized that the prediction of pairs of T-RFs containing both fluorescence-labeled primers, using a matrix of correlation coefficients instead of narrowing down the intersection or subset of a combination of 16S rRNA fragments generated by several restriction enzymes digests, could overcome the difficulty of estimating the origin of each terminal fragment. Furthermore, the proportional composition of bacterial species in all samples can also be estimated. The method is efficient for analyzing more than 50 samples, but unfortunately it cannot be used for analyzing only a few samples. However, even a couple of samples can be analyzed by mixing with other T-RFLP data if they have a similar microfloral composition. Two species (*Abiotrophia defectiva* and *Streptococcus infantis*) were missed in the correlation coefficient matrix method but were identified by using six restriction enzymes in combination, suggesting that the method based on

Figure 4. T-RFLP patterns of DNA fragment amplified with Taq or KOD DNA polymerase. A - DNA fragments amplified with the FAM-labeled primer F8 and Taq polymerase from the 16S rRNA of P. gingivalis; B - DNA fragments amplified under the same conditions, except for the use of the KOD polymerase.

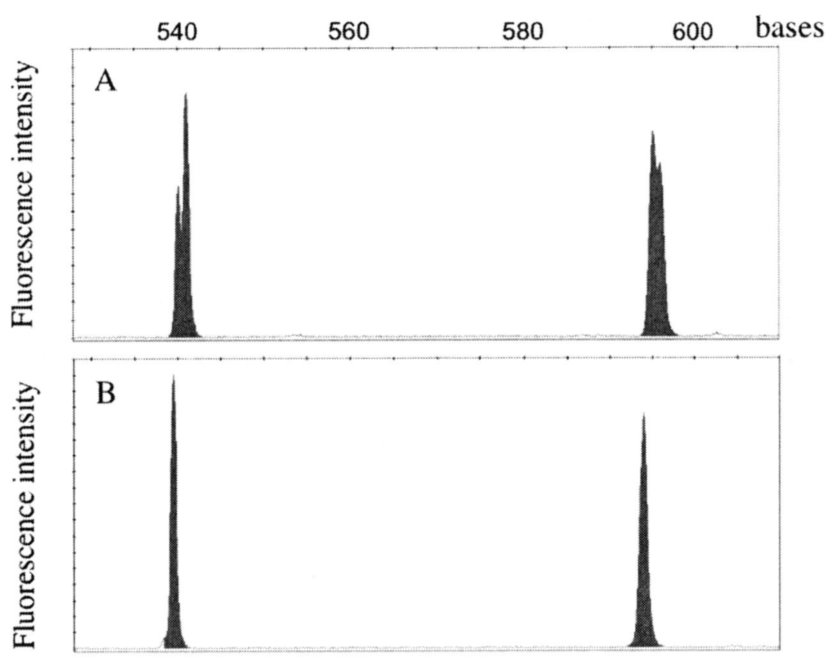

correlation coefficients between peak areas of both terminal fragments is not sufficiently thorough. We need to further explore every possibility for a more sophisticated procedure to understand the complex composition of floral communities.

Essential Support for the Informatics Approach

Based on the technical advances of microbial community analysis described previously, understanding population structures of numerous complex microbial communities simultaneously becomes feasible. The facts imply that in the near future we will have enormous data sets that represent the abundance distribution of more than 700 bacterial species in thousands of microbial community samples. However, such extensive data sets are too complex to be analyzed subjectively. To clarify the relationship with oral health or disease, the support of statistical methods, especially multivariate analysis, is indispensable.

Cluster analysis is an effective approach for exploring the flora pattern associated with oral health or disease. This method is based on computing the dissimilarities between all profiles and allows for the grouping of bacterial communities with similar structure patterns. Comparing the clinical parameters of infected subjects helps to identify the characteristics of the bacterial community composition associated with oral health or diseases. In our recent study, the bacterial composition in stimulated saliva from 200 subjects aged 15–40 years was analyzed using the previously modified T-RFLP method (Takeshita et al., 2009). The data set, which represents the abundance distribution of 110 distinct peaks in the 200 T-RFLP profiles that were obtained, and the subjects were classified into three clusters (I, II, and III) by partitioning into medoids clustering based on their T-RFLP profiles (Figure 5). As predicted from the T-RFs sizes, the more predominant members of each cluster were *Prevotella* and *Veillonella* species in cluster I; *Streptococcus* species in cluster II; and *Neisseria*, *Haemophilus*, or *Aggregatibacter* species and *Porphyromonas* species in cluster III. When the clinical oral health parameters were compared among clusters, the parameters associated with periodontal disease were significantly different. Clusters I and II had a higher percentage of sites in periodontal pockets >4 mm, and cluster I most often contained sites that exhibited bleeding on probing; no significant differences were observed for other parameters, including dental caries. The clustering of the T-RFLP profiles in this study was based mainly on differences in the abundance distribution of the dominant T-RFs detected in most of the subjects, suggesting that the commensal bacteria in saliva are strongly correlated with periodontal health and might influence an individual's susceptibility to periodontal disease. A comprehensive environment composed of indigenous oral bacterial species seems to affect oral health. In this study, the bacterial compositions were classified into only three clusters because the sample size was relatively small (200 subjects). An increase in the number of the subjects would allow for a more detailed classification of the bacterial composition associated with oral health.

Therefore, cluster analysis is useful for obtaining characteristics from numerous complex data. It is difficult to say that this method has been sufficiently optimized and estimated for the comparative analysis of bacterial communities. For example, many different distance measures evaluate the similarity between bacterial community samples. Whereas we used Euclidean distance as the similarity index, which incorporates the abundance of each peak, indexes that utilize only the presence or absence of the peak (such as Dice's coefficient) have been used in other studies. In addition, various clustering methods exist, such as hierarchical clustering, k-means clustering, partitioning around medoids clustering, and the model-based method. The choice of clustering method is affected by the results of the analysis, including the subsequent data normalization. The

Figure 5. T-RFLP peak patterns from 200 subjects (rows) visualized by a gel-like image. From Takeshita et al. (2009). The patterns were sorted into three clusters, separated based on the nearest neighbor of each cluster, and ordered according to each silhouette width (measures the degree of fitness of an object to its cluster) within the cluster. The silhouette width of each sample (displayed as color code bars) and the nearest neighbor cluster are indicated to the left of the image. The area proportion of each T-RFLP profile (6-carboxyfluorescein [6-FAM] and hexachlorofluorescein [HEX]) of the individual peaks (69 6-FAM peaks and 41 HEX peaks; columns) is represented as a color code in each grid. The percentage of sites with periodontal pockets (pocket depths over 4–6 mm) in all surveyed sites of each subject is displayed as color code bars to the right of the image.

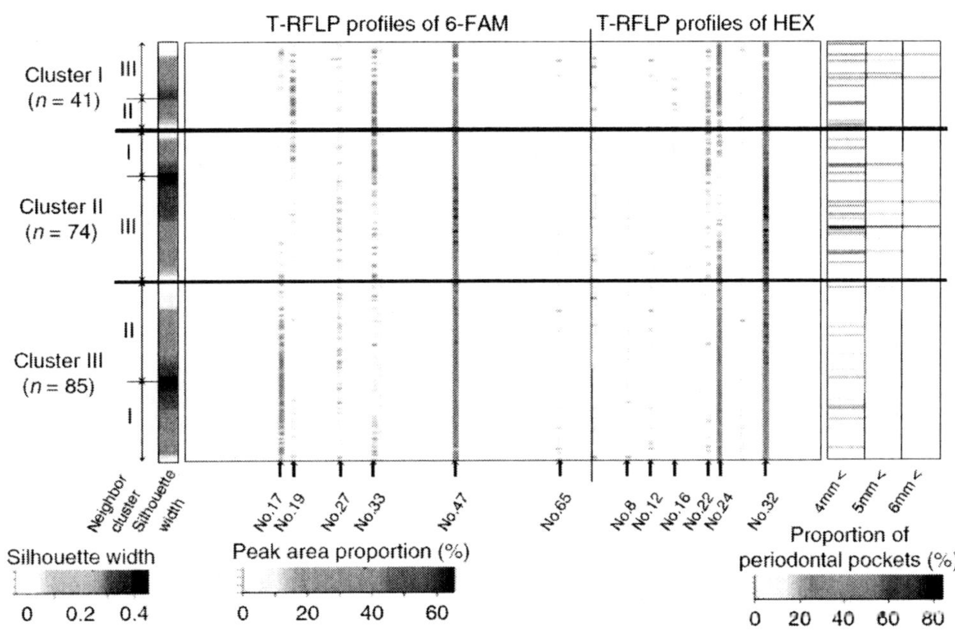

method must be carefully suited to the structure of the data obtained for the appropriate assessment of oral microbial communities.

Following the characterization of the flora pattern associated with oral health or disease, future studies must identify the key bacterial species complex as well as the single pathogenic bacteria. The combinations of the more than 700 bacterial species are too numerous to investigate individually. The incorporation of computer technology in the detection of bacterial complex communities is essential for understanding the significance of these bacteria to oral health.

CONCLUSION

A wealth of technical development presently exists in terms of microbial community analyses. For these technologies to reach their full potential, advances in data analysis are also required. These advances will greatly increase the available evidence concerning the relationship between oral microbes and oral health.

REFERENCES

Aas, J. A., Paster, B. J., Stokes, L. N., Olsen, I., & Dewhirst, F. E. (2005). Defining the normal bacterial flora of the oral cavity. *Journal of Clinical Microbiology*, *43*(11), 5721–5732. doi:10.1128/JCM.43.11.5721-5732.2005

Albandar, J. M., Brown, L. J., & Loe, H. (1997). Clinical features of early-onset periodontitis. *The Journal of the American Dental Association*, *128*(10), 1393–1399.

American_Academy_of_Pediatrics. (2009). Retrieved May 25, 2009, from http://www.aap.org/oralhealth/cme/page4.htm

Bratthall, D. (1970). Demonstration of five serological groups of streptococcal strains resembling Streptococcus mutans. *Odontologisk Revy*, *21*(2), 143–152.

Elgin, M. (2006). There may be strict empirical laws in biology, after all. *Biology and Philosophy*, *21*(1), 119–134. doi:10.1007/s10539-005-3177-z

Health_and_Welfare_Statistics_Association. (2003). *Kokumin Eisei no Doko (Trends in Nation's Health, Japan)*. Tokyo: Health and Welfare Statistics Association (in Japanese).

Kaplan, C. W., & Kitts, C. L. (2003). Variation between observed and true Terminal Restriction Fragment length is dependent on true TRF length and purine content. *Journal of Microbiological Methods*, *54*(1), 121–125. doi:10.1016/S0167-7012(03)00003-4

Keijser, B. J., Zaura, E., Huse, S. M., van der Vossen, J. M., Schuren, F. H., & Montijn, R. C. (2008). Pyrosequencing analysis of the oral microflora of healthy adults. *Journal of Dental Research*, *87*(11), 1016–1020. doi:10.1177/154405910808701104

Kent, A. D., Smith, D. J., Benson, B. J., & Triplett, E. W. (2003). Web-based phylogenetic assignment tool for analysis of terminal restriction fragment length polymorphism profiles of microbial communities. *Applied and Environmental Microbiology*, *69*(11), 6768–6776. doi:10.1128/AEM.69.11.6768-6776.2003

Kolenbrander, P. E., Palmer, R. J. Jr, Rickard, A. H., Jakubovics, N. S., Chalmers, N. I., & Diaz, P. I. (2006). Bacterial interactions and successions during plaque development. *Periodontology 2000*, *42*, 47–79. doi:10.1111/j.1600-0757.2006.00187.x

Kreth, J., Merritt, J., Shi, W., & Qi, F. (2005). Competition and coexistence between Streptococcus mutans and Streptococcus sanguinis in the dental biofilm. *Journal of Bacteriology*, *187*(21), 7193–7203. doi:10.1128/JB.187.21.7193-7203.2005

Kroes, I., Lepp, P. W., & Relman, D. A. (1999). Bacterial diversity within the human subgingival crevice. *Proceedings of the National Academy of Sciences of the United States of America*, *96*(25), 14547–14552. doi:10.1073/pnas.96.25.14547

Kumar, P. S., Leys, E. J., Bryk, J. M., Martinez, F. J., Moeschberger, M. L., & Griffen, A. L. (2006). Changes in periodontal health status are associated with bacterial community shifts as assessed by quantitative 16S cloning and sequencing. *Journal of Clinical Microbiology*, *44*(10), 3665–3673. doi:10.1128/JCM.00317-06

Kuramitsu, H. K., Chen, W., & Ikegami, A. (2005). Biofilm formation by the periodontopathic bacteria Treponema denticola and Porphyromonas gingivalis. *Journal of Periodontology*, *76*(11 Suppl), 2047–2051. doi:10.1902/jop.2005.76.11-S.2047

Li, Y., Ismail, A. I., Ge, Y., Tellez, M., & Sohn, W. (2007). Similarity of bacterial populations in saliva from African-American mother-child dyads. *Journal of Clinical Microbiology*, *45*(9), 3082–3085. doi:10.1128/JCM.00771-07

Liu, W. T., Marsh, T. L., Cheng, H., & Forney, L. J. (1997). Characterization of microbial diversity by determining terminal restriction fragment length polymorphisms of genes encoding 16S rRNA. *Applied and Environmental Microbiology*, *63*(11), 4516–4522.

Loesche, W. J. (1986). Role of Streptococcus-Mutans in Human Dental Decay. *Microbiological Reviews*, *50*(4), 353–380.

Luckey, J. A., & Smith, L. M. (1993). A model for the mobility of single-stranded DNA in capillary gel electrophoresis. *Electrophoresis*, *14*(5-6), 492–501. doi:10.1002/elps.1150140176

Marsh, T. L. (2005). Culture-independent microbial community analysis with terminal restriction fragment length polymorphism. *Methods in Enzymology*, *397*, 308–329. doi:10.1016/S0076-6879(05)97018-3

Marsh, T. L., Saxman, P., Cole, J., & Tiedje, J. (2000). Terminal restriction fragment length polymorphism analysis program, a web-based research tool for microbial community analysis. *Applied and Environmental Microbiology*, *66*(8), 3616–3620. doi:10.1128/AEM.66.8.3616-3620.2000

McNab, R., Ford, S. K., El-Sabaeny, A., Barbieri, B., Cook, G. S., & Lamont, R. J. (2003). LuxS-based signaling in Streptococcus gordonii: autoinducer 2 controls carbohydrate metabolism and biofilm formation with Porphyromonas gingivalis. *Journal of Bacteriology*, *185*(1), 274–284. doi:10.1128/JB.185.1.274-284.2003

Muyzer, G., de Waal, E. C., & Uitterlinden, A. G. (1993). Profiling of complex microbial populations by denaturing gradient gel electrophoresis analysis of polymerase chain reaction-amplified genes coding for 16S rRNA. *Applied and Environmental Microbiology*, *59*(3), 695–700.

Nakano, Y., Takeshita, T., Kamio, N., Shiota, S., Shibata, Y., & Yasui, M. (2008). Development and application of a T-RFLP data analysis method using correlation coefficient matrices. *Journal of Microbiological Methods*, *75*(3), 501–505. doi:10.1016/j.mimet.2008.08.002

Nakano, Y., Takeshita, T., & Yamashita, Y. (2006). TRFMA: a web-based tool for terminal restriction fragment length polymorphism analysis based on molecular weight. *Bioinformatics (Oxford, England)*, *22*(14), 1788–1789. doi:10.1093/bioinformatics/btl186

Nascimento, M. M., Gordan, V. V., Garvan, C. W., Browngardt, C. M., & Burne, R. A. (2009). Correlations of oral bacterial arginine and urea catabolism with caries experience. *Oral Microbiology and Immunology*, *24*(2), 89–95.

Nishikawara, F., Katsumura, S., Ando, A., Tamaki, Y., Nakamura, Y., & Sato, K. (2006). Correlation of cariogenic bacteria and dental caries in adults. *Journal of Oral Science*, *48*(4), 245–251. doi:10.2334/josnusd.48.245

Ota, F., Ota, M., Mahmud, Z. H., Mohammad, A., Yamato, M., & Kassu, A. (2006). Serological diversity demonstrable by a set of monoclonal antibodies to eight serotypes of the mutans streptococci. *Caries Research*, *40*(1), 6–14. doi:10.1159/000088899

Pace, N. R. (1997). A molecular view of microbial diversity and the biosphere. *Science*, *276*(5313), 734–740. doi:10.1126/science.276.5313.734

Paster, B. J., Bartoszyk, I. M., & Dewhirst, F. E. (1998). Identification of oral streptococci using PCR-based, reverse-capture, checkerboard hybridization. *Methods in Cell Science*, (20): 223–231. doi:10.1023/A:1009715710555

Paster, B. J., Boches, S. K., Galvin, J. L., Ericson, R. E., Lau, C. N., & Levanos, V. A. (2001). Bacterial diversity in human subgingival plaque. *Journal of Bacteriology*, *183*(12), 3770–3783. doi:10.1128/JB.183.12.3770-3783.2001

Paster, B. J., Olsen, I., Aas, J. A., & Dewhirst, F. E. (2006). The breadth of bacterial diversity in the human periodontal pocket and other oral sites. *Periodontology 2000*, *42*, 80–87. doi:10.1111/j.1600-0757.2006.00174.x

Petersen, P. E. (2003). The World Oral Health Report 2003: continuous improvement of oral health in the 21st century--the approach of the WHO Global Oral Health Programme. *Community Dentistry and Oral Epidemiology*, *31*(Suppl 1), 3–23. doi:10.1046/j..2003.com122.x

Rasiah, I. A., Wong, L., Anderson, S. A., & Sissons, C. H. (2005). Variation in bacterial DGGE patterns from human saliva: over time, between individuals and in corresponding dental plaque microcosms. *Archives of Oral Biology*, *50*(9), 779–787. doi:10.1016/j.archoralbio.2005.02.001

Ritz, H. L. (1967). Microbial population shifts in developing human dental plaque. *Archives of Oral Biology*, *12*(12), 1561–1568. doi:10.1016/0003-9969(67)90190-2

Socransky, S. S., Haffajee, A. D., Cugini, M. A., Smith, C., & Kent, R. L. Jr. (1998). Microbial complexes in subgingival plaque. *Journal of Clinical Periodontology*, *25*(2), 134–144. doi:10.1111/j.1600-051X.1998.tb02419.x

Socransky, S. S., Smith, C., Martin, L., Paster, B. J., Dewhirst, F. E., & Levin, A. E. (1994). "Checkerboard" DNA-DNA hybridization. *BioTechniques*, *17*(4), 788–792.

Staley, J. T., & Konopka, A. (1985). Measurement of in situ activities of nonphotosynthetic microorganisms in aquatic and terrestrial habitats. *Annual Review of Microbiology*, *39*, 321–346. doi:10.1146/annurev.mi.39.100185.001541

Takeshita, T., Nakano, Y., Kumagai, T., Yasui, M., Kamio, N., & Shibata, Y. (2009). The ecological proportion of indigenous bacterial populations in saliva is correlated with oral health status. *The ISME Journal*, *3*(1), 65–78. doi:10.1038/ismej.2008.91

Takeshita, T., Nakano, Y., & Yamashita, Y. (2007). Improved accuracy in terminal restriction fragment length polymorphism phylogenetic analysis using a novel internal size standard definition. *Oral Microbiology and Immunology*, *22*(6), 419–428. doi:10.1111/j.1399-302X.2007.00384.x

Tong, H., Chen, W., Merritt, J., Qi, F., Shi, W., & Dong, X. (2007). Streptococcus oligofermentans inhibits Streptococcus mutans through conversion of lactic acid into inhibitory H2O2: a possible counteroffensive strategy for interspecies competition. *Molecular Microbiology*, *63*(3), 872–880. doi:10.1111/j.1365-2958.2006.05546.x

KEY TERMS AND DEFINITIONS

16S rRNA Gene: A composition of prokaryotic ribosomal RNA (rRNA), which is the central component of the ribosome. 16S rRNA gene diversity has been extensively analyzed and is used as a phylogenetic tool for describing the evolutionary relationships among prokaryotes.

Biofilm: Microorganisms growing on a solid substrate, which consist of numerous bacteria and archaea living within an extracellular matrix of polymeric substances. This matrix protects the cells within it and facilitates communication among them through chemical and physical signals.

Cariogenic Bacteria: A group of oral streptococci (or mutant streptococci) thought to be the main cause of dental caries in infants. It is unknown whether other acid-producing oral species are involved in cariogenicity, especially in the adult bacterial etiology of dental caries.

Comparative Analysis of Microbial Community: Such studies are performed to understand the similarity among different microbial communities but do not identify the species that characterize the microbial community.

Floral Analysis: The identification of individual species and their occupation rate within the entire floral community.

Multifactorial Disease: There is no doubt that dental caries and periodontal diseases are infectious diseases. However, it is difficult to explain the onset of these diseases solely by the infection of oral bacteria. Host susceptibility and habitat can affect the oral environment and strongly influence the process of both dental caries and periodontal diseases, which exhibit some characteristics of a multifactorial disease.

Necrotizing Ulcerative Periodontitis: The disease presents itself as "blunting" at interdental papillae but rapidly progresses to the destruction of the underlying alveolar bone or periodontium. It is usually associated with severe pain and spontaneous bleeding, which serves as an indicator of severe immunosuppression.

Phylogenetic Information: Information on the position of the corresponding species in a taxonomic hierarchy. Bacteria are classified according to the seven main taxonomic ranks: kingdom, phylum, class, order, family, genus, and species.

Putative Periodontopathogens: Periodontopathogens have not yet been clearly elucidated. Although some anaerobic Gram-negative bacteria are thought to be involved in periodontitis, the association might be derived from species that can adapt to the anaerobic conditions in the deep pocket of the periodontal lesion.

Pyrosequencing Analyses: A multi-sequencing technique using a pyrosequencer (the DNA sequencer of the next generation) that can provide sequences from more than 10,000 samples simultaneously without the need for a clone library.

Restriction Fragment Length Polymorphism (RFLP) Analysis: A DNA fragment amplified by a polymerase chain reaction is characterized using a restriction enzyme digest. The digested fragment exhibits a typical pattern that represents the origin of the template DNA.

Taxonomic Classification: The hierarchical organization of living beings into categories and subcategories that reveal their likenesses.

Section 5
Informatic Tools in the Management of Dental Care

Chapter 16
Automated Telephone Services in Dentist Appointment Management

Reima Suomi
Helsinki University of Technology Lahti Center, Finland

Ari Serkkola
Helsinki University of Technology Lahti Center, Finland

Markku Mikkonen
Social and Health Affairs department in the City of Lahti, Finland

ABSTRACT

Reservation of health care service appointments has traditionally been performed through telephone. This takes a lot of time and resources at both ends of the transaction, and can be error-prone. Especially dentist appointments are standard as compared to many other health service provision activities, and are thus a natural candidate for rationalization through modern information technology. Appointments can of course be made through the Internet, but using phones, especially mobile phones, adds flexibility to the performing of the transaction. In this article we take a look how the middle-sized Finnish city of Lahti has taken a comprehensive approach to develop new innovative services in dentist appointment management.

INTRODUCTION

Dentist health services are very transaction intensive. As related to the actual care-taking activity, transactional activities such as reserving, cancelling and rescheduling activities consume a lot of the patient and staff time, as compared to many other fields of health-care. Visiting a dentist is maybe the most routine and frequent healthcare activity most healthy people in the working age perform. All this has made dentist appointment scheduling a good candidate for automation and re-engineering efforts through telephone-based innovations. This article reports on two systems that have been implemented in the City of Lahti, a 100 000 inhabitant city in Finland, to take care of dentist appointment management activities.

DOI: 10.4018/978-1-60566-733-1.ch016

RELATED TECHNOLOGIES

Appointment scheduling for dental care can be seen as a call center. The efficient handling of the large masses of calls and other contacts would be impossible without good computer-telephony integration . Next we shortly discuss these two concepts that form the cornerstones for the applications in Lahti.

Call Center Management

A call center is an organizational department responsible for handling customer service issues by telephone and other channels (Laudon and Laudon 2006, 97). The British Call Center Association defines a call center as follows (Call Center Association 1999): "a physical or virtual operation within an organisation in which a managed group of people spend most of their time doing business by telephone, usually working in a computer-automated setting." The Pennsylvanian administrative office for public safety radio services has the following definition for a call center (Public Safety Radio Services 2008): "A call center is a central place where customer and other telephone calls are handled by an organization, usually with some amount of computer automation. Typically, a call center has the ability to handle a considerable volume of calls at the same time, to screen calls and forward them to someone qualified to handle them, and to log calls."

Call center operations are divided to inbound and outbound activities. As the name says, inbound call centers handle incoming phone calls. Typical inbound call centres are help desks. Outbound call centers themselves take the contact, often for example in marketing purposes. Performing surveys and other type of research over the telephone is also a typical task.

Stolz (2004) defines a call centre as follows: "an organisation or a unit, located at a geographical distance from its customers and/or principals, that handles inbound or outbound calls in order to answer questions from customers or clients or in order to gather information for a certain activity. Communication with customers includes the use of telephones as well as modern communication media, such as e-mail and chat. Further, call centre activities can be performed either in-house, which refers to services that are provided internally within an organisation, or outsourced, which means that the call centre attends to other organisation's tasks."

The academic and professional discussion on call centers is concentrating very much on working methods in call centers, and on the viability of call centers as working places . A dominant conclusion seems to be that badly managed call centers can be frustrating working places . Thus, automatic speech recognition might be a very good idea, in order to free workforce from boring routine tasks often available in call centers. However, the adoption and acceptance of call centers and especially computerized speech recognition by customers seems to be very scarcely studied in academic literature.

Computer-Telephony Integration

Computer-Telephony Integration (CTI) refers to systems that enable a computer to act as a call center, accepting incoming calls and routing them to the appropriate device or person. These systems can handle a variety of incoming and outgoing communications, including phone calls, faxes, and Internet messages (Public Safety Radio Services 2008).

Call centers are supported by computer-telephony integration, which is integrated and works together with the following technologies too, among others (Yarberry 2000):

- Automatic call distribution (ACD)
- Interactive voice processing
- Workflow
- Predictive dialers
- Image processing

Figure 1. The process of reallocating dentist appointments

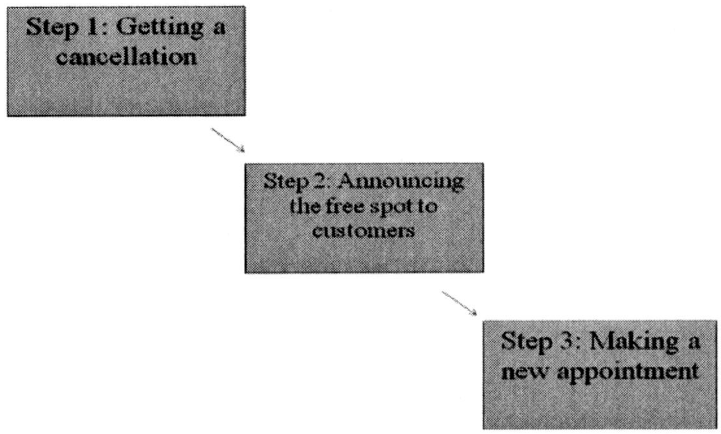

- E-mail processing
- Video/multimedia interaction
- Audio text and announcer
- Fax on demand
- Management reporting

The general opinion is, that computer-telephony integration is still today a burdensome task, as computer and telephone systems have such a diverge history behind them. New digital telephony, and especially Internet telephony, is going to bring some alleviation to this problem.

THE LAHTI PILOT PROJECTS

Introduction to the Environment

The City of Lahti in Finland with 99 800 residents offers its inhabitants the possibility to obtain oral health care services at public dental clinics. The oral health care is provided by 29 dentists, 17 oral hygiene specialists, and 46 dental assistants and receptionists. In addition, about 60 full- or part-time private dentists work in the city. There are 20 dental clinics for the use of clients in different parts of the city.

Dental care has become a market where customers have a choice. There is evidence that the availability of different communication channels with health care professionals and efficient scheduling solutions are key selection factors, as customers select their health care providers .

Both systems presented here support the same goal: dentist appointments should be in effective use, and drop-outs from service by customers should be eliminated. The voice-recognition -based appointment cancellation and rescheduling system makes rescheduling and cancelling of appointments easy for the patients. The GSM-based appointment rescheduling system makes the filling of the empty slots more easy and effective. The systems also support each other in the management of appointments, the voice-recognition -based appointment cancellation and rescheduling being active in step 1, the GSM-based appointment rescheduling system being active in steps 2 and 3 (see Figure 1).

A centralised contact centre has been set up for oral health care in the City of Lahti. Customers entering the service for a first time call directly to a human agent. Customers wishing to inquire, reschedule or cancel their appointment are encouraged to use a number, where a speech recognition system answers.

A customer who calls the contact centre human agent will access one of the following services: an oral health advisor, an emergency duty office,

Figure 2. An example message from the GSM-based appointment rescheduling system

> Cancelled appointment time at Laune Dental Clinic,
>
> Launeenkatu 74 B, 31 March at 12.00.
>
> Please reply IMMEDIATELY: write HA and
>
> send to the number 18444.
>
> Wait for confirmation!

or will be given an appointment with an oral hygienist to assess the need for treatment. Urgent cases are directed from the contact centre to a duty office, where they have access to treatment the same day.

Some 30 percent of dentist appointments in Lahti need rescheduling or cancellation. With the new system using speech recognition the clients can do this activity 24 hour a day at any time, and the system is able to answer several simultaneous calls, an activity not possible for a human answerer. It is of great importance that people really cancel the times they do not want to use: this will save a lot of the dentist resources as free spots can be reallocated in a good time .

The speech recognition system as well as other appointment management services needs joint, agreed-on processes. A crucial decision was to put up a joint patient database, and building a joint queue based on it. There is just one patient queue that all clinics work on.

Secondly, a joint electronic time reservation system is needed. In this reservation system, each clinic has its own calender, where resources are marked. Appointments are provided by the contact center and by the individual clinics.

GSM-Based Appointment Rescheduling System

Before the GSM appointment reservation system, clients were put on a waiting list at a specific dental clinic, and eventually appointments were distributed from there to the other dental clinics manually. This process was rather laborious to handle. Clients on the waiting list were invited to the clinics either by telephone or by letter. A particular problem was posed by appointments that were cancelled the same day. These often remained unfilled.

When managing the appointments and the reservations by GSM, the dental clinic informs clients on the waiting list by SMS-messages about the cancelled appointment time. The GSM-based reservation in this application concerns cancelled appointment times that are reallocated within the same day (2-8 hours) or days before. In the database, the clients may be grouped into either one waiting list or several, depending on the grouping principle. The basis for the grouping may be, for example, the treatment unit, the medical priority, the waiting time, or the local area. Clients can be added or removed from the waiting list according to need. The opportunity for GSM reservation is presented to clients who wish to accept cancelled appointment times by mobile phone.

A receptionist or dental assistant sends the cancelled, available appointment time by one press of a button to five clients simultaneously. The first of the five clients to reply to the text message can reserve the free appointment time. The other four clients are informed that the appointment has been filled, and they return to the top of the list to await the next time that becomes available. The content of the text message invitation corresponds to the following formula as in Figure 2.

Speech Recognition-Based Appointment Cancellation and Rescheduling

The system introduced here is not used for the first and primary scheduling of a dentist appointment, but rather in consequent phases of the customer interaction process:

- When the customer wants to check his/her appointment time
- When the customer wants to cancel his/her appointment
- When the customer wants to reschedule his/her appointment.

Speech recognition leans on the services provided by a system for electronic patient records, in Lahti the used system is WinHIT. Especially the patient database is in the hearth of activities, and it is joint for all the 20 dental clinics in Lahti.

An example discussion flow of the application is as follows (of course in Finnish). The answering solution first asks *"Do you want to change or cancel your appointment, or do you want to do something else?"* The patient is expected to answer one of the alternatives, for example to say "I *cancel my appointment"*. A key feature of the application is the identification of the caller, where the Finnish social security number (of structure ddmmyyyy-123*, for example 05121946-145H) is being questioned. The caller is expected to deliver the social security number sign by sign. When the identification is done, the appointment can be sought from the database. Two questions from the application are needed: *"Is your social security number 05121946-145H"* (example). After a positive confirmation by the caller, a further question can be made. "*Do you want to cancel the time allocated to you on 14.5.2009?* (example). After a positive answer by the client, the transaction is confirmed: "Y*our appointment is cancelled*". The transaction is finished.

In Table 1 we can see some pioneering use statistics from the system from the two first usage months of the system. From the table we can see that the system has processed 44.1 percent of the incoming calls, and that it has been possible to

Table 1. Pioneering period system usage statistics

Classification criteria for the call		Calculation basis	Number of calls	% of all calls
All phone calls together	A		8694	100
Unidentified calls	B		2290	26.3
Processed calls together	C	A - B	6404	73.7
Calls forwarded to human agent in total	D	E + G	4179	48.1
Of these forwarded to human agent without the identification of the patient	E		2573	29.6
Calls processed by the speech recognition system	F	G + H	3831	44.1
Of these forwarded to the human agent after the identification of the patient	G		1606	18.5
Of these automatically handled with connections to the electronic patient records	H	J + K + L	2225	25.5
Transaction types in automatic handling:				
Question about appointment time	J		1589	18.3
Rescheduing of appointment time	K		392	4.5
Canceltion of appontment time	L		244	2.8

process 25.5 percent of the incoming calls with the system. The drop-out rate from this service is 26.3 percent, also so many have aborted their phone call before any transaction could be accomplished.

The changes and cancellations of appointment times mean high labour costs for the clinics. About 30% of appointments in Lahti are subject to changes or cancellations. The pioneering system presented in this article should make the customer's operations easier as it comes to rescheduling and cancelling of appointments, and they should be able to do the activities without interaction with staff. As staff time can be more effectively allocated to activities needing real human interaction, the total resources or the clinics are in more effective use.

Through the speech recognition system, answering times and service level can be somewhat improved in peak hours of operation. More customers can be served simultaneously than in the case of human agents. Waiting times on the phone are almost totally eliminated. The computerized services are available 24 hour a day in every day of the week, which adds to the reachability of the services. The documentation on the care need frees the nurses to take part in other activities, such as helping dentists.

The system at hand seems to be robust and usable. It has served successfully the big general audience, and the system can be used to free dentist clinic appointment service resources for other, maybe more productive activities.

CONCLUSION

Table 2 summarizes the results from the two pioneering appointment management applications in use in Lahti. In addition to these, some other applications are too in use, as for example a reminder service of approaching appointments using SMS-messages, especially productive and handy in the case of school eleven.

Our discussion shows, that a computer system for the management of the dentist appointments cannot be implemented on a flimsy basis. Renewing of both governance structures as well as processes is important. In the case of Lahti, a critical decision was to put all clinics to use just one queue for care. This affects both governance structures as well as processes.

Cancelling and rescheduling dentist appointments needs careful engineering. Cancellation and rescheduling should be made easy for the

Table 2. A summary of the two implemented innovations

	GSM-based appointment rescheduling	**Voice-recognition based appointment cancellation and rescheduling**
Basis technology	GSM-based SMS-messages	Voice recognition
System into use	2006	2008
Activity owner	The health care clinic	The customer
Main idea	Reallocating cancelled appointments fast and efficiently	Making it easy for the patients to cancel and reschedule dentist appointments
Innovations on the background	Queue management Computer-telephone integration	Queue management Computer-telephone integration
Benefits to the customer	Possibility to get to care in short time	Possibility to cancel/question/reschedule dental appointments at any time
Benefits to the clinic	More effective resource usage in appointment management activities More effective resource usage in the core health care activity	More effective resource usage in appointment management activities

citizen, but not too easy so that they do not begin to feel that a dentist appointment is a worthless commodity.

The used technologies can be used in many other application areas too. The technology of appointment rescheduling, GSM-messaging, can be used in the health care setting for example to calling in vacant nurses or doctors, when staff shortage suddenly should occur.

Another growth area could be that of other, more complicated health-care operations, such as daytime surgery. However, in more complicated settings, queues are shorter, and the preconditions that must be met in order to make the operation successful are more detailed and complicated.

Our two examples however manifest, that appointment management can be improved with modern ICT-technologies. A critical success factor is the approval of the services by customers, and how this is going to succeed remains to be seen.

REFERENCES

Batt, R., & Moynihan, L. (2006). The viability of alternative call centre production models. *Human Resource Management Journal, 12*(4), 14–34. doi:10.1111/j.1748-8583.2002.tb00075.x

Call Center Association. (1999). *Definition of call center*. London.

Gopalakrishna, P., & Mummaleni, V. (1993). Influencing satisfaction for dental services. *Journal of Health Care Marketing, 13*(1), 16–22.

Holman, D. (2006). Employee wellbeing in call centres. *Human Resource Management Journal, 12*(4), 35–50. doi:10.1111/j.1748-8583.2002.tb00076.x

Kinder, T. (2001). The use of Call Centres by local public administrations. *Futures, 33*(10), 837–860. doi:10.1016/S0016-3287(01)00022-2

Laudon, K. C., & Laudon, J. P. (2006). *Essentials of business information systems*. Upper Saddle River, NJ: Pearson Education, Prentice-Hall.

Public Safety Radio Services (2008). *Definition of term "Computer-Telephony Integration"*.

Schulzrinne, H., & Rosenberg, J. (2008). Internet Telephony: Architecture and Protocols an IETF Perspective. *Computer Networks, 31*, 237–255. doi:10.1016/S0169-7552(98)00265-7

Stoltz, C. (2004). Calling for Call Centres - A study of Call Centre Locations in a Swedish Rural Region. *Economic Information Systems, Department of Computer and information Science*. Linköping, Sweden: Linköping University.

Suomi, R., & Serkkola, A. (2007). Rescheduling Dental Care with GSM-Based Text Messages. In L. Al-Hakim (Ed.), *Web Mobile-Based Applications for Healthcare Management*, (pp. 335-353). Hershey, PA: IRM Press.

Suomi, R., & Serkkola, A. (2007). GSM-based SMS Time Reservation System for Dental Care. *International Journal of Technology and Human Interaction, 3*(3), 54–68.

Taylor, P., & Bain, P. (2003). 'An assembly line in the head': work and employee relations in the call centre. *Phil Taylor & Peter Bain, 30*(2), 101–117.

Yarberry, W. A., Jr. (2000). *Computer Telephony Integration*. Boca Raton, FL: CRC Press LLC.

KEY TERMS AND DEFINITIONS

Automatic Call Distribution (ACD): The process of distributing incoming (or outgoing) calls to different service agents by an automated system

Call Center: An organizational department responsible for handling customer service issues by telephone and other channels

Call Center Management: The process and governance structure of running a call center

Computer-Telephony Integration (CTI): Systems that enable a computer to act as a call center, accepting incoming calls and routing them to the appropriate device or person

Dentist Appointment: Dental health care service transaction between a dentist and a customer

Dentist Appointment Management: The process of matching demand and supply in dental health care, both at macro and micro levels

Speech Recognition: Speech recognition is computer recognition of human voice

WinHIT: A Finnish Electronic Patient Record (EPR) System

Compilation of References

Aas, J. A., Paster, B. J., Stokes, L. N., Olsen, I., & Dewhirst, F. E. (2005). Defining the normal bacterial flora of the oral cavity. *Journal of Clinical Microbiology*, *43*(11), 5721–5732. doi:10.1128/JCM.43.11.5721-5732.2005

Abell, F., Krams, M., Ashburner, J., Passingham, R., Friston, K., & Frackowiak, R. (1999). The neuroanatomy of autism: a voxel-based whole brain analysis of structural scans. *Neuroreport*, *10*(8), 1647–1651. doi:10.1097/00001756-199906030-00005

Aderem, A. (2005). Systems biology: its practice and challenges. *Cell*, *121*(4), 511–513. doi:10.1016/j.cell.2005.04.020

Aebersold, R., & Mann, M. (2003). Mass spectrometry-based proteomics. *Nature*, *422*, 198–207. doi:10.1038/nature01511

Ahmed, S., & Nawshad, A. (2007). Complexity in interpretation of embryonic epithelial-mesenchymal transition in response to transforming growth factor-beta signaling. *Cells, Tissues, Organs*, *185*(1-3), 131–145. doi:10.1159/000101314

Ajdic, D., McShan, W. M., McLaughlin, R. E., Savic, G., Chang, J., & Carson, M. B. (2002). Genome sequence of Streptococcus mutans UA159, a cariogenic dental pathogen. *Proceedings of the National Academy of Sciences of the United States of America*, *99*(22), 14434–14439. doi:10.1073/pnas.172501299

Albandar, J. M., Brown, L. J., & Loe, H. (1997). Clinical features of early-onset periodontitis. *The Journal of the American Dental Association*, *128*(10), 1393–1399.

Alliez, P., Cohen-Steiner, D., Yvinec, M., & Desbrun, M. (2005). Variational tetrahedral meshing. *ACM Transactions on Graphics*, *24*(3), 617–625. doi:10.1145/1073204.1073238

Amann, R. I., Ludwig, W., & Schleifer, K. H. (1995). Phylogenetic identification and in situ detection of individual microbial cells without cultivation. *Microbiological Reviews*, *59*, 143–169.

American_Academy_of_Pediatrics. (2009). Retrieved May 25, 2009, from http://www.aap.org/oralhealth/cme/page4.htm

Analoui, M. (2001). Radiographic image enhancement. Part I: spatial domain techniques. *Dento Maxillo Facial Radiology*, *30*(1), 1–9. doi:10.1038/sj.dmfr.4600562

Anderson, L., & Hunter, C. L. (2006). Quantitative mass spectrometric multiple reaction monitoring assays for major plasma proteins. *Molecular & Cellular Proteomics*, *5*, 573–588. doi:10.1074/mcp.M500331-MCP200

Andersson, M., Carlsson, L., Persson, M., & Bergman, B. (1996). Accuracy of machine milling and spark erosion with a CAD/CAM system. *The Journal of Prosthetic Dentistry*, *76*(2), 187–193. doi:10.1016/S0022-3913(96)90305-4

Apostol, L., Boudousq, V., Basset, O., Odet, V., Yot, S., & Tabary, J. (2006). Relevance of 2D radiographic texture analysis for the assessment of 3D bone micro-architecture. *Medical Physics*, *33*(9), 3546–3556. doi:10.1118/1.2211727

Arbag, H., Korkmaz, H. H., Ozturk, K., & Uyar, Y. (2008). Comparative evaluation of different miniplates for internal fixation of mandible fractures using finite element analysis. *Journal of Oral and Maxillofacial Surgery, 66*(6), 1225–1232. doi:10.1016/j.joms.2005.11.092

Arbuckle, M. R., McClain, M. T., Rubertone, M. V., Scofield, R. H., Dennis, G. J., & James, J. A. (2003). Development of autoantibodies before the clinical onset of systemic lupus erythematosus. *The New England Journal of Medicine, 349*, 1526–1533. doi:10.1056/NEJMoa021933

Armitage, G. C., Research, Science and Therapy Committee of the American Academy of Periodontology. (2003). Diagnosis of periodontal diseases. *Journal of Periodontology, 74*(8), 1237–1247. doi:10.1902/jop.2003.74.8.1237

Arvisenet, G., Billy, L., Poinot, P., Vigneau, E., Bertrand, D., & Prost, C. (2008). Effect of apple particle state on the release of volatile compounds in a new artificial mouth device. *Journal of Agricultural and Food Chemistry, 56*, 3245–3253. doi:10.1021/jf073145z

Arvisenet, G., Billy, L., Royer, G., & Prost, C. (2006). Role of mastication on the release of apple volatile compounds in a model mouth system. In: Flavour Science. Recent advances and trends. Eds. Bredie W. L. P. and Petersen M. A., Elsevier, 465-468.

Ashburner, J., & Friston, K. (2000). Voxel-based morphometry--the methods. *NeuroImage, 11*(6 pt. 1), 805–821. doi:10.1006/nimg.2000.0582

Ashburner, M., Ball, C. A., Blake, J. A., Botstein, D., Butler, H., & Cherry, J. M. (2000). Gene Ontology: tool for the unification of biology. *Nature Genetics, 25*, 25–29. doi:10.1038/75556

Assuma, R., Oates, T., Cochran, D., Amar, S., & Graves, D. T. (1998). IL-1 and TNF antagonists inhibit the inflammatory response and bone loss in experimental periodontitis. *Journal of Immunology (Baltimore, MD.: 1950), 160*, 403–409.

Audette, M., Delingette, H., Fuchs, A., Burgert, O., & Chinzei, K. (2007). A topologically faithful, tissue-guided, spatially varying meshing strategy for computing patient-specific head models for endoscopic pituitary surgery simulation. *Computer Aided Surgery, 12*(1), 43–52. doi:10.1080/10929080601167413

Auf dem Keller, U., Doucet, A., & Overall, C. M. (2007). Protease research in the era of systems biology. *Biological Chemistry, 388*(11), 1159–1162. doi:10.1515/BC.2007.146

Avila-Campos, M. J., Sacchi, C. T., Whitney, A. M., Steigerwalt, A. G., & Mayer, L. W. (1999). Arbitrarily primed-polymerase chain reaction for identification and epidemiologic subtyping of oral isolates of *Fusobacterium nucleatum*. *Journal of Periodontology, 70*, 1202–1208. doi:10.1902/jop.1999.70.10.1202

Bäckhed, F., Ley, R. E., Sonnenburg, J. L., Peterson, D. A., & Gordon, J. I. (2005). Host-bacterial mutualism in the human intestine. *Science, 307*, 1915–1920. doi:10.1126/science.1104816

Baker, G. C., Smith, J. J., & Cowan, D. A. (2003). Review and re-analysis of domain-specific 16S primers. *Journal of Microbiological Methods, 55*, 541–555. doi:10.1016/j.mimet.2003.08.009

Baldini, C., Giusti, L., Bazzichi, L., Lucacchini, A., & Bombardieri, S. (2008). Proteomic analysis of the saliva: a clue for understanding primary from secondary Sjögren's syndrome? *Autoimmunity Reviews, 7*, 185–191. doi:10.1016/j.autrev.2007.11.002

Balkowiec, A., & Katz, D. M. (2000). Activity-dependent release of endogenous brain-derived neurotrophic factor from primary sensory neurons detected by ELISA in situ. *The Journal of Neuroscience, 20*, 7417–7423.

Balkowiec, A., & Katz, D. M. (2002). Cellular mechanisms regulating activity-dependent release of native brain-derived neurotrophic factor from hippocampal neurons. *The Journal of Neuroscience, 22*, 10399–10407.

Balkowiec-Iskra, E., Kurkowska-Jastrzebska, I., Joniec, I., Ciesielska, A., Czlonkowska, A., & Czlonkowski, A. (2007a). Dopamine, serotonin and noradrenaline changes in the striatum of C57BL mice following myelin oligodendrocyte glycoprotein (MOG) 35-55 and complete Freund adjuvant (CFA) administration. *Acta Neurobiologiae Experimentalis, 67*, 379–388.

Balkowiec-Iskra, E., Kurkowska-Jastrzebska, I., Joniec, I., Ciesielska, A., Muszynska, A., & Przybylkowski, A. (2007b). MPTP-induced central dopamine depletion exacerbates experimental autoimmune encephalomyelitis (EAE) in C57BL mice. *Inflammation Research, 56*, 311–317. doi:10.1007/s00011-007-6128-0

Balkowiec-Iskra, E., Kurkowska-Jastrzebska, I., Joniec, I., Czlonkowska, A., & Czlonkowski, A. (2003). Post intoxicative therapeutic immunization with myelin oligodendrocyte glycoproteine (MOG 35-55) suppresses spontaneous regeneration of dopaminergic neurons injured with 1-methyl-4 phenyl-1,2,3,6-tetrahydropiridine (MPTP). *Acta Neurobiologiae Experimentalis, 63*, 109–115.

Bandtlow, C., Zachleder, T., & Schwab, M. E. (1990). Oligodendrocytes arrest neurite growth by contact inhibition. *The Journal of Neuroscience, 10*, 3837–3848.

Bassiouny, M. A., & Grant, A. A. (1976). Radiographic assessment of infrabony pocket topography. *Journal of Periodontology, 47*(8), 440–443.

Batt, R., & Moynihan, L. (2006). The viability of alternative call centre production models. *Human Resource Management Journal, 12*(4), 14–34. doi:10.1111/j.1748-8583.2002.tb00075.x

Becker, A. (2007). *The orthodontic treatment of impacted teeth,* (2nd Ed.). Hampshire, UK: Thompson Publishing Services.

Becker, F. (2008). Lasersintern versus Gusstechnik. *Dent Lab, 56*(1), 39–48.

Beek, M., Koolstra, J. H., van Ruijven, L. J., & van Eijden, T. M. (2000). Three-dimensional finite element analysis of the human temporomandibular joint disc. *Journal of Biomechanics, 33*(3), 307–316. doi:10.1016/S0021-9290(99)00168-2

Beek, M., Koolstra, J. H., van Ruijven, L. J., & van Eijden, T. M. (2001). Three-dimensional finite element analysis of the cartilaginous structures in the human temporomandibular joint. *Journal of Dental Research, 80*(10), 1913–1918. doi:10.1177/00220345010800101001

Benzley, S., Perry, E., Merkley, K., Clark, B., & Sjaardema, G. (1995). A Comparison of All Hexagonal and All Tetrahedral Finite Element Meshes for Elastic and Elasto-plastic Analysis. In *Proceedings, 4th International Meshing Roundtable* (pp. 179-191).

Berar, M., Desvignes, M., Bailly, G., & Payan, Y. (2004). 3D Meshes Registration: Application to Statistical Skull Model. *Image Analysis and Recognition, 3112*, 100–107.

Berg, E., Davik, G., Hegdahl, T., & Gjerdet, N. R. (1996). Hardness, strength, and ductility of prefabricated titanium rods used in the manufacture of spark erosion crowns. *The Journal of Prosthetic Dentistry, 75*(4), 419–425. doi:10.1016/S0022-3913(96)90035-9

Berkhout, W. E., Beuger, D. A., Sanderink, G. C., & van der Stelt, P. F. (2004). The dynamic range of digital radiographic systems: dose reduction or risk of overexposure? *Dento Maxillo Facial Radiology, 33*(1), 1–5. doi:10.1259/dmfr/40677472

Birkfellner, W., Solar, P., Gahleitner, A., Huber, K., Kainberger, F., & Kettenbach, J. (2001). In-vitro assessment of a registration protocol for image guided implant dentistry. *Clinical Oral Implants Research, 12*(1), 69–78. doi:10.1034/j.1600-0501.2001.012001069.x

Bishara, S. E. (1992). Impacted maxillary canines: a review. *American Journal of Orthodontics and Dentofacial Orthopedics, 101*, 159–171. doi:10.1016/0889-5406(92)70008-X

Bjerklin, K., & Ericson, S. (2006). How a computerized tomography examination changed the treatment plans of 80 children with retained and ectopically positioned maxillary canines. *The Angle Orthodontist*, *76*(1), 43–51.

Blöchl, A., & Thoenen, H. (1995). Characterization of nerve growth factor (NGF) release from hippocampal neurons: evidence for a constitutive and an unconventional sodium-dependent regulated pathway. *The European Journal of Neuroscience*, *7*, 1220–1228. doi:10.1111/j.1460-9568.1995.tb01112.x

Blöchl, A., & Thoenen, H. (1996). Localization of cellular storage compartments and sites of constitutive and activity-dependent release of nerve growth factor (NGF) in primary cultures of hippocampal neurons. *Molecular and Cellular Neurosciences*, *7*, 173–190. doi:10.1006/mcne.1996.0014

Bobetsis, Y. A., Barros, S. P., Lin, D. M., Weidman, J. R., Dolinoy, D. C., & Jirtle, R. L. (2007). Bacterial infection promotes DNA hypermethylation. *Journal of Dental Research*, *86*(2), 169–174. doi:10.1177/154405910708600212

Boelrijk, A. E. M., Weel, K. G. C., Burger, J. J., Verschueren, M., Gruppen, H., Voragen, A. G. J., & Smit, G. (2006). The artificial throat: a new device to simulate swallowing and *in vivo* aroma release in the throat. The effect of emulsion properties on release in relation to sensory intensity. In: Flavour Science. Recent advances and trends. Eds. Bredie W. L. P. and Petersen M. A., Elsevier, 565-568.

Bonet, J., & Wood, R. (1997). *Nonlinear Continuum Mechanics for Finite Element Analysis*. Cambridge, UK: Cambridge University Press.

Borg, E., Attaelmanan, A., & Gröndahl, H. G. (2000). Subjective image quality of solid-state and photostimulable storage phosphor systems for digital intra-oral radiography. *Dento Maxillo Facial Radiology*, *29*(2), 70–75. doi:10.1038/sj.dmfr.4600501

Borg, E., Gröndahl, K., & Gröndahl, H. G. (1997). Marginal bone level buccal to mandibular molars in digital radiographs from charge-coupled device and storage phosphor systems. An in vitro study. *Journal of Clinical Periodontology*, *24*(5), 306–312. doi:10.1111/j.1600-051X.1997.tb00762.x

Bork, P., & Serrano, L. (2005). Towards cellular systems in 4D. *Cell*, *121*(4), 507–509. doi:10.1016/j.cell.2005.05.001

Boughner, J. C., & Hallgrimsson, B. (2008). Biological spacetime and the temporal integration of functional modules: a case study of dento-gnathic developmental timing. *Developmental Dynamics*, *237*(1), 1–17. doi:10.1002/dvdy.21383

Bradley, E. (1979). Bootstrap Methods . *Another Look at the Jackknife.*, *7*, 1–27.

Brägger, U. (2005). Radiographic parameters: biological significance and clinical use. *Periodontology 2000*, *39*, 73–90. doi:10.1111/j.1600-0757.2005.00128.x

Bratthall, D. (1970). Demonstration of five serological groups of streptococcal strains resembling Streptococcus mutans. *Odontologisk Revy*, *21*(2), 143–152.

Bressem, J. (2006). Laserschmelzen. *dent lab*, *54*(10), 1337-1340.

Bressem, J. (2007). Laser Melting. *Dent Lab Internat*, *3*(1), 29–32.

Brogden, K. A., Guthmiller, J. M., & Taylor, C. E. (2004). Human polymicrobial infections. *Lancet*, *365*, 253–255.

Brosenitsch, T. A., & Katz, D. M. (2001). Physiological patterns of electrical stimulation can induce neuronal gene expression by activating N-type calcium channels. *The Journal of Neuroscience*, *21*, 2571–2579.

Buettner, A., Beer, A., Hannig, C., & Settles, M. (2001). Observation of the Swallowing Process by Application of Videofluoroscopy and Real-time Magnetic Resonance Imaging-Consequences for Retronasal Aroma Stimulation. *Chemical Senses*, *26*, 1211–1219. doi:10.1093/chemse/26.9.1211

Buettner, A., Beer, A., Hannig, C., Settles, M., & Schieberle, P. (2002). Physiological and analytical studies on flavor perception dynamics as induced by the eating and swallowing process. *Food Quality and Preference*, *13*, 497–504. doi:10.1016/S0950-3293(02)00052-6

Buldyrev, I., Tanner, N. M., Hsieh, H. Y., Dodd, E. G., Nguyen, L. T., & Balkowiec, A. (2006). Calcitonin gene-related peptide enhances release of native brain-derived neurotrophic factor from trigeminal ganglion neurons. *Journal of Neurochemistry*, *99*, 1338–1350. doi:10.1111/j.1471-4159.2006.04161.x

Bunin, G. (2006). Non-Local Topological Clean-Up. In *Proceedings, 15th International Meshing Roundtable*, (pp. 3-20).

Cadieux, N., Lebel, P., & Brousseau, R. (1993). Use of a triplex polymerase chain reaction for the detection and differentiation of *Mycoplasma pneumoniae* and Mycoplasma genitalium in the presence of human DNA. *Journal of General Microbiology*, *139*, 2431–2437.

Call Center Association. (1999). *Definition of call center*. London.

Canossa, M., Gartner, A., Campana, G., Inagaki, N., & Thoenen, H. (2001). Regulated secretion of neurotrophins by metabotropic glutamate group I (mGluRI) and Trk receptor activation is mediated via phospholipase C signalling pathways. *The EMBO Journal*, *20*, 1640–1650. doi:10.1093/emboj/20.7.1640

Carey, J.P., Craig, M., Kerstein, R.B., Radke, J. (2007). Determining a relationship between applied occlusal load and articulating paper mark area. *The Open Dentistry Journal*, (1), 1-7

Carossa, S., Lojacono, A., Schierano, G., & Pera, P. (2000). Evaluation of occlusal contacts in the dental laboratory: influence of strip thickness and operator experience. *The International Journal of Prosthodontics*, *13*(3), 201–204.

Castellano-Smith, A., Hartkens, T., Schnabel, J., Hose, R., Liu, H., Hall, W., et al. (2001). Constructing Patient Specific Models for Correcting Intraoperative Brain Deformation. In *MICCAI* (pp. 1091-109).

Chapple, I. L., & Matthews, J. B. (2007). The role of reactive oxygen and antioxidant species in periodontal tissue destruction. *Periodontology 2000*, *43*, 160–232. doi:10.1111/j.1600-0757.2006.00178.x

Chattopadhyay, A. (1993). AgNORs in tumoral pathology. Review of literature and observations on the technic and reaction in normal oral epithelium. *Indian Journal of Dental Research*, *4*(2), 47–53.

Chattopadhyay, A. (2010). *Oral Health Epidemiology: Principles and Practice*. Sudbury, MA: Jones & Bartlett Publishers.

Chattopadhyay, A., & Ray, J. G. (2008). AgNOR cut-point to distinguish mild and moderate epithelial dysplasia. *Journal of Oral Pathology & Medicine*, *37*(2), 78–82.

Chattopadhyay, A., Chawda, J. G., & Doshi, J. J. (1994). Silver-binding nucleolar organizing regions: a study of oral leukoplakia and squamous cell carcinoma. *International Journal of Oral and Maxillofacial Surgery*, *23*(6 Pt 1), 374–377. doi:10.1016/S0901-5027(05)80060-8

Chattopadhyay, A., Gray, L. R., Patton, L. L., Caplan, D. J., Slade, G. D., & Tien, H. C. (2004). Salivary secretory leukocyte protease inhibitor and oral candidiasis in human immunodeficiency virus type 1-infected persons. *Infection and Immunity*, *72*(4), 1956–1963. doi:10.1128/IAI.72.4.1956-1963.2004

Chattopadhyay, A., Ray, J. G., & Caplan, D. J. (2002). AgNOR count as objective marker for dysplastic features in oral leukoplakia. *Journal of Oral Pathology & Medicine*, *31*(9), 512–517. doi:10.1034/j.1600-0714.2002.00153.x

Chaushu, S., Brin, I., Ben-Bassat, Y., Zilberman, Y., & Becker, A. (2002). Periodontal status following surgical-orthodontic alignment of impacted central incisors with an open-eruption technique. *American Journal of Orthodontics and Dentofacial Orthopedics*, *122*, 9–14.

Chaushu, S., Dykstein, N., Ben-Bassat, Y., & Becker, A. (2009). Periodontal status of impacted maxillary incisors uncovered by 2 different surgical techniques. *Journal of Oral and Maxillofacial Surgery*, *67*, 120–124. doi:10.1016/j.joms.2008.08.012

Chelius, D., & Bondarenko, P. V. (2002). Quantitative profiling of proteins in complex mixtures using liquid chromatography and mass spectrometry. *Journal of Proteome Research*, *1*, 317–323. doi:10.1021/pr025517j

Chen, J., & Xu, L. (1994). A finite element analysis of the human temporomandibular joint. *Journal of Biomechanical Engineering*, *116*(4), 401–407. doi:10.1115/1.2895790

Chen, J., He, Q. Y., Yuen, A. P. W., & Chiu, J. F. (2004). Proteomics of buccal squamous cell carcinoma: The involvement of multiple pathways in tumorigenesis. *Proteomics*, *4*, 2465–2475. doi:10.1002/pmic.200300762

Chen, K., Neimark, H., Rumore, P., & Steinman, C. R. (1989). Broad range DNA probes for detecting and amplifying eubacterial nucleic acids. *FEMS Microbiology Letters*, *48*, 19–24. doi:10.1111/j.1574-6968.1989.tb03213.x

Chen, L., & XU, J. (2004). Optimal Delaunay triangulations. *Journal of Computational Mathematics*, *22*(2), 299–308.

Chernyaev, E. (1995). *Marching cubes 33: Construccion of topologically correct isosurfaces*, (Technical Report CN/95-17).

Chesney, J. (2006). 6-phosphofructo-2-kinase/fructose-2,6-bisphosphatase and tumor cell glycolysis. *Current Opinion in Clinical Nutrition and Metabolic Care*, *9*(5), 535–539. doi:10.1097/01.mco.0000241661.15514.fb

Cheverud, J. M. (2007). The relationship between development and evolution through heritable variation. *Novartis Foundation Symposium*, *284*, 55–65. doi:10.1002/9780470319390.ch4

Cohen-Steiner, D., Alliez, P., & Desbrun, M. (2004). Variational Shape Approximation. In *ACM Transanctions on Graphics (SIGGRAPH)* (pp. 905-914).

Colett, A. R. (2000). Conservative management of lower second premolar impaction. *Australian Dental Journal*, *45*, 279–281. doi:10.1111/j.1834-7819.2000.tb00264.x

Coll, N., Guerrieri, M., & Sellares, J. (2006). Mesh Modification Under Local Domain Changes. In *Proceedings, 15th International Meshing Roundtable*, (pp. 39-56).

Conrads, G. (2002). DNA probes and primers in dental practice. *Clinical Infectious Diseases*, *35*, 72–77. doi:10.1086/341924

Cotin, S., Delingette, H., & Ayache, N. (1996). Real Time Volumetric Deformable Models for Surgery Simulation. *VBC*, (pp. 535-540).

Couteau, B., Payan, Y., & Lavallee, S. (2000). The mesh-matching algorithm: an automatic 3D mesh generator for finite element structures. *Journal of Biomechanics*, *33*(8), 1005–1009. doi:10.1016/S0021-9290(00)00055-5

Cox, S. W., Rodriguez-Gonzalez, E. M., Booth, V., & Eley, B. M. (2006). Secretory leukocyte protease inhibitor and its potential interactions with elastase and cathepsin B in gingival crevicular fluid and saliva from patients with chronic periodontitis. *Journal of Periodontal Research*, *41*(5), 477–485. doi:10.1111/j.1600-0765.2006.00891.x

Cramer von Clausbruch, S. (2003). Zirkon und Zirkonium. *dent lab*, *51*(7), 1137-1142.

Cramer von Clausbruch, S. (2006). Zurück in die Zukunft? *dental lab*, *54*(9), 1169-1180.

Cramer von Clausbruch, S. (2008). Kopierfräsen als verlässliches Verfahren in der Zahntechnik. *Die Quintessenz der Zahntechnik*, *34*(3), 332–342.

Cummings, C. A., & Relman, D. A. (2000). Using DNA microarrays to study host-microbe interactions. *Emerging Infectious Diseases*, *6*, 513–525. doi:10.3201/eid0605.000511

Dachi, S. F., & Howell, F. V. (1961). A survey of 3, 874 routine full-month radiographs. II. A study of impacted teeth. *Oral Surgery, Oral Medicine, and Oral Pathology*, *14*, 1165–1169. doi:10.1016/0030-4220(61)90204-3

Davies, A. M. (1988). The trigeminal system: an advantageous experimental model for studying neuronal development. *Development*, *103*(Supplement), 175–183.

Davies, A. M. (1997). Studies of neurotrophin biology in the developing trigeminal system. *Journal of Anatomy*, *191*, 483–491. doi:10.1046/j.1469-7580.1997.19140483.x

DeGaravilla, L., Greco, M. N., Sukumar, N., Chen, Z. W., Pineda, A. O., & Mathews, F. S. (2005). A novel, potent dual inhibitor of the leukocyte proteases cathepsin G and chymase: molecular mechanisms and anti-inflammatory activity in vivo. *The Journal of Biological Chemistry*, *280*(18), 18001–18007. doi:10.1074/jbc.M501302200

De Koninck, P., Carbonetto, S., & Cooper, E. (1993). NGF induces neonatal rat sensory neurons to extend dendrites in culture after removal of satellite cells. *The Journal of Neuroscience*, *13*, 577–585.

De Pablo, P., Chapple, I. L. C., Buckley, C. D., & Dietrich, T. (2009). Periodontitis in systemic rheumatic diseases. *Nature Reviews Rheumatology, 5*, 218 – 224. Retrieved from doi: 10.1038/nrrheum.2009.28

Deibler, K. D., Lavin, E. H., Linforth, R. S. T., Taylor, A. J., & Acree, T. E. (2001). Verification of a mouth simulator by in-vivo measurement. *Journal of Agricultural and Food Chemistry*, *49*, 1388–1393. doi:10.1021/jf0012401

Delaunay, B. (1934). Sur la sphere vide. *Izvestia Akademii Nauk SSSR . Otdelenie Matematicheskikh i Estestvennykh Nauk*, *7*, 793–800.

Delingette, H. (1999). General Object Reconstruction based on Simplex Meshes. *International Journal of Computer Vision*, *32*(2), 111–146. doi:10.1023/A:1008157432188

Demmer, R. T., Behle, J. H., Wolf, D. L., Handfield, M., Kebschull, M., & Celenti, R. (2008). Transcriptomes in healthy and diseased gingival tissues. *Journal of Periodontology*, *79*, 2112–2124. doi:10.1902/jop.2008.080139

DeSouza, L. V., Romaschin, A. D., Colgan, T. J., & Siu, K. W. (2009). Absolute quantification of potential cancer markers in clinical tissue homogenates using multiple reaction monitoring on a hybrid triple quadrupole/linear ion trap tandem mass spectrometer. *Analytical Chemistry*, *81*, 3462–3470. doi:10.1021/ac802726a

Desvarieux, M., Demmer, R. T., Rundek, T., Boden-Albala, B., & Jacobs, D. R. Jr (2005). Periodontal microbiota and carotid intima-media thickness: the Oral Infections and Vascular Disease Epidemiology Study (INVEST). *Circulation*, *111*, 576–582. doi:10.1161/01.CIR.0000154582.37101.15

Desvarieux, M., Schwahn, C., Volzke, H., Demmer, R. T., & Ludemann, J. (2004). Gender differences in the relationship between periodontal disease, tooth loss, and atherosclerosis. *Stroke*, *35*, 2029–2035. doi:10.1161/01.STR.0000136767.71518.36

DIN_EN_ISO_10271. (2001). *Dentale metallische Werkstoffe Korrosionsprüfverfahren*. Berlin: Beuth Verlag.

DIN_EN_ISO_9693. (2001). *Metall-Keramik-Systeme für zahnärztliche Restaurationen*. Berlin: Beuth Verlag.

Dreiseidler, T., Mischkowski, R. A., Neugebauer, J., Ritter, L., & Zöller, J. E. (2009). Comparison of Cone-Beam Imaging with Orthopantomography and Computerized Tomography for Assessment in Presurgical Implant Dentistry. *The International Journal of Oral & Maxillofacial Implants*, *24*(2), 216–225.

Dreiseidler, T., Neugebauer, J., Ritter, L., Lingohr, T., Rothamel, D., & Mischkowski, R. A. (2009). Accuracy of a newly developed integrated system for dental implant planning. *Clinical Oral Implants Research*, *20*(11), 1191–1199. doi:10.1111/j.1600-0501.2009.01764.x

Du Tré, F., Jacobs, R., Styven, S., & van Steenberghe, D. (2006). Development of a novel digital subtraction technique for detecting subtle changes in jawbone density. *Clinical Oral Investigations*, *10*(3), 235–248. doi:10.1007/s00784-006-0055-2

Duret, F. (1992). Dental CAD/CAM. *The Journal of the American Dental Association*, *123*(6), 11–14.

Duret, F. (1993). The practical dental CAD/CAM in 1993. *J Can Dent Assoc*, *59*(5), 445–453.

Duret, F., & Preston, J. D. (1991). CAD/CAM imaging in dentistry. *Current Opinion in Dentistry*, *1*, 150–154.

Duret, F., Blouin, J.-L., & Duret, B. (1988). CAD-CAM in Dentistry. *The Journal of the American Dental Association, 117*(11), 715–720.

Dzink, J. L., Socransky, S. S., & Haffajee, A. D. (1988). The predominant cultivable microbiota of active and inactive lesions of destructive periodontal diseases. *Journal of Clinical Periodontology, 15*, 316–323. doi:10.1111/j.1600-051X.1988.tb01590.x

Edwards, U., Rogall, T., Blocker, H., Emde, M., & Bottger, E. C. (1989). Isolation and direct complete nucleotide determination of entire genes. Characterization of a gene coding for 16S ribosomal RNA. *Nucleic Acids Research, 17*, 7843–7853. doi:10.1093/nar/17.19.7843

Egger, G., Liang, G., Aparicio, A., & Jones, P. A. (2004). Epigenetics in human disease and prospects for epigenetic therapy. *Nature, 429*(6990), 457–463. doi:10.1038/nature02625

Eickholz, P., & Hausmann, E. (2000). Accuracy of radiographic assessment of interproximal bone loss in intrabony defects using linear measurements. *European Journal of Oral Sciences, 108*(1), 70–73. doi:10.1034/j.1600-0722.2000.00729.x

Eickholz, P., Riess, T., Lenhard, M., Hassfeld, S., & Staehle, H. J. (1999). Digital radiography of interproximal bone loss: validity of different filters. *Journal of Clinical Periodontology, 26*(5), 294–300. doi:10.1034/j.1600-051X.1999.260506.x

Eidenbenz, S., & Schärer, P. (1994). Das Kopierschleifen keramischer Formkörper. *Phillip Journal, 11*(3), 91–95.

Eisen, M., & Hinterseher, J. (2008). SLM-Verfahren: Mehr Formgenauigkeit - weniger Eigenspannung. *Zahntech Mag, 12*(10), 626–632.

Eley, B. M., & Cox, S. W. (1998). Advances in periodontal diagnosis. 3. Assessing potential biomarkers of periodontal disease activity. *British Dental Journal, 184*(3), 109–113. doi:10.1038/sj.bdj.4809556

Elgin, M. (2006). There may be strict empirical laws in biology, after all. *Biology and Philosophy, 21*(1), 119–134. doi:10.1007/s10539-005-3177-z

Ericson, S., & Kurol, J. (1987). Radiographic examination of ectopically erupting maxillary canines. *American Journal of Orthodontics, 91*, 483–492.

Ericson, S., & Kurol, J. (1988). Early treatment of palatally erupting maxillary canines by extraction of primary canines. *European Journal of Orthodontics, 10*, 283–295.

Espy, M. J., Uhl, J. R., Sloan, L. M., Buckwalter, S. P., Jones, M. F., & Vetter, E. A. (2006). Real-time PCR in clinical microbiology: applications for routine laboratory testing. *Clinical Microbiology Reviews, 19*, 165–256. doi:10.1128/CMR.19.1.165-256.2006

Farah, J. W., Craig, R. G., & Meroueh, K. A. (1988). Finite element analysis of a mandibular model. *Journal of Oral Rehabilitation, 15*(6), 615–624. doi:10.1111/j.1365-2842.1988.tb00199.x

Farrelly, V., Rainey, F. A., & Stackebrandt, E. (1995). Effect of genome size and rrn gene copy number on PCR amplification of 16S rRNA genes from a mixture of bacterial species. *Applied and Environmental Microbiology, 61*, 2798–2801.

Fedorov, A., Chrisochoides, N., Kikinis, R., & Warfield, S. (2005). Tetrahedral mesh generation for medical Imaging. *Insight Journal - MICCAI Open Source Workshop.*

Feichtinger, M., Mossbock, R., & Karcher, H. (2007). Assessments of bone resorption after secondary alveolar bone grafting using three-dimensional computed tomography: a three-year study. *The Cleft Palate-Craniofacial Journal, 44*(2), 142–148. doi:10.1597/06-047.1

Feng, Z., & Weinberg, A. (2006). Role of bacteria in health and disease of periodontal tissues. *Periodontology 2000, 40*, 50–76. doi:10.1111/j.1600-0757.2005.00148.x

Fernández, J. R., Gallas, M., Burguera, M., & Viaño, J. M. (2003). A three-dimensional numerical simulation of mandible fracture reduction with screwed miniplates. *Journal of Biomechanics, 36*(3), 329–337. doi:10.1016/S0021-9290(02)00416-5

Ferrant, M., Warfield, S., Guttmann, C., Mulkern, R., Jolesz, F., & Kikinis, R. (1999). 3D Image Matching Using a Finite Element Based Elastic Deformation Model. In *Medical Image Computing and Computer--Assisted Intervention (MICCAI),* (pp. 202-209).

Ferré, J. C., Legoux, R., Helary, J. L., Albugues, F., Le Floc'h, C., & Bouteyre, J. (1985). Study of the deformations of the isolated mandible under static constraints by simulations on physcomathematical model. *Anatomia Clinica, 7*(3), 183–192. doi:10.1007/BF01654640

Finkel, R., & Bentley, J. (1974). Quad Trees: A Data Structure for Retrieval on Composite Keys. *Acta Informatica, 4*(1), 1–9. doi:10.1007/BF00288933

Fisher, J., & Henzinger, T. A. (2007). Executable cell biology. *Nature Biotechnology, 25*(11), 1239–1249. doi:10.1038/nbt1356

Fitch, P. M., Roghanian, A., Howie, S. E., & Sallenave, J. M. (2006). Human neutrophil elastase inhibitors in innate and adaptive immunity. *Biochemical Society Transactions, 34*(Pt 2), 279–282. doi:10.1042/BST20060279

Forrester, J. W. (1985). 'The Model' Versus a Modeling 'Process'. *System Dynamics Review, 1*(1 & 2), 133–134. doi:10.1002/sdr.4260010112

Fortin, T., Champleboux, G., Bianchi, S., Buatois, H., & Coudert, J. L. (2002). Precision of transfer of preoperative planning for oral implants based on cone-beam CT-scan images through a robotic drilling machine. *Clinical Oral Implants Research, 13*(6), 651–656. doi:10.1034/j.1600-0501.2002.130612.x

Frank, C. A. (2000). Treatment options for impacted teeth. *The Journal of the American Dental Association, 131*, 623–632.

Frank, J. A., Reich, C. I., Sharma, S., Weisbaum, J. S., Wilson, B. A., & Olsen, G. J. (2008). Critical evaluation of two primers commonly used for amplification of bacterial 16S rRNA genes. *Applied and Environmental Microbiology, 74*, 2461–2470. doi:10.1128/AEM.02272-07

Fraser, I. D., & Germain, R. N. (2009). Navigating the network: signaling cross-talk in hematopoietic cells. *Nature Immunology, 10*(4), 327–331. doi:10.1038/ni.1711

Frasse, P., Lambert, S., Levesque, C., Melcion, D., Richard-Molard, D., & Chiron, H. (1992). The influence of fermentation on volatile compounds in French bread crumb. *Lebensmittel Wisstercraft und Technologie, 25*, 66–70.

Freitag, L. (1997). On combining Laplacian and optimization-based mesh smoothing techniques, In *Proc. Symp. Trends in Unstructured Mesh Generation*, (pp.37-43).

Frey, P. (2004). Generation and adaptation of computational surface meshes from discrete anatomical data. *International Journal for Numerical Methods in Engineering, 60*, 1049–1074. doi:10.1002/nme.992

Friboulet, A., & Thomas, D. (2005). Systems Biology-an interdisciplinary approach. *Biosensors & Bioelectronics, 20*(12), 2404–2407. doi:10.1016/j.bios.2004.11.014

Fuhrmann, R. A., Bücker, A., & Diedrich, P. R. (1997). Furcation involvement: comparison of dental radiographs and HR-CT slices in human specimens. *Journal of Periodontal Research, 32*(5), 409–418. doi:10.1111/j.1600-0765.1997.tb00553.x

Gal, J. Y., Fovet, Y., & Adib-Yadzi, M. (2001). About a synthetic saliva for in vitro studies. *Talanta, 53*, 1103–1115. doi:10.1016/S0039-9140(00)00618-4

Gallas, M., & Fernández, J. R. (2004). A three-dimensional computer model of the human mandible in two simulated standard trauma situations. *Journal of Cranio-Maxillo-Facial Surgery, 32*(5), 303–307. doi:10.1016/j.jcms.2004.04.008

Gärtner, A., & Staiger, V. (2002). Neurotrophin secretion from hippocampal neurons evoked by long-term-potentiation-inducing electrical stimulation patterns. *Proceedings of the National Academy of Sciences of the United States of America, 99*, 6386–6391. doi:10.1073/pnas.092129699

Gebhardt, A. (2000). *Rapid prototyping: Werkzeuge für die schnelle Produktentstehung* (2. Auflage ed.). München - Wien: Hanser.

Geng, J.-P., Tan, K. B. C., & Lui, G.-R. (2001). Application of finite element analysis in implant dentistry: a review of the literature. *The Journal of Prosthetic Dentistry, 85*(6), 585–598. doi:10.1067/mpr.2001.115251

Gentleman, R. C., Carey, V. J., Bates, D. M., Bolstad, B., Dettling, M., & Dudoit, S. (2004). Bioconductor: Open software development for computational biology and bioinformatics. *Genome Biology, 5*, R80. doi:10.1186/gb-2004-5-10-r80

Ghosh, A., Carnahan, J., & Greenberg, M. E. (1994). Requirement for BDNF in activity-dependent survival of cortical neurons. *Science, 263*, 1618–1623. doi:10.1126/science.7907431

Gibbs, S. J. (2000). Effective dose equivalent and effective dose: comparison for common projections in oral and maxillofacial radiology. *Oral Surgery, Oral Medicine, Oral Pathology, Oral Radiology, and Endodontics, 90*(4), 538–545. doi:10.1067/moe.2000.109189

Gopalakrishna, P., & Mummaleni, V. (1993). Influencing satisfaction for dental services. *Journal of Health Care Marketing, 13*(1), 16–22.

Graham, K. L., Vaysberg, M., Kuo, A., & Utz, P. J. (2006). Autoantigen arrays for multiplex analysis of antibody isotypes. *Proteomics, 6*, 5720–5724. doi:10.1002/pmic.200600345

Graves, D. (2008). Cytokines that promote periodontal tissue destruction. *Journal of Periodontology, 79*, 1585–1591. doi:10.1902/jop.2008.080183

Griesbeck, O., Canossa, M., Campana, G., Gärtner, A., Hoener, M. C., & Nawa, H. (1999). Are there differences between the secretion characteristics of NGF and BDNF? Implications for the modulatory role of neurotrophins in activity-dependent neuronal plasticity. *Microscopy Research and Technique, 45*, 262–275. doi:10.1002/(SICI)1097-0029(19990515/01)45:4/5<262::AID-JEMT10>3.0.CO;2-K

Grimard, B. A., Hoidal, M. J., Mills, M. P., Mellonig, J. T., Nummikoski, P. V., & Mealy, B. L. (2009). Comparison of clinical, periapical radiograph, and cone-beam volume tomography measurement techniques for assessing bone level changes following regenerative periodontal therapy. *Journal of Periodontology, 80*(1), 48–55. doi:10.1902/jop.2009.080289

Grover, P. S., & Lorton, L. (1985). The incidence of unerupted permanent teeth and related clinical cases. *Oral Surg Oral Med Oral Pathol, 59*, 420-425. Hechler, S.L. (2008). Cone-beam CT: Applications in orthodontics. *Dental Clinics of North America, 52*, 809–823.

Guo, T., Rudnick, P. A., Wang, W., Lee, C. S., Devoe, D. L., & Balgley, B. M. (2006). Characterization of the human salivary proteome by capillary isoelectric focusing/nanoreversed-phase liquid chromatography coupled with ESI-tandem MS. *Journal of Proteome Research, 5*, 1469–1478. doi:10.1021/pr060065m

Gygi, S. P., Rist, B., Gerber, S. A., Turecek, F., Gelb, M. H., & Aebersold, R. (1999). Quantitative analysis of complex protein mixtures using isotope-coded affinity tags. *Nature Biotechnology, 17*, 994–999. doi:10.1038/13690

Haines, D. E. (2000). *Neuroanatomy: An Atlas of Structures, Sections, and Systems*, (5th Ed.) (pp. 175, 193). Baltimore, MD: Lippincott, William and Wilkins.

Hamp, S. E., Nyman, S., & Lindhe, J. (1975). Periodontal treatment of multirooted teeth. Results after 5 years. *Journal of Clinical Periodontology, 2*(3), 126–135. doi:10.1111/j.1600-051X.1975.tb01734.x

Han, Y. W., Shi, W., Huang, G. T., Kinder, S., Haake, N. H., & Park, H. (2000). Interactions between periodontal bacteria and human oral epithelial cells: *Fusobacterium nucleatum* adheres to and invades epithelial cells. *Infection and Immunity, 68*, 3140–3146. doi:10.1128/IAI.68.6.3140-3146.2000

Handfield, M., Mans, J. J., Zheng, G., Lopez, M. C., Mao, S., & Progulske-Fox, A. (2005). Distinct transcriptional profiles characterize oral epithelium-microbiota interactions. *Cellular Microbiology, 7*(6), 811–823. doi:10.1111/j.1462-5822.2005.00513.x

Hansen, K. C., Schmitt-Ulms, G., Chalkley, R. J., Hirsch, J., Baldwin, M. A., & Burlingame, A. L. (2003). Mass spectrometric analysis protein mixtures at low levels using cleavable 13C-isotope-coded affinity tag and multidimensional chromatography. *Molecular & Cellular Proteomics*, *2*, 299–314.

Hansson, A., Giannouli, P., & van Ruth, S. M. (2003). The influence of gel strength on aroma release from pectin gels in a model mouth and in vivo, monitored with proton-transfer-reaction mass spectrometry. *Journal of Agricultural and Food Chemistry*, *51*, 4732–4740. doi:10.1021/jf030050y

Harris, D., Buser, D., Dula, K., Grondahl, K., Haris, D., & Jacobs, R. (2002). E.A.O. guidelines fo the use of diagnostic imaging in implant dentistry. A consensus workshop organized by the European Association for Osseointegration in Trinity College Dublin. *Clinical Oral Implants Research*, *13*(5), 566–570. doi:10.1034/j.1600-0501.2002.130518.x

Hartmann, M., Heumann, R., & Lessmann, V. (2001). Synaptic secretion of BDNF after high-frequency stimulation of glutamatergic synapses. *The EMBO Journal*, *20*, 5887–5897. doi:10.1093/emboj/20.21.5887

Hartroth, B., Seyfarth, I., & Conrads, G. (1999). Sampling of periodontal pathogens by paper points: evaluation of basic parameters. *Oral Microbiology and Immunology*, *14*, 326–330. doi:10.1034/j.1399-302X.1999.140510.x

Hasegawa, Y., Mans, J. J., Song, M., Lopez, M. C., Baker, H. V., Handfield, M., & Lamont, R. J. (2007). Gingival epithelial cell transcriptional responses to commensal and opportunistic oral microbial specie. *Infection and Immunity*, *75*(5), 2540–2547. doi:10.1128/IAI.01957-06

Hasegawa, Y., Tribble, G. D., Baker, H. V., & Mans, J. J. (2008). Role of Porphyromonas gingivalis SerB in gingival epithelial cell cytoskeletal remodeling and cytokine production. *Infection and Immunity*, *76*(6), 2420–2427. doi:10.1128/IAI.00156-08

Hassfeld, S., & Muhling, J. (2000). Comparative examination of the accuracy of a mechanical and an optical system in CT and MRT based instrument navigation. *International Journal of Oral and Maxillofacial Surgery*, *29*(6), 400–407. doi:10.1016/S0901-5027(00)80069-7

Hausmann, E., & Allen, K. (1997). Reproducibility of bone height measurements made on serial radiographs. *Journal of Periodontology*, *68*(9), 839–841.

He, Q. Y., Chen, J., Kung, H. F., Yuen, A. P. W., & Chiu, J. F. (2004). Identification of tumor-associated proteins in oral tongue squamous cell carcinoma by proteomics. *Proteomics*, *4*, 271–278. doi:10.1002/pmic.200300550

Health_and_Welfare_Statistics_Association. (2003). *Kokumin Eisei no Doko (Trends in Nation's Health, Japan)*. Tokyo: Health and Welfare Statistics Association (in Japanese).

Hefti, A. F. (1997). Periodontal probing. *Critical Reviews in Oral Biology and Medicine*, *8*(3), 336–356. doi:10.1177/10454411970080030601

Heid, C. A., Stevens, J., Livak, K. J., & Williams, P. M. (1996). Real time quantitative PCR. *Genome Research*, *6*, 986–994. doi:10.1101/gr.6.10.986

Hennessey, P. T., Westra, W. H., & Califano, J. A. (2009). Human papillomavirus and head and neck squamous cell. *Journal of Dental Research*, *88*(4), 300–306. doi:10.1177/0022034509333371

Heo, M. S., Choi, D. H., Benavides, E., Huh, K. H., Yi, W. J., Lee, S. S., & Choi, S. C. (2009). Effect of bit depth and kVp of digital radiography for detection of subtle differences. *Oral Surgery, Oral Medicine, Oral Pathology, Oral Radiology, and Endodontics*, *108*(2), 278–283. doi:10.1016/j.tripleo.2008.12.053

Herrmann, I., Lekholm, U., Holm, S., & Kultje, C. (2005). Evaluation of patient and implant characteristics as potential prognostic factors for oral implant failures. *The International Journal of Oral & Maxillofacial Implants*, *20*(2), 220–230.

Hettne, K. M., Weeber, M., Laine, M. L., Cate, H., & Boyer, S. (2007). Automatic mining of the literature to generate new hypotheses for the possible link between periodontitis and atherosclerosis: lipopolysaccharide as a case study. *Journal of Clinical Periodontology, 34*, 1016–1024. doi:10.1111/j.1600-051X.2007.01152.x

Heymach, J. V., Krüttgen, A., Suter, U., & Shooter, E. M. (1996). The regulated secretion and vectorial targeting of neurotrophins in neuroendocrine and epithelial cells. *The Journal of Biological Chemistry, 271*, 25430–25437. doi:10.1074/jbc.271.41.25430

Hirose, M., Tanaka, E., Tanaka, M., Fujita, R., Kuroda, Y., & Yamano, E. (2006). Three-dimensional finite-element model of the human temporomandibular joint disc during prolonged clenching. *European Journal of Oral Sciences, 114*(5), 441–448. doi:10.1111/j.1600-0722.2006.00389.x

Hirsch, E., Wolf, U., Heinicke, F., & Silva, M. A. (2008). Dosimetry of the cone beam computed tomography Veraviewepocs 3D compared with the 3D Accuitomo in different fields of view. *Dento Maxillo Facial Radiology, 37*, 268–273. doi:10.1259/dmfr/23424132

Hitschfeld, N. (2005). Generation of 3D mixed-element meshes using a flexible refinement approach. *Engineering with Computers, 21*, 101–114. doi:10.1007/s00366-005-0306-x

Hitschfeld, N., Navarro, G., & Farias, R. (2000). Tessellations of cuboids with Steiner points. In *Proceedings, 9th International Meshing Roundtable*, (pp. 275-282).

Holland, P. M., Abramson, R. D., Watson, R., & Gelfand, D. H. (1991). Detection of specific polymerase chain reaction product by utilizing the 5'-3' exonuclease activity of Thermus aquaticus DNA polymerase. *Proceedings of the National Academy of Sciences of the United States of America, 88*, 7276–7280. doi:10.1073/pnas.88.16.7276

Holman, D. (2006). Employee wellbeing in call centres. *Human Resource Management Journal, 12*(4), 35–50. doi:10.1111/j.1748-8583.2002.tb00076.x

Hong, J. H., Duncan, S. E., Dietrich, A. M., & O'Keefe, S. F. (2006). Effect of copper on the volatility of aroma compounds in a model mouth system. *Journal of Agricultural and Food Chemistry, 54*, 9168–9175. doi:10.1021/jf061229m

Horz, H.-P., Scheer, S., Huenger, F., Vianna, M. E., & Conrads, G. (2008). Selective isolation of bacterial DNA from human clinical specimens. *Journal of Microbiological Methods, 72*, 98–102. doi:10.1016/j.mimet.2007.10.007

Horz, H.-P., Vianna, M. E., Gomes, B. P., & Conrads, G. (2005). Evaluation of universal probes and primer sets for assessing total bacterial load in clinical samples: general implications and practical use in endodontic antimicrobial therapy. *Journal of Clinical Microbiology, 43*, 5332–5337. doi:10.1128/JCM.43.10.5332-5337.2005

Hsu, K. L., Gildersleeve, J. C., & Mahal, L. K. (2008). A simple strategy for the creation of a recombinant lectin microarray. *Molecular BioSystems, 4*, 654–662. doi:10.1039/b800725j

Hu, S., & Wong, D. (2009). Lectin microarray. *Proteomics Clinical Applications, 3*, 148–154. doi:10.1002/prca.200800153

Hu, S., Arellano, M., Boontheung, P., Wang, J., Zhou, H., & Jiang, J. (2008). Salivary proteomics for oral cancer biomarker discovery. *Clinical Cancer Research, 14*, 6246–6252. doi:10.1158/1078-0432.CCR-07-5037

Hu, S., Wang, J., Meijer, J., Ieong, S., Xie, Y., & Yu, T. (2007). Salivary proteomic and genomic biomarkers for primary Sjögren's syndrome. *Arthritis and Rheumatism, 56*, 3588–3600. doi:10.1002/art.22954

Hu, S., Yu, T., Xie, Y., Yang, Y., Li, Y., & Zhou, X. (2007). Discovery of oral fluid biomarkers for human oral cancer by mass spectrometry. *Cancer Genomics & Proteomics, 4*, 55–64.

Hu, S., Zhou, M., Jiang, J., Wang, J., Elashoff, D., & Gorr, S. (2009). Systems biology analysis of Sjögren's syndrome and mucosa-associated lymphoid tissue lymphoma in parotid glands. *Arthritis and Rheumatism, 60*, 81–92. doi:10.1002/art.24150

Hua, Y., Nackaerts, O., Duyck, J., Maes, F., & Jacobs, R. (2009). Bone quality assessment based on cone beam computed tomography imaging. *Clinical Oral Implants Research*, *20*(8), 767–771. doi:10.1111/j.1600-0501.2008.01677.x

Huang, H. K., & Ledley, R. S. (1969). Numerical experiments with a linear force-displacements tooth model. *Journal of Dental Research*, *48*(1), 32–37.

Hudson, M. E., Pozdnyakova, I., Haines, K., Mor, G., & Snyder, M. (2007). Identification of differentially expressed proteins in ovarian cancer using high-density protein microarrays. *Proceedings of the National Academy of Sciences of the United States of America*, *104*, 17494–17499. doi:10.1073/pnas.0708572104

Hugenholtz, P. (2002). Exploring prokaryotic diversity in the genomic era. *Genome Biology*, *3*, 1–8. doi:10.1186/gb-2002-3-2-reviews0003

Hughes, T. (1987). *The Finite element method: Linear static and dynamic Finite element analysis*, (pp. 292-294). Upper Saddle River, NJ: Prentice-Hall.

Ichikawa, H., Yabuuchi, T., Jin, H. W., Terayama, R., Yamaai, T., & Deguchi, T. (2006). Brain-derived neurotrophic factor-immunoreactive primary sensory neurons in the rat trigeminal ganglion and trigeminal sensory nuclei. *Brain Research*, *1081*, 113–118. doi:10.1016/j.brainres.2006.01.027

Ideker, T. (2004). Systems biology 101--what you need to know. *Nature Biotechnology*, *22*(4), 473–475. doi:10.1038/nbt0404-473

Idoji, Y., Watanabe, Y., Yamashita, A., Yamanishi, K., Nishiguchi, S., & Shimada, K. (2008). In silico study of whey-acidic-protein domain containing oral protease inhibitors. *International Journal of Molecular Medicine*, *21*(4), 461–468.

Ingham, K. E., Linforth, R. S. T., & Taylor, A. J. (1995). The effect of eating on aroma release from strawberries. *Food Chemistry*, *54*, 283–288. doi:10.1016/0308-8146(95)00048-N

Institute for systems biology (2009). *Premise of Systems Biology*. Last accessed June 13, 2009 from http://www.systemsbiology.org/Systems_Biology_in_Depth/Premise_of_Systems_Biology

Iyengar, S. S. (1998). Introduction. In S.S. Iyengar (Ed). *Computer modeling and simulations of complex biological systems*. Boca Raton, FL: CRC Press.

Jacobs, S. G. (1987). The surgical exposure of teeth – simplest, safest and best? *Australian Orthodontic Journal*, *10*, 5–11.

Jacobs, S. G. (1999). Radiographic localization of unerupted maxillary anterior teeth using the vertical tube shift technique: the history and application of the method with some case reports. *American Journal of Orthodontics and Dentofacial Orthopedics*, *116*, 415–423. doi:10.1016/S0889-5406(99)70226-X

Jana, N. K., Gray, L. R., & Shugars, D. C. (2005). Human immunodeficiency virus type 1 stimulates the expression and production of secretory leukocyte protease inhibitor (SLPI) in oral epithelial cells: a role for SLPI in innate mucosal immunity. *Journal of Virology*, *79*(10), 6432–6440. doi:10.1128/JVI.79.10.6432-6440.2005

Januario, A. L., Barriviera, M., & Duarte, W. R. (2008). Soft tissue cone-beam computed tomography: a novel method for the measurement of gingival tissue and the dimensions of the dentogingival unit. *Journal of Esthetic and Restorative Dentistry*, *20*(6), 366–373. doi:10.1111/j.1708-8240.2008.00210.x

Jeffcoat, M. K., & Reddy, M. S. (1991). Progression of probing attachment loss in adult periodontitis. *Journal of Periodontology*, *62*(3), 185–189.

Jeffcoat, M. K., Reddy, M. S., van den Berg, H. R., & Bertens, E. (1992). Quantitative digital subtraction radiography for the assessment of peri-implant bone change. *Clinical Oral Implants Research*, *3*(1), 22–27. doi:10.1034/j.1600-0501.1992.030104.x

Jemal, A., Siegel, R., Ward, E., Hao, Y., Xu, J., & Murray, T. (2008). Cancer statistics, 2008. *CA: a Cancer Journal for Clinicians*, *58*, 71–96. doi:10.3322/CA.2007.0010

Jenkins, G. N. (1978). The physiology and biochemistry of the mouth. 4th ed. Blackwell Scientific, Oxford.

Jenner, R. G., & Young, R. A. (2005). Insights into host responses against pathogens from transcriptional profiling. *Nature Reviews Microbiology*, *3*, 281–294. doi:10.1038/nrmicro1126

Jensen, K. D., Beck, H. C., Jeppesen, L., Norrelykke, M. R., & Hansen, A. M. (2003). A new system for dynamic measurements of flavour release: A combined artificial mouth and membrane inlet mass spectrometer. In: Flavour research at the dawn of the twenty-first century. Eds. Le Quéré J. L. and Etievant P., Lavoisier, London, Paris, New York, 228-231.

Jernvall, J., & Salazar-Ciudad, I. (2007). The economy of tinkering mammalian teeth. *Novartis Foundation Symposium*, *284*, 207–216. doi:10.1002/9780470319390.ch14

Jernvall, J., & Thesleff, I. (2000). Reiterative signaling and patterning during mammalian tooth morphogenesis. *Mechanisms of Development*, *92*(1), 19–29. doi:10.1016/S0925-4773(99)00322-6

Jo, S., Juhasz, A., Zhang, K., Ruel, C., Loera, S., & Wilczynski, S. P. (2009). Human Papillomavirus Infection as a Prognostic Factor in Oropharyngeal Squamous Cell Carcinomas Treated in a Prospective Phase II Clinical Trial. *Anticancer Research*, *29*, 1467–1474.

Jorgenson, T., Masood, F., Beckerley, J. M., Burqin, C., & Parker, D. E. (2007). Comparison of two imaging modalities: F-speed film and digital images for detection of osseous defects in patients with interdental vertical bone loss. *Dento Maxillo Facial Radiology*, *36*(8), 500–505. doi:10.1259/dmfr/29704550

Ju, T., Losasso, F., Schaefer, S., & Warren, J. (2002). Dual Contouring of Hermite Data. In *ACM SIGGRAPH*, (pp. 339-346).

Kaepller, G., Vogel, A., & Axmann-Krcmar, D. (2000). Intra-oral storage phosphor and conventional radiography in the assessment of alveolar bone structures. *Dento Maxillo Facial Radiology*, *29*(6), 362–367. doi:10.1038/sj.dmfr.4600556

Kaiser, T., Wittke, S., Just, I., Krebs, R., Bartel, S., & Fliser, D. (2004). Capillary electrophoresis coupled to mass spectrometer for automated and robust polypeptide determination in body fluids for clinical use. *Electrophoresis*, *25*, 2044–2055. doi:10.1002/elps.200305788

Kaltenboeck, B., & Wang, C. (2005). Advances in real-time PCR: Application to clinical laboratory diagnostics. *Advances in Clinical Chemistry*, *40*, 219–259. doi:10.1016/S0065-2423(05)40006-2

Kaplan, C. W., & Kitts, C. L. (2003). Variation between observed and true Terminal Restriction Fragment length is dependent on true TRF length and purine content. *Journal of Microbiological Methods*, *54*(1), 121–125. doi:10.1016/S0167-7012(03)00003-4

Kaplan, R. C., & Frishman, W. H. (2001). Systemic inflammation as a cardiovascular disease risk factor and as a potential target for drug therapy. *Heart Disease*, *3*, 326–332. doi:10.1097/00132580-200109000-00009

Kappert, H. F., & Krah, M. (2001). Keramiken - eine Übersicht. *Die Quintessenz der Zahntechnik*, *27*(6), 668–704.

Karn, K. W., Shockett, H. P., Moffitt, W. C., & Gray, J. L. (1984). Topographic classification of deformities of the alveolar process. *Journal of Periodontology*, *55*(6), 336–340.

Kassebaum, D. K., Nummikoski, P. V., Triplett, R. G., & Langlais, R. P. (1990). Cross-sectional radiography for implant site assessment. *Oral Surgery, Oral Medicine, and Oral Pathology*, *70*(5), 674–678. doi:10.1016/0030-4220(90)90421-N

Kau, C. H., Richmond, S., Palomo, J. M., & Hans, M. G. (2005). Three-dimensional cone beam computerized tomography in orthodontics. *Journal of Orthodontics*, *32*, 282–293. doi:10.1179/146531205225021285

Keijser, B. J., Zaura, E., Huse, S. M., van der Vossen, J. M., Schuren, F. H., & Montijn, R. C. (2008). Pyrosequencing analysis of the oral microflora of healthy adults. *Journal of Dental Research*, *87*(11), 1016–1020. doi:10.1177/154405910808701104

Kent, A. D., Smith, D. J., Benson, B. J., & Triplett, E. W. (2003). Web-based phylogenetic assignment tool for analysis of terminal restriction fragment length polymorphism profiles of microbial communities. *Applied and Environmental Microbiology*, *69*(11), 6768–6776. doi:10.1128/AEM.69.11.6768-6776.2003

Kerstein, R. (2001). Current Applications of Computerized Occlusal Analysis in Dental Medicine. *General Dentistry*, *49*(5), 521–530.

Kerstein, R. B. (1992). Disocclusion time-reduction therapy with immediate complete anterior guidance development to treat chronic myofascial pain-dysfunction syndrome. *Quintessence International*, *23*(11), 735–747.

Kerstein, R. B. (1993). A Comparison of Traditional Occlusal Equilibration and Immediate Complete Anterior Guidance Development. *Cranio*, *11*(2), 126–140.

Kerstein, R. B. (1994). Disclusion time measurement studies, Part 2: A comparison of disclusion time length of 49 chronic myofascial pain dysfunction syndrome patients to 40 non - patients. A population analysis. *The Journal of Prosthetic Dentistry*, *72*(5), 473–480. doi:10.1016/0022-3913(94)90117-1

Kerstein, R. B. (1994). Disclusion Time Measurement Studies: Stability of disclusion time. a 1 year follow - up study. *The Journal of Prosthetic Dentistry*, *72*(2), 164–168. doi:10.1016/0022-3913(94)90075-2

Kerstein, R. B. (1995). Treatment of myofascial pain dysfunction syndrome with occlusal therapy to reduce lengthy disclusion time - a recall study. *Cranio*, *13*(2), 105–115.

Kerstein, R. B. (1999). Computerized Occlusal Management of a Fixed/ Detachable Implant Prosthesis. *Pract Periodontol Aesthet Dent*, *11*(9 November/December), 1093-1102.

Kerstein, R. B. (2004). Combining Technologies: A Computerized Occlusal Analysis System Synchronized with a Computerized Electromyography System. *Cranio*, *22*(2), 96–109.

Kerstein, R. B., & Radke, J. (2006). The effect of Disclusion Time Reduction on maximal clench muscle activity level. *Cranio*, *24*(3), 156–165.

Kerstein, R. B., & Wilkerson, D. (2001). Locating the Centric Relation Prematurity with a Computerized Occlusal Analysis System. *Compend Contin Educ Dent*, *22*(6), 525–532.

Kerstein, R. B., & Wright, N. (1991). An electromyographic and computer analysis of patients suffering from chronic myofascial pain dysfunction syndrome; pre and post - treatment with immediate complete anterior guidance development. *The Journal of Prosthetic Dentistry*, *66*(5), 677–686. doi:10.1016/0022-3913(91)90453-4

Kerstein, R. B., Chapman, R., & Klein, M. (1997). A Comparison of ICAGD (Immediate Complete Anterior Guidance Development) to Mock ICAGD for Symptom Reductions in Chronic Myofascial Pain Dysfunction Syndrome Patient. *Cranio*, *5*(1), 21–37.

Kerstein, R.B., & Lowe, M., Harty, Radke, J. (2006). A Force reproduction analysis of two recording sensors of a computerized occlusal analysis system. *Cranio*, *24*(1), 15–24.

Kerstein, RB Grundset, K. (2001). Obtaining Measurable Bilateral Simultaneous Occlusal Contacts with Computer-Analyzed and Guided Occlusal Adjustments. *Quintessence International, January*, *32*(1), 7-18.

Khader, Y. S., Albashaireh, Z. S., & Alomari, M. A. (2004). Periodontal diseases and the risk of coronary heart and cerebrovascular diseases: a meta-analysis. *Journal of Periodontology*, *75*(8), 1046–1053. doi:10.1902/jop.2004.75.8.1046

Kinder, T. (2001). The use of Call Centres by local public administrations. *Futures*, *33*(10), 837–860. doi:10.1016/S0016-3287(01)00022-2

Kirches, M., Pack, N., & Schoofs, R. (2000). Die Komponenten des dualen Legierungssystems Vigo Liberty im Vergleich. *dent lab*, *48*(4), 555-564.

Klaassen, C. H., Prinsen, C. F., de Vals, H. A., Horrevorts, A. M., Jeunink, M. A., & Thunnissen, F. B. (2004). DNA microarray format for detection and subtyping of human papillomavirus. *Journal of Clinical Microbiology*, *42*, 2152–2160. doi:10.1128/JCM.42.5.2152-2160.2004

Klappenbach, J. A., Dunbar, J. M., & Schmidt, T. M. (2000). rRNA operon copy number reflects ecological strategies of bacteria. *Applied and Environmental Microbiology*, *66*, 1328–1333. doi:10.1128/AEM.66.4.1328-1333.2000

Klemetti, E., Kolmakov, S., Heiskanen, P., Vainio, P., & Lasilla, V. (1993). Panoramic mandibular index and bone mineral densities in postmenopausal women. *Oral Surgery, Oral Medicine, and Oral Pathology*, *75*(6), 774–779. doi:10.1016/0030-4220(93)90438-A

Klipp, E., Herwig, R., Kowald, A., Wierling, C., & Lehrach, H. (2005). *Biology in Practice*. Hoboken, NJ: Wiley-VCH.

Knoell, A. C. (1977). A mathematical model of an in vitro human mandible. *Journal of Biomechanics*, *10*(3), 159–166. doi:10.1016/0021-9290(77)90054-9

Kobbelt, K., Botsch, M., Schwanecke, U., & Seidel, H. (2001). Feature-sensitive surface extraction from volume data. In *ACM SIGGRAPH*, (pp. 57-66).

Kober, C., Stübinger, S., Hellmich, C., Sader, R., & Zeilhofer, H. F. (2008). Mandibular finite element simulation as a tool for trauma surgery. *International Journal of Computerized Dentistry*, *11*(3-4), 175–181.

Koch, A., Macherel, J. M., Wirth, T., de Groot, P. M., Ducourant, T., Couder, D., et al. (2001). *Detective quantum efficiency of an x-ray image intensifier chain as a benchmark for amorphous silicon flat-panal detectors* (Vol. 4320).

Kokich, V. G., & Mathews, D. P. (1993). Surgical and orthodontic management of impacted teeth. *Dental Clinics of North America*, *37*, 181–204.

Kolch, W., Neusüss, C., Pelzing, M., & Mischak, H. (2005). Capillary electrophoresis-mass spectrometry as a powerful tool in clinical diagnosis and biomarker discovery. *Mass Spectrometry Reviews*, *24*, 959–977. doi:10.1002/mas.20051

Kolenbrander, P. E., Palmer, R. J. Jr, Rickard, A. H., Jakubovics, N. S., Chalmers, N. I., & Diaz, P. I. (2006). Bacterial interactions and successions during plaque development. *Periodontology 2000*, *42*, 47–79. doi:10.1111/j.1600-0757.2006.00187.x

Koolstra, J. H., van Eijden, T. M., Weijs, W. A., & Naeije, M. (1988). A three-dimensional mathematical model of the human masticatory system predicting maximum possible bite forces. *Journal of Biomechanics*, *21*(7), 563–576. doi:10.1016/0021-9290(88)90219-9

Korioth, T. W. P., & Versluis, A. (1997). Modeling the mechanical behavior of the jaws and their related structures by finite element (FE) analysis. *Critical Reviews in Oral Biology and Medicine*, *8*(1), 90–104. doi:10.1177/10454411970080010501

Korioth, T. W., Romilly, D. P., & Hannam, A. G. (1992). Three-dimensional finite element stress analysis of the dentate human mandible. *American Journal of Physical Anthropology*, *88*(1), 69–96. doi:10.1002/ajpa.1330880107

Korkmaz, H. H. (2007). Evaluation of different miniplates in fixation of fractured human mandible with the finite element method. *Oral Surgery, Oral Medicine, Oral Pathology, Oral Radiology, and Endodontics*, *103*(6), e1–e13. doi:10.1016/j.tripleo.2006.12.016

Kreth, J., Merritt, J., Shi, W., & Qi, F. (2005). Competition and coexistence between Streptococcus mutans and Streptococcus sanguinis in the dental biofilm. *Journal of Bacteriology*, *187*(21), 7193–7203. doi:10.1128/JB.187.21.7193-7203.2005

Kroes, I., Lepp, P. W., & Relman, D. A. (1999). Bacterial diversity within the human subgingival crevice. *Proceedings of the National Academy of Sciences of the United States of America*, *96*(25), 14547–14552. doi:10.1073/pnas.96.25.14547

Krüttgen, A., Möller, J. C., Heymach, J. V., & Shooter, E. M. (1998). Neurotrophins induce release of neurotrophins by the regulated secretory pathway. *Proceedings of the National Academy of Sciences of the United States of America*, *95*, 9614–9619. doi:10.1073/pnas.95.16.9614

Kuhls-Gilcrist, A., Yadava, G., Patel, V., Jain, A., Bednarek, D. R., & Rudin, S. (2008). The Solid-State X-Ray Image Intensifier (SSXII): An EMCCD-Based X-Ray Detector. *Proc Soc Photo Opt Instrum Eng, 6913*, nihpa68284.

Kumar, P. S., Leys, E. J., Bryk, J. M., Martinez, F. J., Moeschberger, M. L., & Griffen, A. L. (2006). Changes in periodontal health status are associated with bacterial community shifts as assessed by quantitative 16S cloning and sequencing. *Journal of Clinical Microbiology*, *44*(10), 3665–3673. doi:10.1128/JCM.00317-06

Künzel, A., Scherkowski, D., Willers, R., & Becker, J. (2003). Visually detectable resolution of intraoral dental films. *Dento Maxillo Facial Radiology*, *32*(6), 385–389. doi:10.1259/dmfr/22478778

Kuo, W. P. (2003). Overview of bioinformatics and its application to oral genomics. *Advances in Dental Research*, *17*, 89–94. doi:10.1177/154407370301700121

Kuo, W. P., Hasina, R., Ohno-Machado, L., & Lingen, M. W. (2003). Classification and identification of genes associated with oral cancer based on gene expression profiles. A preliminary study. *The New York State Dental Journal*, *69*(2), 23–26.

Kuramitsu, H. K., Chen, W., & Ikegami, A. (2005). Biofilm formation by the periodontopathic bacteria Treponema denticola and Porphyromonas gingivalis. *Journal of Periodontology*, *76*(11Suppl), 2047–2051. doi:10.1902/jop.2005.76.11-S.2047

Kurkowska-Jastrzebska, I., Balkowiec-Iskra, E., Ciesielska, A., Joniec, I., Cudna, A., Zaremba, M. M., et al. (2009). Decreased inflammation and augmented expression of trophic factors correlate with MOG-induced neuroprotection of the injured nigrostriatal system in the murine MPTP model of Parkinson's disease. *International Immunopharmacology*.

Kurkowska-Jastrzebska, I., Balkowiec-Iskra, E., Joniec, I., Litwin, T., Czlonkowski, A., & Czlonkowska, A. (2005). Immunization with myelin oligodendrocyte glycoprotein and complete Freund adjuvant partially protects dopaminergic neurons from 1-methyl-4-phenyl-1,2,3,6-tetrahydropyridine-induced damage in mouse model of Parkinson's disease. *Neuroscience*, *131*, 247–254. doi:10.1016/j.neuroscience.2004.10.027

Lamont, R. J., & Jenkinson, H. F. (1998). Life below the gum line: pathogenic mechanisms of *Porphyromonas gingivalis*. *Microbiology and Molecular Biology Reviews*, *62*, 1244–1263.

Laudon, K. C., & Laudon, J. P. (2006). *Essentials of business information systems*. Upper Saddle River, NJ: Pearson Education, Prentice-Hall.

Ledley, R. S., & Huang, H. K. (1968). Linear model of tooth displacement by applied forces. *Journal of Dental Research*, *47*(3), 427–432.

Lee, W. E. III. (1986). A suggested instrumental technique for studying dynamic flavour release from food products. *Journal of Food Science*, *51*, 249–250. doi:10.1111/j.1365-2621.1986.tb10888.x

Lee, Y. H. (2008). Associations between FCGr3A polymorphisms and rheumatoid arthritis susceptibility: a metaanalysis. *The Journal of Rheumatology*, *35*, 2129–2135. doi:10.3899/jrheum.080186

Lee, Y. H. (2009). Association between interleukin 1 polymorphisms and rheumatoid arthritis susceptibility: a metaanalysis. *The Journal of Rheumatology*, *36*(1), 12–15.

Lekholm, U., & Zarb, G. A. (1985). Patient selection and preparation. In P. I. Brånemark, G. A. Zarb, T. Albrekttson, (Ed.), *Tissue-integrated prostheses: osseointegration in clinical dentistry*, (pp. 1-356). Chicago: Quintessence Publishing.

Lemos, J. A., & Burne, R. A. (2008). A model of efficiency: stress tolerance by Streptococcus mutans. *Microbiology*, *154*(Pt 11), 3247–3255. doi:10.1099/mic.0.2008/023770-0

Lerner, U. H. (2006). Inflammation-induced bone remodelling in periodontal disease and the influence of postmenopausal osteoporosis. *Journal of Dental Research*, *85*(7), 596–607. doi:10.1177/154405910608500704

Lever, I. J., Bradbury, E. J., Cunningham, J. R., Adelson, D. W., Jones, M. G., & McMahon, S. B. (2001). Brain-derived neurotrophic factor is released in the dorsal horn by distinctive patterns of afferent fiber stimulation. *The Journal of Neuroscience*, *21*, 4469–4477.

Li, G., Engström, P. E., Nasström, K., Lü, Z. Y., Sanderink, G., & Welander, U. (2007). Marginal bone levels measured in film and digital radiographs corrected for attenuation and visual response: an in-vitro study. *Dento Maxillo Facial Radiology*, *36*(1), 7–11. doi:10.1259/dmfr/28315324

Li, X., & Freitag. L. (1999). *Optimization-based quadrilateral and hexahedral mesh untangling and smoothing techniques*. Tech. Report, Argonne National Laboratory, a contract Laboratory of the United States Department of Energy.

Li, Y., Ismail, A. I., Ge, Y., Tellez, M., & Sohn, W. (2007). Similarity of bacterial populations in saliva from African-American mother-child dyads. *Journal of Clinical Microbiology*, *45*(9), 3082–3085. doi:10.1128/JCM.00771-07

Liang, X., Jacobs, R., Hassan, B., Li, L., Pauwels, R., Corpas, L., Souza, P. C., Martens, W., et al. (2009). A comparative evaluation of Cone Beam Computed Tomography (CBCT) and Multi-Slice CT (MSCT) Part I. On subjective image quality. *Eur J Radiol*, (e-pub ahead of print).

Lichanska., et al. (2005). Retrieved from http://www.ebi.ac.uk/microarray-as/ae/ (E-GEOD-2525)

Lillesaar, C., Eriksson, C., & Fried, K. (2001). Rat tooth pulp cells elicit neurite growth from trigeminal neurones and express mRNAs for neurotrophic factors in vitro. *Neuroscience Letters*, *308*, 161–164. doi:10.1016/S0304-3940(01)01997-8

Lindh, C., Horner, K., Jonasson, G., Olsson, P., Rohlin, M., & Jacobs, R. (2008). The use of visual assessment of dental radiographs for identifying women at risk of having osteoporosis: the OSTEODENT project. *Oral Surgery, Oral Medicine, Oral Pathology, Oral Radiology, and Endodontics*, *106*(2), 285–293. doi:10.1016/j.tripleo.2007.09.008

Lindh, C., Petersson, A., & Rohlin, M. (1996). Assessment of the trabecular pattern before endosseous implant treatment: diagnostic outcome of periapical radiography in the mandible. *Oral Surgery, Oral Medicine, Oral Pathology, Oral Radiology, and Endodontics*, *82*(3), 335–343. doi:10.1016/S1079-2104(96)80363-5

Linforth, R., & Taylor, A. J. (2000). Persistence of volatile compounds in the breath after their consumption in aqueous solutions. *Journal of Agricultural and Food Chemistry*, *48*, 5419–5423. doi:10.1021/jf000488n

Liu, E. T. (2005). Systems biology, integrative biology, predictive biology. *Cell*, *121*(4), 505–506. doi:10.1016/j.cell.2005.04.021

Liu, W. T., Marsh, T. L., Cheng, H., & Forney, L. J. (1997). Characterization of microbial diversity by determining terminal restriction fragment length polymorphisms of genes encoding 16S rRNA. *Applied and Environmental Microbiology*, *63*(11), 4516–4522.

Lobos, C., & Hitschfeld, N. (2006). 3D NOffset mixed-element mesh generator approach, *The 14th International Conference in Central Europe on Computer Graphics, Visualization and Computer Vision (WSCG)*, (pp. 47-52).

Lobos, C., Bucki, M., Hitschfeld, N., & Payan, Y. (2007). Mixed-element mesh for an intra-operative modeling of the brain tumor extraction. In *Proceedings, 16th International Meshing Roundtable*, (pp. 387-404).

Loesche, W. J. (1986). Role of Streptococcus-Mutans in Human Dental Decay. *Microbiological Reviews*, *50*(4), 353–380.

Lofthag-Hansen, S., Huumonen, S., Gröndahl, K., & Gröndahl, H. G. (2007). Limited cone-beam CT and intraoral radiography for the diagnosis of periapical pathology. *Oral Surgery, Oral Medicine, Oral Pathology, Oral Radiology, and Endodontics*, *103*, 114–119. doi:10.1016/j.tripleo.2006.01.001

Loos, B., Nylund, K., Claffey, N., & Egelberg, J. (1989). Clinical effects of root debridement in molar and non-molar teeth. A 2-year follow-up. *Journal of Clinical Periodontology*, *16*(8), 498–504. doi:10.1111/j.1600-051X.1989.tb02326.x

Lorensen, W., & Cline, H. (1987). Marching Cubes: A high resolution 3D surface construction algorithm. *Computer Graphics*, *21*(4), 163–169. doi:10.1145/37402.37422

Lovald, S. T., Khraishi, T., Wagner, J., Baack, B., Kelly, J., & Wood, J. (2006). Comparison of plate-screw systems used in mandibular fracture reduction: finite element analysis. *Journal of Biomechanical Engineering*, *128*(5), 654–662. doi:10.1115/1.2244575

Low, K., Dula, K., Bürgin, W., & von Arx, T. (2008). Comparison of periapical radiography and limited cone-beam tomography in posterior maxillary teeth referred for apical surgery. *Journal of Endodontics*, *34*, 557–562. doi:10.1016/j.joen.2008.02.022

Luboz, V., Chabanas, M., Swider, P., & Payan, Y. (2005). Orbital and Maxillofacial Computer Aided Surgery: Patient-Specific Finite Element Models To Predict Surgical Outcomes. *Computer Methods in Biomechanics and Biomedical Engineering*, *8*(4), 259–265. doi:10.1080/10255840500289921

Luboz, V., Payan, Y., & Couteau, B. (2001). Automatic 3D Finite Element mesh generation: an atlas fitted onto patient data. In *Proceedings of the Fifth international Symposium on Computer Methods in Biomechanics and Biomedical Engineering.*

Luckey, J. A., & Smith, L. M. (1993). A model for the mobility of single-stranded DNA in capillary gel electrophoresis. *Electrophoresis*, *14*(5-6), 492–501. doi:10.1002/elps.1150140176

Ludlow, J. B., & Ivanovic, M. (2008). Comparative dosimetry of dental CBCT devices and 64-slice CT for oral and maxillofacial radiology. *Oral Surgery, Oral Medicine, Oral Pathology, Oral Radiology, and Endodontics*, *106*(1), 106–114. doi:10.1016/j.tripleo.2008.03.018

Ludlow, J. B., Davies-Ludlow, L. E., & Brooks, S. L. (2003). Dosimetry of two extraoral direct digital imaging devices: NewTom cone beam CT and Orthophos Plus DS panoramic unit. *Dento Maxillo Facial Radiology*, *32*, 229–234. doi:10.1259/dmfr/26310390

Ludlow, J. B., Davies-Ludlow, L. E., & White, S. C. (2008). Patient risk related to common dental radiographic examinations: the impact of 2007 International Commission on Radiological Protection recommendations regarding dose calculation. *The Journal of the American Dental Association*, *139*(9), 1237–1243.

Ludwig, J. A., & Weinstein, J. N. (2005). Biomarkers in cancer staging, prognosis and treatment selection. *Nature Reviews. Cancer*, *5*, 845–856. doi:10.1038/nrc1739

Lundberg, J. M., Rudehill, A., Sollevi, A., Fried, G., & Wallin, G. (1989). Co-release of neuropeptide Y and noradrenaline from pig spleen *in vivo*: importance of subcellular storage, nerve impulse frequency and pattern, feedback regulation and resupply by axonal transport. *Neuroscience*, *28*, 475–486. doi:10.1016/0306-4522(89)90193-0

Luthard, R., Rudolph, H., Sandkuhl, O., & Walter, M. (2001). Aktuelle CAD/CAM-Systeme zur Herstellung von keramischen Zahnersatz Teil 1: Systeme ohne zusätzliche Sinterung des keramischen Grundmaterials. *Zahnärztliche Welt*, *110*(11), 747–754.

Luthardt, R., Rudolph, H., Sandkuhl, O., & Walter, M. (2001). Aktuelle CAD/CAM-Systeme zur Herstellung von keramischen Zahnersatz Teil 2: Systeme mit zusätzlicher Sinterung des keramischen Grundmaterials. *Zahnärztliche Welt*, *110*(12), 797–802.

Luukko, K., Suvanto, P., Saarma, M., & Thesleff, I. (1997). Expression of GDNF and its receptors in developing tooth is developmentally regulated and suggests multiple roles in innervation and organogenesis. *Developmental Dynamics*, *210*, 463–471. doi:10.1002/(SICI)1097-0177(199712)210:4<463::AID-AJA9>3.0.CO;2-E

Maarse, H. (1991). Volatile compounds in foods and beverages. Eds. Maarse H., Dekker Inc.: New York, Basel, Hong Kong.

Machiels, D., van Ruth, S. M., Posthumus, M. A., & Istasse, L. (2003). Gas chromatography-olfactometry analysis of the volatile compounds of two commercial Irish beef meats. *Talanta*, *60*, 755–764. doi:10.1016/S0039-9140(03)00133-4

MacPhedran, S. E., & Hall, A. K. (2001). Influence of non-neuronal cells on establishment of neuropeptide Y expression by sympathetic neurons in vitro. *Developmental Neuroscience*, *23*, 307–317. doi:10.1159/000048714

Maness, W. L. (1988). Force Movie: A Time and Force View of Occlusal Contacts. *Compend Contin Educ Dent*, *10*(7), 404–408.

Maness, W. L. (1993). Computerized Occlusal Analysis, Hi-Tech, Hi-Care. *Dental Journal*, *59*(8).

Maness, W. L., Benjamin, M., Podoloff, R., Bobick, A., & Golden, R. F. (1987). Computerized occlusal analysis: a new technology. *Quintessence International*, *18*(4), 287–292.

Mann, M., Højrup, P., & Roepstorff, P. (1993). Use of mass spectrometric molecular weight information to identify proteins in sequence databases. *Biological Mass Spectrometry*, *22*, 338–345. doi:10.1002/bms.1200220605

Mans, J. J., Baker, H. V., Oda, D., Lamont, R. J., & Handfield, M. (2006). Distinctive characteristics of transcriptional profiles from two epithelial cell lines upon interaction with *Actinobacillus actinomycetemcomitans*. *Oral Microbiology and Immunology*, *21*, 261–267. doi:10.1111/j.1399-302X.2006.00281.x

Mans, J. J., Lamont, R. J., & Handfield, M. (2006). Microarray analysis of human epithelial cell responses to bacterial interaction. *Infectious Disorders Drug Targets*, *6*, 299–309. doi:10.2174/187152606778249926

Marsh, P. D. (2003). Are dental diseases examples of ecological catastrophes? *Microbiology*, *149*, 279–294. doi:10.1099/mic.0.26082-0

Marsh, T. L. (2005). Culture-independent microbial community analysis with terminal restriction fragment length polymorphism. *Methods in Enzymology*, *397*, 308–329. doi:10.1016/S0076-6879(05)97018-3

Marsh, T. L., Saxman, P., Cole, J., & Tiedje, J. (2000). Terminal restriction fragment length polymorphism analysis program, a web-based research tool for microbial community analysis. *Applied and Environmental Microbiology*, *66*(8), 3616–3620. doi:10.1128/AEM.66.8.3616-3620.2000

Martin, H. (1991). Cleanliness, disinfection, and sterilization of the root canal. *Current Opinion in Dentistry*, *1*, 734–736.

Martin, J. L., Jenkins, V. K., Hsieh, H.-Y., & Balkowiec, A. (2009). Brain-derived neurotrophic factor in arterial baroreceptor pathways: Implications for activity-dependent plasticity at baroafferent synapses. *Journal of Neurochemistry*, *108*, 450–464. doi:10.1111/j.1471-4159.2008.05781.x

Mathew, J. P., Taylor, B. S., Bader, G. D., Pyarajan, S., Antoniotti, M., & Chinnaiyan, A. M. (2007). From bytes to bedside: data integration and computational biology for translational cancer research. *PLoS Computational Biology*, *3*(2), e12. doi:10.1371/journal.pcbi.0030012

Mayol, A. R., & Acree, T. E. (2001). Advances in Gas Chromatography-Olfactometry. In: Gas-Chromatography-Olfactometry. The state of the art. Eds. Leland J.V., Schieberle P., Buettner A. and Acree T.E., Oxford University Press, 1-10.

Mayr, D., van Ruth, S. M., & Märk, T. D. (2003). Evaluation of the influence of mastication on temporal aroma release of ripe and unripe bananas, using a model mouth system and gas chromatography-olfactometry. *European Food Research and Technology, 217*, 291–295. doi:10.1007/s00217-003-0777-1

McAboy, C. P., Grumet, J. T., Siegel, E. B., & Iacopino, A. M. (2003). Surgical uprighting and repositioning of severely impacted mandibular second molars. *The Journal of the American Dental Association, 134*, 1459–1462.

McCollough, C. H., Primak, A. N., Braun, N., Kofler, J., Yu, L., & Christner, J. (2009). Strategies for reducing radiation dose in CT. *Radiologic Clinics of North America, 47*, 27–40. doi:10.1016/j.rcl.2008.10.006

McDavid, W. D., Welander, U., Pillai, B. K., & Morris, C. R. (1982). The Intrex—a constant-potential x-ray unit for periapical dental radiography. *Oral Surgery, Oral Medicine, and Oral Pathology, 53*(4), 433–436. doi:10.1016/0030-4220(82)90448-0

McGuire, K., & Glass, E. J. (2005). The expanding role of microarrays in the investigation of macrophage responses to pathogens. *Veterinary Immunology and Immunopathology, 105*, 259–275. doi:10.1016/j.vetimm.2005.02.001

McNab, R., Ford, S. K., El-Sabaeny, A., Barbieri, B., Cook, G. S., & Lamont, R. J. (2003). LuxS-based signaling in Streptococcus gordonii: autoinducer 2 controls carbohydrate metabolism and biofilm formation with Porphyromonas gingivalis. *Journal of Bacteriology, 185*(1), 274–284. doi:10.1128/JB.185.1.274-284.2003

Melchers, W. J. (2005). Comparison of two commercial assays for detection of human papillomavirus (HPV) in cervical scrape specimens: validation of the Roche AMPLICOR HPV test as a means to screen for HPV genotypes associated with a higher risk of cervical disorders. *Journal of Clinical Microbiology, 43*, 2662–2667. doi:10.1128/JCM.43.6.2662-2667.2005

Mengel, R., Candir, M., Shiratori, K., & Flores-de-Jacoby, L. (2005). Digital volume tomography in the diagnosis of periodontal defects: an in vitro study on native pig and human mandibles. *Journal of Periodontology, 76*(5), 665–673. doi:10.1902/jop.2005.76.5.665

Meyer, J. M. (1977). Corrosion resistance of nickel -chromium dental casting alloys. *Corrosion Science, 17*, 971–982.

Miller, G., Pave, S., & Walkington, N. (2003). When and Why Ruppert's Algorithm Works. In *Proceedings 12th International Meshing Roundtable*, (pp. 91-102).

Millstein, P., & Maya, A. (2001). An evaluation of occlusal contact marking indicators descriptive quantitative method. *The Journal of the American Dental Association, 132*(9), 1280–1286.

Misch, K. A., Yi, E. S., & Sarment, D. P. (2006). Accuracy of cone beam computed tomography for periodontal defect measurements. *J Peridontol, 77*(7), 1261–1266. doi:10.1902/jop.2006.050367

Mischkowski, R. A., Pulsfort, R., Ritter, L., Neugebauer, J., Brochhagen, H. G., & Keeve, E. (2007). Geometric accuracy of a newly developed cone-beam device for maxillofacial imaging. *Oral Surgery, Oral Medicine, Oral Pathology, Oral Radiology, and Endodontics, 104*(4), 551–559. doi:10.1016/j.tripleo.2007.02.021

Mischkowski, R. A., Zinser, M. J., Ritter, L., Neugebauer, J., Keeve, E., & Zoller, J. E. (2007). Intraoperative navigation in the maxillofacial area based on 3D imaging obtained by a cone-beam device. *International Journal of Oral and Maxillofacial Surgery, 36*(8), 687–694. doi:10.1016/j.ijom.2007.04.001

Miyagi, M., & Rao, K. C. (2007). Proteolytic 18O-labeling strategies for quantitative proteomics. *Mass Spectrometry Reviews, 26*, 121–136. doi:10.1002/mas.20116

Molander, B., Ahlqwist, M., & Gröndhal, A. G. (1995). Panoramic and restrictive intraoral radiography in comprehensive oral radiographic diagnosis. *European Journal of Oral Sciences, 103*(4), 191–198. doi:10.1111/j.1600-0722.1995.tb00159.x

Molino, N., Bridson, R., Teran, J., & Fedkiw, R. (2003). A crystalline, red green strategy for meshing highly deformable objects with tetrahedral. In *Proceedings, 12th International Meshing Roundtable*, (pp. 103-114).

Montagnat, J., & Delingette, H. (1998). Globally constrained deformable models for 3D object reconstruction. [SP]. *Signal Processing, 71*(2), 173–186. doi:10.1016/S0165-1684(98)00143-1

Montagnat, J., & Delingette, H. (2005). 4D deformable models with temporal constraints: application to 4D cardiac image segmentation. [MedIA]. *Medical Image Analysis, 9*(1), 87–100. doi:10.1016/j.media.2004.06.025

Montgomery, M., & Kerstein, R. B. (2000). Mapping Occlusal Forces on Rebuilt Anterior Guidance. *Contemporary Esthetics, 4*(4), 68–72.

Motamedi, M. H., Tabatabaie, F. A., Navi, F., Shafeie, H. A., Fard, B. K., & Hayati, Z. (2009). Assessment of radiographic factors affecting surgical exposure and orthodontic alignment of impacted canines of the palate: A 15-year retrospective study. *Oral Surgery, Oral Medicine, Oral Pathology, Oral Radiology, and Endodontics, 107*, 772–775. doi:10.1016/j.tripleo.2008.12.022

Moutsopoulos, N. M., Greenwell-Wild, T., & Wahl, S. M. (2006). Differential mucosal susceptibility in HIV-1 transmission and infection. *Advances in Dental Research, 19*(1), 52–56. doi:10.1177/154407370601900111

Mozzo, P., Procacci, C., Tacconi, A., Martini, P. T., & Andreis, I. A. (1998). A new volumetric CT machine for dental imaging based on the cone-beam technique: preliminary results. *European Radiology, 8*(9), 1558–1564. doi:10.1007/s003300050586

Mullis, K. B., & Faloona, F. A. (1987). Specific synthesis of DNA in vitro via a polymerase-catalyzed chain reaction. *Methods in Enzymology, 155*, 335–350. doi:10.1016/0076-6879(87)55023-6

Munoz, N., Bosch, F. X., de Sanjose, S., Herrero, R., Castellsague, X., & Shah, K. V. (2003). Epidemiologic classification of human papillomavirus types associated with cervical cancer. *The New England Journal of Medicine, 348*, 518–527. doi:10.1056/NEJMoa021641

Muyzer, G., de Waal, E. C., & Uitterlinden, A. G. (1993). Profiling of complex microbial populations by denaturing gradient gel electrophoresis analysis of polymerase chain reaction-amplified genes coding for 16S rRNA. *Applied and Environmental Microbiology, 59*(3), 695–700.

Nadkarni, M. A., Martin, F. E., Jacques, N. A., & Hunter, N. (2002). Determination of bacterial load by real-time PCR using a broad-range (universal) probe and primers set. *Microbiology, 148*, 257–266.

Nadler, S. T., Stoehr, J. P., Schueler, K. L., Tanimoto, G., Yandell, B. S., & Attie, A. D. (2000). The expression of adipogenic genes is decreased in obesity and diabetes mellitus. *Proceedings of the National Academy of Sciences of the United States of America, 97*(21), 11371–11376. doi:10.1073/pnas.97.21.11371

Nakano, Y., Takeshita, T., & Yamashita, Y. (2006). TRFMA: a web-based tool for terminal restriction fragment length polymorphism analysis based on molecular weight. *Bioinformatics (Oxford, England), 22*(14), 1788–1789. doi:10.1093/bioinformatics/btl186

Nakano, Y., Takeshita, T., Kamio, N., Shiota, S., Shibata, Y., & Yasui, M. (2008). Development and application of a T-RFLP data analysis method using correlation coefficient matrices. *Journal of Microbiological Methods, 75*(3), 501–505. doi:10.1016/j.mimet.2008.08.002

Nascimento, M. M., Gordan, V. V., Garvan, C. W., Browngardt, C. M., & Burne, R. A. (2009). Correlations of oral bacterial arginine and urea catabolism with caries experience. *Oral Microbiology and Immunology, 24*(2), 89–95.

Nassl, K., Kropf, F., & Klostermeyer, H. (1995). A method to mimic and to study the release of compounds from chewed food. *Lebensmittel Untersuchung und Forshung, 201*, 62–68. doi:10.1007/BF01193202

Nazmul-Hossain, A. N., Patel, K. J., Rhodus, N. L., & Moser, K. L. (2008). Microarrays: applications in dental research. *Oral Diseases, 14*(1), 25–29.

Negrel, D. (2006). Chromes with CAD/CAM. *The Dental Technician, 70*, 25–30.

Nesme, M. (2008). *Milieu mecanique deformable multiresolution pour la simulation Interactive*. Universite Joseph Fourier.

Ng, Y. L., Spratt, D., Sriskantharajah, S., & Gulabivala, K. (2003). Evaluation of protocols for field decontamination before bacterial sampling of root canals for contemporary microbiology techniques. *Journal of Endodontics*, *29*, 317–320. doi:10.1097/00004770-200305000-00001

Niemann, P. (2003). Laser-Sinterverfahren in der CAD/CAM-Technik. *Die Quintessenz der Zahntechnik*, *29*(1), 38–42.

Nilsson, M., & Kopp, S. (2008). Gingivitis and periodontitis are related to repeated high levels of circulating tumor necrosis factor-alpha in patients with rheumatoid arthritis. *Journal of Periodontology*, *79*, 1689–1696. doi:10.1902/jop.2008.070599

Nishikawara, F., Katsumura, S., Ando, A., Tamaki, Y., Nakamura, Y., & Sato, K. (2006). Correlation of cariogenic bacteria and dental caries in adults. *Journal of Oral Science*, *48*(4), 245–251. doi:10.2334/josnusd.48.245

Nosrat, C. A., Fried, K., Ebendal, T., & Olson, L. (1998). NGF, BDNF, NT3, NT4 and GDNF in tooth development. *European Journal of Oral Sciences*, *106*(Supplement 1), 94–99.

Nyman, S., & Lindhe, J. (1997). Examination of patients with periodontal disease. In J. Lindhe, T. Karring, N. P. Lang (Ed.), *Clinical periodontology and implant dentistry, 3* (pp. 383-395). Copenhagen: Munksgard.

Odake, S., Roozen, J. P., & Burger, J. J. (1998). Effect of saliva dilution on the release of diacetyl and 2-heptanone from cream style dressings. *Die Nahrung*, *42*, 385–391. doi:10.1002/(SICI)1521-3803(199812)42:06<385::AID-FOOD385>3.0.CO;2-B

Odake, S., Roozen, J. P., & Burger, J. J. (2000). Flavor release of diacetyl and 2-heptanone from cream style dressings in three model mouth systems. *Bioscience, Biotechnology, and Biochemistry*, *64*, 2523–2529. doi:10.1271/bbb.64.2523

Offenbacher, S., Barros, S. P., & Beck, J. D. (2008). Rethinking periodontal inflammation. *Journal of Periodontology*, *79*(8Suppl), 1577–1584. doi:10.1902/jop.2008.080220

Oh, T. J., Kim, C. J., Woo, S. K., Kim, T. S., Jeong, D. J., & Kim, M. S. (2004). Development and clinical evaluation of a highly sensitive DNA microarray for detection and genotyping of human papillomaviruses. *Journal of Clinical Microbiology*, *42*, 3272–3280. doi:10.1128/JCM.42.7.3272-3280.2004

Ohman, I., & Ohman, A. (1980). The eruption tendency and changes of direction of impacted teeth following surgical exposure. *Oral Surgery, Oral Medicine, and Oral Pathology*, *49*, 383–389. doi:10.1016/0030-4220(80)90279-0

Oliveira Costa, F., Cota, L. O., Costa, J. E., & Pordeus, I. A. (2007). Periodontal disease progression among young subjects with no preventive dental care: a 52-month follow-up study. *Journal of Periodontology*, *78*(2), 198–203. doi:10.1902/jop.2007.060150

Onda, T., Uzawa, K., Nakashima, D., Saito, K., Iwadate, Y., & Seki, N. (2007). Lin-7C/VELI3/MALS-3: an essential component in metastasis of human squamous cell carcinoma. *Cancer Research*, *67*, 9643–9648. doi:10.1158/0008-5472.CAN-07-1911

Ong, S. E., Blagoev, B., Kratchmarova, I., Kristensen, D. B., Steen, H., & Pandey, A. (2002). Stable isotope labeling by amino acids in cell culture, SILAC, as a simple and accurate approach to expression proteomics. *Molecular & Cellular Proteomics*, *1*, 376–386. doi:10.1074/mcp.M200025-MCP200

Ooshima, T., Ishida, R., Mishima, K., & Sobue, S. (1996). The prevalence of developmental anomalies of teeth and their association with tooth size in the primary and permanent dentitions of 1650 Japanese children. *International Journal of Paediatric Dentistry*, *6*, 87–94.

Oppacher, R. (2000). Alle guten Dinge sind drei: eine Keramik auf zwei unterschiedlichen Legierungen - erste Erfahrungen mit Vigo Liberty. *Die Quintessenz der Zahntechnik*, *26*(5), 429–438.

Ota, F., Ota, M., Mahmud, Z. H., Mohammad, A., Yamato, M., & Kassu, A. (2006). Serological diversity demonstrable by a set of monoclonal antibodies to eight serotypes of the mutans streptococci. *Caries Research*, *40*(1), 6–14. doi:10.1159/000088899

Ott, S. J., El Mokhtari, N. E., Musfeldt, M., Hellmig, S., & Freitag, S. (2006). Detection of diverse bacterial signatures in atherosclerotic lesions of patients with coronary heart disease. *Circulation*, *113*, 929–937. doi:10.1161/CIRCULATIONAHA.105.579979

Pace, N. R. (1997). A molecular view of microbial diversity and the biosphere. *Science*, *276*(5313), 734–740. doi:10.1126/science.276.5313.734

Pages, A., Sermesant, M., & Frey, P. (2005). Generation of computational meshes from MRI and CT-scan data. In *ESAIM: Proceedings*, (pp. 213-223).

Palomo, J. M., Rao, P. S., & Hans, M. G. (2008). Influence of exposure conditions on radiation dose. *Oral Surgery, Oral Medicine, Oral Pathology, Oral Radiology, and Endodontics*, *105*(6), 773–782. doi:10.1016/j.tripleo.2007.12.019

Papapanou, P. N., Sedaghatfar, M. H., Demmer, R. T., Wolf, D. L., Yang, J., & Roth, G. A. (2007). Periodontal therapy alters gene expression of peripheral blood monocytes. *Journal of Clinical Periodontology*, *34*(9), 736–747. doi:10.1111/j.1600-051X.2007.01113.x

Pappin, D. J., Hojrup, P., & Bleasby, A. J. (1993). Rapid identification of proteins by peptide-mass fingerprinting. *Current Biology*, *3*, 327–332. doi:10.1016/0960-9822(93)90195-T

Paraskevas, S., Huizinga, J. D., & Loos, B. G. (2008). A systematic review and meta-analyses on C-reactive protein in relation to periodontitis. *Journal of Clinical Periodontology*, *35*, 277–290. doi:10.1111/j.1600-051X.2007.01173.x

Paster, B. J., Bartoszyk, I. M., & Dewhirst, F. E. (1998). Identification of oral streptococci using PCR-based, reverse-capture, checkerboard hybridization. *Methods in Cell Science*, (20): 223–231. doi:10.1023/A:1009715710555

Paster, B. J., Boches, S. K., Galvin, J. L., Ericson, R. E., Lau, C. N., & Levanos, V. A. (2001). Bacterial diversity in human subgingival plaque. *Journal of Bacteriology*, *183*(12), 3770–3783. doi:10.1128/JB.183.12.3770-3783.2001

Paster, B. J., Olsen, I., Aas, J. A., & Dewhirst, F. E. (2006). The breadth of bacterial diversity in the human periodontal pocket and other oral sites. *Periodontology 2000*, *42*, 80–87. doi:10.1111/j.1600-0757.2006.00174.x

Patel, V., Hood, B. L., Molinolo, A. A., Lee, N. H., Conrads, T. P., & Braisted, J. C. (2008). Proteomic analysis of laser-captured paraffin-embedded tissues: a molecular portrait of head and neck cancer progression. *Clinical Cancer Research*, *14*, 1002–1014. doi:10.1158/1078-0432.CCR-07-1497

Payne, B., & Toga, A. (1990). Surface mapping brain function on 3d models. *IEEE Computer Graphics and Applications*, *10*(5), 33–41. doi:10.1109/38.59034

Pecoraro, M., Azadivatan-le, N., Janal, M., & Khocht, A. (2005). Comparison of observer reliability in assessing alveolar bone height on direct digital and conventional radiographs. *Dento Maxillo Facial Radiology*, *34*(5), 279–284. doi:10.1259/dmfr/13900561

Peluso, G., De Santis, M., Inzitari, R., Fanali, C., Cabras, T., & Messana, I. (2007). Proteomic study of salivary peptides and proteins in patients with Sjögren's syndrome before and after pilocarpine treatment. *Arthritis and Rheumatism*, *56*, 2216–2222. doi:10.1002/art.22738

Pepelassi, E. A., & Diamanti-Kipioti, A. (1997). Selection of the most accurate method of conventional radiography for the assessment of periodontal osseous destruction. *Journal of Clinical Periodontology*, *24*(8), 557–567. doi:10.1111/j.1600-051X.1997.tb00229.x

Petersen, P. E. (2003). The World Oral Health Report 2003: continuous improvement of oral health in the 21st century--the approach of the WHO Global Oral Health Programme. *Community Dentistry and Oral Epidemiology*, *31*(Suppl 1), 3–23. doi:10.1046/j..2003.com122.x

Pfeifer, G. M., & Riquier, R. (2006). Outsourcing oder Fertigung? *Die Quintessenz der Zahntechnik*, *32*(12), 1451–1456.

Picinbono, G., Delingette, H., & Ayache, N. (2003). Non-Linear Anisotropic Elasticity for Real-Time Surgery Simulation. *Graphical Models*, *65*(5), 305–321. doi:10.1016/S1524-0703(03)00045-6

Piggott, J. R., & Schaschke, C. J. (2001). Release cells, breath analysis and in-mouth analysis in flavour research. *Biomolecular Engineering*, *17*, 129–136. doi:10.1016/S1389-0344(01)00071-5

Pionnier, E., Chabanet, C., Mioche, L., Le Quéré, J. L., & Salles, C. (2004). 1. In vivo aroma release during eating of a model cheese: relationships with oral parameters. *Journal of Agricultural and Food Chemistry*, *52*, 557–564. doi:10.1021/jf030544v

Pishwa, L., Freesmeyer, W. B., & Blumenrath, B. (2007). Verblendkronen aus CAD/CAM-Laser-gesinterten Gerüsten - eine Anwendungsbeobachtung. *Deutsche Zahnarztliche Zeitschrift*, *62*(7), 470–477.

Preda, L., Di Maggio, E. M., Dore, R., La Fianza, A., Solcia, M., & Schifino, M. R. (1997). Use of spiral computed tomography for multiplanar dental reconstruction. *Dento Maxillo Facial Radiology*, *26*(6), 327–331. doi:10.1038/sj.dmfr.4600290

Priami, C., & Quaglia, P. (2004). Modelling the dynamics of biosystems. *Briefings in Bioinformatics*, *5*(3), 259–269. doi:10.1093/bib/5.3.259

Public Safety Radio Services (2008). *Definition of term "Computer-Telephony Integration"*.

Quirynen, M., Callens, A., van Steenberghe, D., & Nys, M. (1993). Clinical evaluation of a constant force electronic probe. *Journal of Periodontology*, *64*(1), 35–39.

R Development Core Team. (2005). *R: A Language and Environment for Statistical Computing.* Vienna, Austria: R Foundation for Statistical Computing.

Rabe, S., Krings, U., & Berger, R. G. (2004 a). In vitro study of the influence of physiological parameters on dynamic in-mouth flavour release from liquids. *Chemical Senses*, *29*, 153–162. doi:10.1093/chemse/bjh020

Rabe, S., Krings, U., Banavara, D. S., & Berger, R. G. (2002). Computerized apparatus for measuring dynamic flavor release from liquid food matrices. *Journal of Agricultural and Food Chemistry*, *50*, 6440–6447. doi:10.1021/jf020231k

Rabe, S., Linforth, R. S. T., Krings, U., Taylor, A. J., & Berger, R. G. (2004 b). Volatile release from liquids: Comparison of in vivo APCI-MS, in mouth headspace trapping and in vitro Mouth Model Data. *Chemical Senses*, *29*, 263–173.

Rajab, L. D., & Hamdan, M. A. (2002). Supernumerary teeth: review of the literature and a survey of 152 cases. *International Journal of Paediatric Dentistry*, *12*, 244–254. doi:10.1046/j.1365-263X.2002.00366.x

Ralhan, R., Desouza, L. V., Matta, A., Chandra Tripathi, S., Ghanny, S., & Dattagupta, S. (2009). iTRAQ-multidimensional liquid chromatography and tandem mass spectrometry-based identification of potential biomarkers of oral epithelial dysplasia and novel networks between inflammation and premalignancy. *Journal of Proteome Research*, *8*, 300–309. doi:10.1021/pr800501j

Ramadan, A. B., & Mitchell, D. F. (1962). A roentgenographic study of experimental bone desctruction. *Oral Surgery, Oral Medicine, and Oral Pathology*, *15*, 934–943. doi:10.1016/0030-4220(62)90087-7

Ramakers, C., Ruijter, J. M., Lekanne-Deprez, R. H., & Moorman, A. F. M. (2003). Assumption-free analysis of quantitative real-time polymerase chain reaction (PCR) data. *Neuroscience Letters*, *339*, 62–66. doi:10.1016/S0304-3940(02)01423-4

Rams, T. E., Listgarten, M. A., & Slots, J. (1994). Utility of the radiographic crestal lamina dura for predictiong periodontitis disease-activity. *Journal of Clinical Periodontology*, *21*(9), 571–576. doi:10.1111/j.1600-051X.1994.tb00745.x

Rasche, A., Al-Hasani, H., & Herwig, R. (2008). Meta-Analysis Approach identifies Candidate Genes and associated Molecular Networks for Type-2 Diabetes Mellitus. *BMC Genomics*, *9*, 310. doi:. doi:10.1186/1471-2164-9-310

Rasiah, I. A., Wong, L., Anderson, S. A., & Sissons, C. H. (2005). Variation in bacterial DGGE patterns from human saliva: over time, between individuals and in corresponding dental plaque microcosms. *Archives of Oral Biology*, *50*(9), 779–787. doi:10.1016/j.archoralbio.2005.02.001

Raul, J. S., Baumgartner, D., Willinger, R., & Ludes, B. (2006). Finite element modelling of human head injuries caused by a fall. *International Journal of Legal Medicine*, *120*(4), 212–218. doi:10.1007/s00414-005-0018-1

Raul, J. S., Deck, C., Willinger, R., & Ludes, B. (2008). Finite-element models of the human head and their applications in forensic practice. *International Journal of Legal Medicine*, *122*(5), 359–366. doi:10.1007/s00414-008-0248-0

Reiber, T., Fuhr, K., & Hartmann, H. (1989). Recording pattern of occlusal indicators, influence of indicator thickness, pressure, and surface morphology. *Deutsche Zahnarztliche Zeitschrift*, *44*(2), 90–93.

Rekow, D. (1987). Computer-aided design and manufacturing in dentistry: A review of the state of the art. *The Journal of Prosthetic Dentistry*, *58*(4), 512–516. doi:10.1016/0022-3913(87)90285-X

Rekow, E. D. (1991). CAD/CAM in dentistry. *The Alpha Omegan*, *84*(4), 41–44.

Rekow, E. D., & Erdmann, A. G. (1985). Comparison of techniques for aquiring high-precision tree-dimensional computer-based geometric data directly from the human mouth. *Ceramics in Bioengenering*, 139-140.

Rekow, E. D., Erdmann, A. G., & Speidel, T. M. (1985). Computer-Assisted System to Automate Production of Posterior Dental Restorations. *Biostereometrics*, *602*, 204–210.

Ribeiro-Rotta, R. F., Lindh, C., & Rohlin, M. (2007). Efficacy of clinical methods to assess jaw bone tissue prior to and during endosseus dental implant placement: a systematic literature review. *The International Journal of Oral & Maxillofacial Implants*, *22*(2), 289–300.

Richard, H. (1992). Connaissance de la nature des arômes alimentaires. In: Les Arômes Alimentaires. Eds. Richard H., Multon J.L., Tec & Doc, Lavoisier, Paris, 22-40.

Ries, L. A. G., Melbert, D., Krapcho, M., Stinchcomb, D. G., Howlader, N., Horner, M. J., et al. (Eds.). (2008). *SEER Cancer Statistics Review*, 1975-2005, National Cancer Institute. Bethesda, MD, http://seer.cancer.gov/csr/1975_2005/, based on November 2007 SEER data submission, posted to the SEER website.

Rinke, S., Hüls, A., & Chafizadeh, A. (1995). Vergleichende Qualitätsbeurteilung kopiergefräster vollkeramischer Kronen und Brücken (Celay/In-Ceram). *Deutsche Zahnarztliche Zeitschrift*, *50*, 671–673.

Rinke, S., Markgraf, G., Jahn, L., & Hüls, A. (1994). Qualitätsbeurteilung von kopiergefrästen vollkeramischen Kronengerüsten (Celay/In-Ceram). *Schweiz Mschr Zahnmed*, *104*, 1495.

Riquier, R. (2006). Frästechnik versus Lasersintern. *Die Quintessenz der Zahntechnik*, *32*(5), 534–546.

Ritz, H. L. (1967). Microbial population shifts in developing human dental plaque. *Archives of Oral Biology*, *12*(12), 1561–1568. doi:10.1016/0003-9969(67)90190-2

Roberts, D. D., & Acree, T. E. (1995). Simulation of retronasal aroma using a modified headspace technique: investigating the effects of saliva, temperature, shearing and oil on flavour release. *Journal of Agricultural and Food Chemistry*, *43*, 2179–2186. doi:10.1021/jf00056a041

Roberts, D. D., & Acree, T. E. (1996). Effects of heating and cream addition on fresh raspberry aroma using a retronasal aroma simulator and gas chromatography olfactometry. *Journal of Agricultural and Food Chemistry*, *44*, 3919–3925. doi:10.1021/jf950701t

Robinson, W. H., DiGennaro, C., Hueber, W., Haab, B. B., Kamachi, M., & Dean, E. J. (2002). Autoantigen microarrays for multiplex characterization of autoantibody responses. *Nature Medicine*, *8*, 295–301. doi:10.1038/nm0302-295

Rohlin, M., Akesson, L., Hakansson, J., Hakansson, H., & Nasstrom, K. (1989). Comparison between panoramic and periapical radiography in the diagnosis of periodontal bone loss. *Dento Maxillo Facial Radiology*, *18*(2), 72–76.

Ross, P. L., Huang, Y. N., Marchese, J. N., Williamson, B., Parker, K., & Hattan, S. (2004). Multiplexed protein quantitation in saccharomyces cerevisiae using amine-reactive isobaric tagging reagents. *Molecular & Cellular Proteomics*, *3*, 1154–1169. doi:10.1074/mcp.M400129-MCP200

Rudolph, M., Beoeckler, A. F., & Setz, J. M. (2007). Metallkeramikkronen mit lasergeschmolzenem Gerüst: Randspaltmessung und Festigkeitsprüfung - erste Ergebnisse. *Deutsche Zahnarztliche Zeitschrift*, *62*(7), 465–469.

Ruppert, J. (1995). A Delaunay Refinement Algorithm for Quality 2-Dimensional Mesh Generation. *Journal of Algorithms*, *18*(3), 548–585. doi:10.1006/jagm.1995.1021

Ruppin, J., Popovic, A., Strauss, M., Spuntrup, E., Steiner, A., & Stoll, C. (2008). Evaluation of the accuracy of three different computer-aided surgery systems in dental implantology: optical tracking vs. stereolithographic splint systems. *Clinical Oral Implants Research*, *19*(7), 709–716. doi:10.1111/j.1600-0501.2007.01430.x

Rushton, V. E., Horner, K., & Worthington, H. V. (2001). Screening panoramic radiology of adults in general dental practice: radiological findings. *British Dental Journal*, *190*(9), 495–501. doi:10.1038/sj.bdj.4801014a

Rustemeyer, P., Streubuhr, U., & Suttmoeller, J. (2004). Low-dose dental computed tomography: significant dose reduction without loss of image quality. *Acta Radiol*, *45*(8), 847–853. doi:10.1080/02841850410001402

Rychlik, M., & Grosch, W. (1996). Identification and quantification of potent odorants formed by toasting of wheat bread. *Lebensmittel Wisstercraft und Technologie*, *29*, 515–525. doi:10.1006/fstl.1996.0079

Ryu, O. H., Atkinson, J. C., Hoehn, G. T., Illei, G. G., & Hart, T. C. (2006). Identification of parotid salivary biomarkers in Sjogren's syndrome by surface-enhanced laser desorption/ionization time-of-flight mass spectrometry and two-dimensional difference gel electrophoresis. *Rheumatology (Oxford, England)*, *45*, 1077–1086. doi:10.1093/rheumatology/kei212

Saad, M.N., Weiner, Ehrenberg D., et al. (2008). Effects of load and indicator type upon occlusal contact markings. *Journal of Biomedical Materials Research. Part B, Applied Biomaterials*, *85*(1), 18–22. doi:10.1002/jbm.b.30910

Sakr, K., Farag, I. A., & Zeitonum, I. M. (2006). Review of 509 mandibular fractures treated at the University Hospital, Alexandria, Egypt. *The British Journal of Oral & Maxillofacial Surgery*, *44*(2), 107–111. doi:10.1016/j.bjoms.2005.03.014

Salles, C., Tarrega, A., Mielle, P., Maratray, J., Gorria, P., Liaboeuf, J., & Liodenot, J. J. (2007). Development of a chewing simulator for food breakdown and the analysis of in vitro flavor compounds release in a mouth environment. *Journal of Food Engineering*, *82*, 189–198. doi:10.1016/j.jfoodeng.2007.02.008

Saraçoğlu, A., & Ozpinar, B. J. (2002). In vivo and in vitro evaluation of occlusal indicator sensitivity. *The Journal of Prosthetic Dentistry*, *88*(5), 522–526. doi:10.1067/mpr.2002.129064

Saremi, A., Nelson, R. G., Tulloch-Reid, M., Hanson, R. L., & Sievers, M. L. (2005). Periodontal disease and mortality in type 2 diabetes. *Diabetes Care*, *28*, 27–32. doi:10.2337/diacare.28.1.27

Sarment, D. P., Sukovic, P., & Clinthorne, N. (2003). Accuracy of implant placement with a stereolithographic surgical guide. *The International Journal of Oral & Maxillofacial Implants*, *18*(4), 571–577.

Scanlin, H. L., Carroll, E. A., Jenkins, V. K., & Balkowiec, A. (2008). Endomorphin-2 is released from newborn rat primary sensory neurons in a frequency- and calcium-dependent manner. *The European Journal of Neuroscience*, *27*, 2629–2642. doi:10.1111/j.1460-9568.2008.06238.x

Scarfe, W. C., & Farman, A. G. (2008). What is cone-beam CT and how does it work? *Dental Clinics of North America*, *52*, 707–730. doi:10.1016/j.cden.2008.05.005

Schatz, J. P., & Joho, J. P. (1994). Indications of autotransplantation of teeth in orthodontic problem cases. *American Journal of Orthodontics and Dentofacial Orthopedics*, *106*, 351–357. doi:10.1016/S0889-5406(94)70055-9

Scheiner, M. A., & Sampson, W. J. (1997). Supernumerary teeth: a review of the literature and four case reports. *Australian Dental Journal*, *42*, 160–165. doi:10.1111/j.1834-7819.1997.tb00114.x

Schmidt, A., Kellermann, J., & Lottspeich, F. (2005). A novel strategy for quantitative proteomics using isotope-coded protein labels. *Proteomics*, *5*, 4–15. doi:10.1002/pmic.200400873

Schmitt, M., Bravo, I. G., Snijders, P. J. F., Gissmann, L., Pawlita, M., & Waterboer, T. (2006). Bead-based multiplex genotyping of human papillomaviruses. *Journal of Clinical Microbiology*, *44*, 504–512. doi:10.1128/JCM.44.2.504-512.2006

Schnabel, J., Rueckert, D., Quist, M., Blackall, J., Castellano-Smith, A., Hartkens, T., et al. (2001). A Generic Framework for Non-rigid Registration Based on Non-uniform Multi-level Free-Form Deformations. In *MICCAI*, (pp. 573-581).

Schulz, M., Reichart, P. A., Stich, H., Lussi, A., & Bornstein, M. M. (2009). Bilateral malformation of maxillary third molars. *Oral Surgery, Oral Medicine, Oral Pathology, Oral Radiology, and Endodontics*, *108*, e25–e31. doi:10.1016/j.tripleo.2009.04.017

Schulzrinne, H., & Rosenberg, J. (2008). Internet Telephony: Architecture and Protocols an IETF Perspective. *Computer Networks*, *31*, 237–255. doi:10.1016/S0169-7552(98)00265-7

Schwartz, J., Langelier, E., Moisan, C., & Laurendeau, D. (2001). Non-linear Soft Tissue Deformations for the Simulation of Percutaneous Surgeries. In *MICCAI*, (pp. 1271-1272).

Schweiger, J., Erdelt, K.-J., & Beuer, F. (2004). Rapid Prototyping - Technik der Zukunft? *Dent Lab*, *52*(7), 1109–1118.

Seemann, R., Schicho, K., Reichwein, A., Eisenmenger, G., Ewers, R., & Wagner, A. (2007). Clinical evaluation of mechanically optimized plates for the treatment of condylar process-Fractures. *Oral Surgery, Oral Medicine, Oral Pathology, Oral Radiology, and Endodontics*, *104*(6), e1–e4. doi:10.1016/j.tripleo.2007.07.010

Seymour, G. J., Ford, P. J., Cullinan, M. P., Leishman, S., & Yamazaki, K. (2007). Relationship between periodontal infections and systemic disease. *Clinical Microbiology and Infection*, *13*(Suppl 4), 3–10. doi:10.1111/j.1469-0691.2007.01798.x

Shapira, Y., Borell, G., Kuftinec, M. M., Stom, D., & Nahlieli, O. (1996)... *The Journal of the American Dental Association*, *127*, 1075–1078.

Shewchuk, J. (1999). *Lecture notes on Delaunay mesh generation.* Technical Report: Department of Electrical Engineering and Computer Science, University of California, Berkeley.

Shewchuk, J. (2002). What Is a Good Linear Element? Interpolation, Conditioning, and Quality Measures. In *Proceedings of the 11 International Meshing Roundtable*, (pp. 115-126).

Shewchuk, J. (2002a). Delaunay refinement algorithms for triangular mesh generation . *Computational Geometry: Theory and Applications*, *22*(1-3), 21–74.

Shugars, D. C., Watkins, C. A., & Cowen, H. J. (2001). Salivary concentration of secretory leukocyte protease inhibitor, an antimicrobial protein, is decreased with advanced age. *Gerontology*, *47*, 246–253. doi:10.1159/000052808

Slots, J. (2003). Update on general health risk of periodontal disease. *International Dental Journal*, *53*(Suppl 3), 200–207.

Smythe, D. (1990). *A two-pass mesh warping alogrithm for object transformation and image interpolation.* Tech. Report, ILM Computer Graphics Department, Lucasfilm.

Socransky, S. S., Haffajee, A. D., Cugini, M. A., Smith, C., & Kent, R. L. Jr. (1998). Microbial complexes in subgingival plaque. *Journal of Clinical Periodontology, 25*(2), 134–144. doi:10.1111/j.1600-051X.1998.tb02419.x

Socransky, S. S., Smith, C., Martin, L., Paster, B. J., Dewhirst, F. E., & Levin, A. E. (1994). "Checkerboard" DNA-DNA hybridization. *BioTechniques, 17*(4), 788–792.

Song, Y. (2005). PCR-based diagnostics for anaerobic infections. *Anaerobe, 11*, 79–91. doi:10.1016/j.anaerobe.2004.10.006

Sorsa, T. (2006). Matrix metalloproteinases: contribution to pathogenesis, diagnosis and treatment of periodontal inflammation. *Annals of Medicine, 38*, 306–321. doi:10.1080/07853890600800103

Spector, L. (2008). Computer-aided dental implant planning. *Dental Clinics of North America, 52*, 761–775. doi:10.1016/j.cden.2008.05.004

Spisak, S., Tulassay, Z., Molnar, B., & Guttman, A. (2007). Protein microchips in biomedicine and biomarker discovery. *Electrophoresis, 28*, 4261–4373. doi:10.1002/elps.200700539

Springett, M. B., Rozier, V., & Bakker, J. (1999). Use of fiber interface direct mass spectrometry for the determination of volatile flavor release from model food systems. *Journal of Agricultural and Food Chemistry, 47*, 1125–1131. doi:10.1021/jf980199n

Staley, J. T., & Konopka, A. (1985). Measurement of in situ activities of nonphotosynthetic microorganisms in aquatic and terrestrial habitats. *Annual Review of Microbiology, 39*, 321–346. doi:10.1146/annurev.mi.39.100185.001541

Steger, E. (2005). ZirkonZahn für die Grünlingsbearbeitung von Zirkoniumdioxid-Gerüstmaterial. *Die Quintessenz der Zahntechnik, 31*(6), 624–633.

Stock, D. W. (2001). The genetic basis of modularity in the development and evolution of the vertebrate dentition. *Philosophical Transactions of the Royal Society of London. Series B, Biological Sciences, 356*(1414), 1633–1653. doi:10.1098/rstb.2001.0917

Stoltz, C. (2004). Calling for Call Centres - A study of Call Centre Locations in a Swedish Rural Region. *Economic Information Systems, Department of Computer and information Science*. Linköping, Sweden: Linköping University.

Stone, H., & Sidel, J. L. (2004). Introduction to sensory evaluation. In: Sensory evaluation practices. Eds. Stone H. and Sidel J. L., Elsevier Academic Press, 1-16.

Strietzel, R. (2004). Herstellung von metallischen Gerüsten mit Hilfe des BEGO Medifacturing Verfahrens. *Die Quintessenz der Zahntechnik, 30*(4), 406–417.

Strietzel, R. (2005). *Die Werkstoffkunde der Metall-Keramik-Systeme*. München: Verlag Neuer Merkur.

Strietzel, R., & Lahl, C. (2007). *CAD/CAM-Systeme in Labor und Praxis*. München: Verlag Neuer Merkur.

Subramanian, A., Tamayo, P., & Mootha, V. K. (2005). Gene set enrichment analysis: a knowledge-based approach for interpreting genome-wide expression profiles . *Proceedings of the National Academy of Sciences of the United States of America, 102*(43), 15545–15550. doi:10.1073/pnas.0506580102

Sun, Y., Rao, M. S., Zigmond, R. E., & Landis, S. C. (1994). Regulation of vasoactive intestinal peptide expression in sympathetic neurons in culture and after axotomy: the role of cholinergic differentiation factor/leukemia inhibitory factor. *Journal of Neurobiology, 25*, 415–430. doi:10.1002/neu.480250407

Suomi, R., & Serkkola, A. (2007). GSM-based SMS Time Reservation System for Dental Care. *International Journal of Technology and Human Interaction, 3*(3), 54–68.

Suomi, R., & Serkkola, A. (2007). Rescheduling Dental Care with GSM-Based Text Messages. In L. Al-Hakim (Ed.), *Web Mobile-Based Applications for Healthcare Management,* (pp. 335-353).Hershey, PA: IRM Press.

Suttor, D. (2004). Lava zirconia crowns and bridges. *International Journal of Computerized Dentistry*, *7*(1), 67–76.

Suzuki, M. T., & Giovannoni, S. J. (1996). Bias caused by template annealing in the amplification of mixtures of 16S rRNA genes by PCR. *Applied and Environmental Microbiology*, *62*, 625–630.

Suzuki, N., Yoshida, A., & Nakano, Y. (2005). Quantitative analysis of multi-species oral biofilms by TaqMan real-time PCR. *Clinical Medicine & Research*, *3*, 176–185. doi:10.3121/cmr.3.3.176

Swoboda, J. R., Kiyak, H. A., Darveau, R., & Persson, G. R. (2008). Correlates of periodontal decline and biological markers in older adults. *Journal of Periodontology*, *79*(10), 1920–1926. doi:10.1902/jop.2008.080005

Taguchi, A., Asano, A., Ohtsuka, M., Nakamoto, T., Suei, Y., & Tsuda, M. (2008). Observer performance in diagnosing osteoporosis by dental panoramic radiographs: results from the osteoporosis screening project in dentistry (OSPD). *Bone*, *43*(1), 209–213. doi:10.1016/j.bone.2008.03.014

Takada, H., Abe, S., Tamatsu, Y., Mitarashi, S., Saka, H., & Ide, Y. (2006). Three-dimensional bone microstructures of the mandibular angle using micro-CT and finite element analysis: relationship between partially impacted mandibular third molars and angle fractures. *Dental Traumatology*, *22*(1), 18–24. doi:10.1111/j.1600-9657.2006.00368.x

Takeshita, T., Nakano, Y., & Yamashita, Y. (2007). Improved accuracy in terminal restriction fragment length polymorphism phylogenetic analysis using a novel internal size standard definition. *Oral Microbiology and Immunology*, *22*(6), 419–428. doi:10.1111/j.1399-302X.2007.00384.x

Takeshita, T., Nakano, Y., Kumagai, T., Yasui, M., Kamio, N., & Shibata, Y. (2009). The ecological proportion of indigenous bacterial populations in saliva is correlated with oral health status. *The ISME Journal*, *3*(1), 65–78. doi:10.1038/ismej.2008.91

Tanaka, E., & Koolstra, J. H. (2008). Biomechanics of the temporomandibular joint. *Journal of Dental Research*, *87*(11), 989–991. doi:10.1177/154405910808701101

Tanaka, E., Rodrigo, D. P., Tanaka, M., Kawaguchi, A., Shibazaki, T., & Tanne, K. (2001). Stress analysis in the TMJ during jaw opening by use of a three-dimensional finite element model based on magnetic resonance images. *International Journal of Oral and Maxillofacial Surgery*, *30*(5), 421–430. doi:10.1054/ijom.2001.0132

Tanke, H. J. (2007). Genomics and proteomics: the potential role of oral diagnostics. *Annals of the New York Academy of Sciences*, *1098*, 330–334. doi:10.1196/annals.1384.042

Tarnow, D., & Fletcher, P. (1984). Classification of the vertical component of furcation involvement. *Journal of Periodontology*, *55*(5), 283–284.

Tarsa, L., & Balkowiec, A. (2009). Nerve growth factor regulates synaptophysin expression in developing trigeminal ganglion neurons *in vitro*. *Neuropeptides*, *43*, 47–52. doi:10.1016/j.npep.2008.09.009

Taylor, A. J. (1996). Volatile flavor release from foods during eating. *Critical Reviews in Food Science and Nutrition*, *36*, 765–784. doi:10.1080/10408399609527749

Taylor, A. J., & Linforth, R. S. T. (1994). Methodology for measuring volatile profiles in the mouth and nose during eating. In: Trends in Flavour Research. Eds. Maarse H. and van der Heij D. G., Elsevier Science B.V. Amsterdam, 3-14.

Taylor, A. J., Linforth, R. S. T., Harvey, B. A., & Blake, A. (2000). Atmospheric pressure chemical ionisation mass spectrometry for in vivo analysis of volatile flavour release. *Food Chemistry*, *71*, 327–338. doi:10.1016/S0308-8146(00)00182-5

Taylor, G. S. (1972). Characteristics of supernumerary teeth in the primary and permanent dentition. *Dental Practitioner and Dental Record*, *22*, 203–208.

Taylor, P., & Bain, P. (2003). 'An assembly line in the head': work and employee relations in the call centre. *Phil Taylor & Peter Bain*, *30*(2), 101–117.

Thilander, B., & Jakobsson, S. O. (1968). Local factors in impaction of maxillary canines. *Acta Odontologica Scandinavica, 26*, 145–168. doi:10.3109/00016356809004587

Thresher, R. W., & Saito, G. E. (1973). The stress analysis of human teeth. *Journal of Biomechanics, 6*(5), 443–449. doi:10.1016/0021-9290(73)90003-1

Todd, R., Lingen, M. W., & Kuo, W. P. (2002). Gene expression profiling using laser capture microdissection. *Expert Review of Molecular Diagnostics, 2*, 497–507. doi:10.1586/14737159.2.5.497

Tong, H., Chen, W., Merritt, J., Qi, F., Shi, W., & Dong, X. (2007). Streptococcus oligofermentans inhibits Streptococcus mutans through conversion of lactic acid into inhibitory H2O2: a possible counteroffensive strategy for interspecies competition. *Molecular Microbiology, 63*(3), 872–880. doi:10.1111/j.1365-2958.2006.05546.x

Tribble, G. D., Mao, S., James, C. E., & Lamont, R. J. (2006). A *Porphyromonas gingivalis* haloacid dehalogenase family phosphatase interacts with human phosphoproteins and is important for invasion. *Proceedings of the National Academy of Sciences of the United States of America, 103*, 11027–11032. doi:10.1073/pnas.0509813103

Tugnait, A., Clerehugh, V., & Hirschmann, P. N. (2000). The usefulness of radiographs in diagnosis and management of periodontal diseases: a review. *Journal of Dentistry, 28*(4), 219–226. doi:10.1016/S0300-5712(99)00062-7

Tugnait, A., Clerehugh, V., & Hirschmann, P. N. (2004). Use of the basic periodontal examination and radiographs in the assessment of periodontal diseases in general dental practice. *Journal of Dentistry, 32*(1), 17–25. doi:10.1016/S0300-5712(03)00126-X

Turhani, D., Krapfenbauer, K., Thurnher, D., Langen, H., & Fountoulakis, M. (2006). Identification of differentially expressed, tumor-associated proteins in oral squamous cell carcinoma by proteomic analysis. *Electrophoresis, 27*, 1417–1423. doi:10.1002/elps.200500510

Turnbaugh, P. J., Ley, R. E., Hamady, M., Fraser-Ligett, C. M., Knight, R., & Gordon, J. I. (2007). The human microbiome project. *Nature, 449*, 804–809. doi:10.1038/nature06244

Tyndall, D. A., & Rathore, S. (2008). Cone-beam CT diagnoistic applications: caries, periodontal bone assessment, and endodontic applications. *Dental Clinics of North America, 52*, 825–841. doi:10.1016/j.cden.2008.05.002

Van de Brule, A. J., Pol, R., Fransen-Daalmeijer, N., Schouls, L. M., Meijer, C. J., & Snijders, P. J. (2002). GP5+/6+ PCR followed by reverse line blot analysis enables rapid and high-throughput identification of human papillomavirus genotypes. *Journal of Clinical Microbiology, 40*, 779–787. doi:10.1128/JCM.40.3.779-787.2002

Van Ham, M. A., Bakkers, J. M., Harbers, G. K., Quint, W. G., Massuger, L. F., & Melchers, W. J. (2005). Comparison of two commercial assays for detection of human papillomavirus (HPV) in cervical scrape specimens: validation of the Roche AMPLICOR HPV test as a means to screen for HPV genotypes associated with a higher risk of cervical disorders. *Journal of Clinical Microbiology, 43*, 2662–2667. doi:10.1128/JCM.43.6.2662-2667.2005

van Ruth, S. M., & Buhr, K. (2004). Influence of mastication rate on dynamic flavour release analysed by combined model mouth/proton transfer reaction–mass spectrometry. *International Journal of Mass Spectrometry, 239*, 187–192. doi:10.1016/j.ijms.2004.08.009

van Ruth, S. M., & Roozen, J. P. (2000 a). Gas chromatography / sniffing port analysis of aroma compounds released under mouth conditions. *Talanta, 52*, 253–259. doi:10.1016/S0039-9140(00)00325-8

van Ruth, S. M., & Roozen, J. P. (2000 b). Influence of mastication, saliva on aroma release in a model mouth system. *Food Chemistry, 71*, 339–345. doi:10.1016/S0308-8146(00)00186-2

van Ruth, S. M., Roozen, J. P., & Cozijnsen, J. L. (1994). Comparison of dynamic headspace mouth model systems for flavour release from rehydrated bell pepper cuttings. In: Trends in Flavour Research. Eds. Maarse H. and van der Heij D. G., Elsevier Science B.V. Amsterdam, 59-64.

van Ruth, S. M., Roozen, J. P., & Cozijnsen, J. L. (1995 a). Changes in flavour release from rehydrated diced bell peppers (*Capsicum annuum*) by artificial saliva components in three model mouth systems. *Journal of the Science of Food and Agriculture, 37*, 189–196. doi:10.1002/jsfa.2740670208

van Ruth, S. M., Roozen, J. P., & Cozijnsen, J. L. (1995 b). Volatile compounds of rehydrated French beans, bell peppers and leeks. Part 1. Flavour release in the mouth and in three mouth model systems. *Food Chemistry, 53*, 15–22. doi:10.1016/0308-8146(95)95780-A

Vandenberghe, B., Hassan, B., Armellini, D., Maes, F., & Jacobs, R. (2009, July). Volumetric quantification of bone loss for determination of bone grafting accuracy: a pilot study. *Programme and abstract book of the 17th International Congress of Dentomaxillofacial Radiology 2009*, (p. 59).

Vandenberghe, B., Jacobs, R., & Yang, J. (2007). Diagnostic validity (or acuity) of 2D CCD versus 3D CBCT-images for assessing periodontal breakdown. *Oral Surgery, Oral Medicine, Oral Pathology, Oral Radiology, and Endodontics, 104*(3), 395–401. doi:10.1016/j.tripleo.2007.03.012

Vandenberghe, B., Jacobs, R., & Yang, J. (2007). Topographic assessment of periodontal craters and furcation involvements by using 2D digital images versus 3D cone beam CT: an in-vitro study. *The Chinese Journal of Dental Research, 10*(1), 21–29.

Vandenberghe, B., Jacobs, R., & Yang, J. (2008). Detection of periodontal bone loss using digital intra-oral and CBCT images: an in-vitro assessment of bony and/or infrabony defects. *Dento Maxillo Facial Radiology, 37*(5), 252–260. doi:10.1259/dmfr/57711133

Velasco, F., Torres, J., Leon, A., & Soler, F. (2007). Adaptive cube tessellation for topologically correct isosurfaces. In *Proceeding of the computer graphics theory and applications*, (pp. 220-227).

Vianna, M. E., Holtgraeve, S., Seyfarth, I., Conrads, G., & Horz, H.-P. (2008). Quantitative analysis of three hydrogenotrophic microbial groups - methanogenic archaea, sulfate-reducing bacteria, and acetogenic bacteria - within plaque biofilms associated with human periodontal disease. *Journal of Bacteriology, 190*, 3779–3785. doi:10.1128/JB.01861-07

Vianna, M. E., Horz, H.-P., Gomes, B. P., & Conrads, G. (2006). *In vivo* evaluation of microbial reduction after chemo-mechanical preparation of human root canals containing necrotic pulp tissue. *International Endodontic Journal, 39*, 484–492. doi:10.1111/j.1365-2591.2006.01121.x

Völkl, L. (2001). cercon - das CAM-Vollkeramiksystem von Degussa Dental. *Die Quintessenz, 52*(8), 811–814.

von Wintzingerode, F., Goebel, U. B., & Stackebrandt, E. (1997). Determination of microbial diversity in environmental samples: pitfalls of PCR-based rRNA analysis. *FEMS Microbiology Reviews, 21*, 213–229. doi:10.1111/j.1574-6976.1997.tb00351.x

Voo, L., Kumaresan, S., Pintar, F. A., Yoganandan, N., & Sances, A. (1996). Finite-element models of the human head. *Medical & Biological Engineering & Computing, 34*(5), 375–381. doi:10.1007/BF02520009

Wagner, A., Krach, W., Schicho, K., Urdt, S., Ploder, O., & Ewers, R. (2002). A 3-dimensional finite-element analysis investigating the biomechanical behavior of the mandible and plate osteosynthesis in cases of fractures of the condylar process. *Oral Surgery, Oral Medicine, Oral Pathology, Oral Radiology, and Endodontics, 94*(6), 678–686. doi:10.1067/moe.2002.126451

Wallace, J., Woda, B. A., & Pihan, G. (2005). Facile, comprehensive, high-throughput genotyping of human genital papillomaviruses using spectrally addressable liquid bead microarrays. *The Journal of Molecular Diagnostics, 7*, 72–80.

Walter, C., Kaner, D., Berndt, D. C., Weiger, R., & Zitzmann, N. U. (2009). Three-dimensional imaging as a pre-operative tool in decision making for furcation surgery. *Journal of Clinical Periodontology, 36*(3), 250–257. doi:10.1111/j.1600-051X.2008.01367.x

Wang, W., Zhou, H., Lin, H., Roy, S., Shaler, T. A., & Hill, L. R. (2003). Quantification of proteins and metabolites by mass spectrometry without isotopic labeling or spiked standards. *Analytical Chemistry, 75*, 4818–4826. doi:10.1021/ac026468x

Wang, Z., Jiang, L., Huang, C., Li, Z., Chen, L., & Gou, L. (2008). Comparative proteomics approach to screening of potential diagnostic and therapeutic targets for oral squamous cell carcinoma. *Molecular & Cellular Proteomics, 7*, 1639–1650. doi:10.1074/mcp.M700520-MCP200

Washburn, M. P., Wolters, D., & Yates, J. R. III. (2001). Large-scale analysis of the yeast proteome by multidimensional protein identification technology. *Nature Biotechnology, 19*, 242–247. doi:10.1038/85686

Webber, R. L., Horton, R. A., Tyndall, D. A., & Ludlow, J. B. (1997). Tuned-aperture computed tomography (TACT). Theory and application for three-dimensional dento-alveolar imaging. *Dento Maxillo Facial Radiology, 26*(1), 53–62. doi:10.1038/sj.dmfr.4600201

Weel, K. G. C., Boelrijk, A. E. M., Burger, J. J., Verschueren, M., Gruppen, H., Voragen, A. G. J., & Smit, G. (2004). New Device To Simulate Swallowing and in Vivo Aroma Release in the Throat from Liquid and Semiliquid Food Systems. *Journal of the Science of Food and Agriculture, 52*, 6564–6571. doi:10.1021/jf049499x

Weisburg, W. G., Barns, S. M., Pelletier, D. A., & Lane, D. J. (1991). 16S ribosomal DNA amplification for phylogenetic study. *Journal of Bacteriology, 173*, 697–703.

Weng, L. P., Wu, C. C., Hsu, B. L., Chi, L. M., Liang, Y., & Tseng, C. P. (2008). Secretome-based identification of Mac-2 binding protein as a potential oral cancer marker involved in cell growth and motility. *Journal of Proteome Research, 7*, 3765–3775. doi:10.1021/pr800042n

Wenzel, A., Haiter-Neto, F., & Gotfredsen, E. (2007). Influence of spatial resolution and bit depth on detection of small caries lesions with digital receptors. *Oral Surgery, Oral Medicine, Oral Pathology, Oral Radiology, and Endodontics, 103*(3), 418–422. doi:10.1016/j.tripleo.2006.05.016

Whim, M. D., & Lloyd, P. E. (1994). Differential regulation of the release of the same peptide transmitters from individual identified motor neurons in culture. *The Journal of Neuroscience, 14*, 4244–4251.

White, S. C., & Pharoah, M. J. (2008). The evolution and application of dental maxillofacial imaging modalities. *Dental Clinics of North America, 52*, 689–705. doi:10.1016/j.cden.2008.05.006

Widmann, G., & Bale, R. J. (2006). Accuracy in computer-aided implant surgery--a review. *The International Journal of Oral & Maxillofacial Implants, 21*(2), 305–313.

Witkowski, S. (2001). Digitale Workstation und Wachs-Drucker in der dentalen Gußtechnik. *Zahntech Mag, 5*, 244–247.

Wittwer, C. T., Herrmann, M. G., Moss, A. A., & Rasmussen, R. P. (1997). Continuous fluorescence monitoring for rapid cycle DNA amplification. *BioTechniques, 22*, 130–138.

Wolberg, G. (1998). Image morphing: a surrey. *The Visual Computer, 14*(8-9), 360–372. doi:10.1007/s003710050148

Wolf, B., von Bethlenfalvy, E., Hassfeld, S., Staehle, H. J., & Eickholz, P. (2001). Reliability of assessing interproximal bone loss by digital radiography: infrabony defects. *Journal of Clinical Periodontology, 28*(9), 869–878. doi:10.1034/j.1600-051x.2001.028009869.x

Wolf-Yadlin, A., Hautaniemi, S., Lauffenburger, D. A., & White, F. M. (2007). Multiple reaction monitoring for robust quantitative proteomic analysis of cellular signaling networks. *Proceedings of the National Academy of Sciences of the United States of America, 104*, 5860–5865. doi:10.1073/pnas.0608638104

Wolters, D. A., Washburn, M. P., & Yates, J. R. III. (2001). An automated multidimensional protein identification technology for shotgun proteomics. *Analytical Chemistry*, *73*, 5683–5690. doi:10.1021/ac010617e

World Health Organization (WHO). (2005). *Report of the Consultation on human papillomavirus vaccines*. Geneva, April.

Xie, H., Onsongo, G., Popko, J., de Jong, E. P., Cao, J., & Carlis, J. V. (2008). Proteomics analysis of cells in whole saliva from oral cancer patients via value-added three-dimensional peptide fractionation and tandem mass spectrometry. *Molecular & Cellular Proteomics*, *7*, 486–498. doi:10.1074/mcp.M700146-MCP200

Xie, H., Rhodus, N. L., Griffin, R. J., Carlis, J. V., & Griffin, T. J. (2005). A catalogue of human saliva proteins identified by free flow electrophoresis-based peptide separation and tandem mass spectrometry. *Molecular & Cellular Proteomics*, *4*, 1826–1830. doi:10.1074/mcp.D500008-MCP200

Xie, Q., Ainamo, A., & Tilvis, R. (1997). Association of residual ridge resorption with systemic factors in home-living elderly subjects. *Acta Odontologica Scandinavica*, *55*(5), 299–305. doi:10.3109/00016359709114968

Yarberry, W. A., Jr. (2000). *Computer Telephony Integration*. Boca Raton, FL: CRC Press LLC.

Yates, J. R., Speicher, S., Griffin, P. R., & Hunkapiller, T. (1993). Peptide mass maps: a highly informative approach to protein identification. *Analytical Biochemistry*, *214*, 397–408. doi:10.1006/abio.1993.1514

Yettram, A. L., Wright, K. W., & Pickard, H. M. (1976). Finite Element Stress Analysis of the crowns of normal and restored teeth. *Journal of Dental Research*, *55*(6), 1004–1011.

You, L. (2004). Toward computational systems biology. *Cell Biochemistry and Biophysics*, *40*(2), 167–184. doi:10.1385/CBB:40:2:167

Zhang, H., & Zhao, G. (2007). Adaptive hexahedral mesh generation based on local domain curvature and thickness using a modified grid-based method. *Finite Elements in Analysis and Design*, *43*(9), 691–704. doi:10.1016/j.finel.2007.03.001

Zhang, L., Jiang, J., Arellano, M., Zhang, L., Yan, X., & Wong, D. T. (2008). Quantification of serum proteins of metastatic oral cancer patients using LC-MS/MS and iTRAQ labeling. *The Open Proteomics Journal*, *1*, 72–78. doi:10.2174/1875039700801010072

Zhang, Y., & Bajaj, C. (2006). Adaptive and Quality Quadrilateral/Hexahedral Meshing from Volumetric Data. *Computer Methods in Applied Mechanics and Engineering*, *195*(9-12), 942–960. doi:10.1016/j.cma.2005.02.016

Zhou, X., Zhao, Z., Zhao, M., & Fan, Y. (1999). The boundary design of mandibular model by means of the three-dimensional finite element method. *West China J Stomatol*, *17*(4), 1–16.

Ziegler, C. M., Woertche, R., Brief, J., & Hassfeld, S. (2002). Clinical indications for digital volume tomography in oral and maxillofacial surgery. *Dento Maxillo Facial Radiology*, *31*(2), 126–130. doi:10.1038/sj.dmfr.4600680

Zulqarnain, B. J., & Almas, K. (1998). Effect of x-ray beam vertical angulation on radiographic assessment of alveolar crest level. *Indian Journal of Dental Research*, *9*(4), 132–138.

Zuo, X., Lee, K., Ali-Khan, N., & Speicher, D. W. (2005). Protein profiling by microscale solution isoelectrofocusing (MicroSol-IEF). *Current Protocol in Protein Science*, Chapter 22, Unit 22.6.

About the Contributors

Andriani Daskalaki is a dentist and bioinformatician. She presently works in the field of molecular medicine and bioinformatics at the Max Planck Institute for Molecular Genetics in Berlin. She completed her PhD in 2002 on working in the applications of photodynamic therapy in the area of oral medicine from the Free University of Berlin. She received a two-year DAAD scholarship for her research in the field of PDT. Dr. Daskalaki received a MS in Medical Informatics from TFH Berlin with her work in "Development of a documentation software for robot-assisted intraoral operations" and a MS degree in bioinformatics with her work in "Variance analysis of multifactor models in gene expression experiments with application to the identification of genetic markers for hypertension." She received a poster prize for her participation in the International Photodynamic Association Meeting in Nantes. She is the editor of the "Handbook of Research on Systems Biology Applications in Medicine" and has presented many oral presentations at national and international meetings. She is a founding member and committee member of the Greek Dental Laser Association. Her research interest areas include systems biology, PDT, and laser applications in dentistry.

* * *

Gaëlle Arvisenet is assistant professor in Food Aroma Research group, in ENITIAA, an Engineer School in Nantes (France). Her research topics concern the release and perception of food aroma. She uses both instrumental techniques and sensory analyses to better understand the influence of food matrix and food texture on aroma perception. She has studied model matrices as well as several food products. She has been participating to regional and European projects. She is currently the author (or co-author) of 13 papers in international journals and book chapters and 10 scientific communications or lectures in conferences.

Agnieszka Balkowiec is an Assistant Professor of Integrative Biosciences at the Oregon Health & Science University School of Dentistry in Portland, Oregon, USA. A major focus of Dr. Balkowiec's laboratory is the role of neuronal growth factors in development and plasticity of sensory synapses, with the current emphasis on activity-dependent regulation of neurotrophin expression and release. After graduating with M.D. and Ph.D. degrees from the Medical University of Warsaw, she moved in 1997 to Case Western Reserve University, Cleveland, Ohio, to the laboratory of Dr. David Katz, Ph.D. This is where she invented ELISA in situ for quantification of endogenous neurotrophins released from neurons by physiological patterns of electrical field stimulation. Since then, these techniques got advanced in her laboratory, and are now employed to examine the role of neuronal activity patterns in regulation of neurotrophin genes in trigeminal and other sensory neurons. She has served as principal investigator on grants from the National Institutes of Health, American Heart Association, Medical Research Foundation of Oregon, and co-investigator or research sponsor of several other projects funded by the March of Dimes, American Association for Dental Research, American Association of Endodontists, etc.

Ewa Balkowiec-Iskra received her M.D. and Ph.D. degrees from the Medical University of Warsaw, Poland. As an undergraduate student, she followed her instincts and worked in the field of immunology on anti-cancer therapies of melanoma malignum. Owing to this experience, she crystallized her research focus and joined the Department of Experimental and Clinical Pharmacology to study the influence of the nigro-striatal dopaminergic system injury on the experimental autoimmune encephalomyelitis, the project that became her Ph.D. thesis. After graduation in 2004, she joined the faculty of the Department of Experimental and Clinical Pharmacology, where she currently holds the position of Associate Professor. Her current research focuses on the role of inflammation in neurodegenerative diseases and the influence of neurotransmitters on autoimmune reaction in the central nervous system. In 2007, she began a 5-year residency program in the 2nd Department of Neurology, Institute of Psychiatry and Neurology in Warsaw. She also serves as a national consultant for the drug administration of the Office for Registration of Medicinal Products, Medical Devices and Biocidal Products.

Michael Bornstein studied dental medicine at the University of Basel, where he obtained his dental degree (1998) and thesis (Dr. med. dent., 2001). He received his postgraduate training in oral surgery at the Universities of Basel and Bern, and is a board-certified oral surgeon since 2003. In 2004, he was a visiting assistant professor at the Department of Periodontics at the University of Texas Health Science Center at San Antonio, USA, with a grant from the Swiss National Research Foundation. In 2007 he was appointed head of the Section of Dental Radiology and Stomatology at the Department of Oral Surgery and Stomatology, University of Bern. His main fields of research are guided bone regenerative (GBR) procedures with bioresorbable membranes and dental implants, and stomatology/oral medicine.

Amit Chattopadhyay recently joined the National Institute of Dental and Craniofacial Research, Office of Science Policy and Analysis at the National Institutes of Health in Bethesda, Maryland. His varied duties will include serving as oral epidemiologist, faculty to the dental public health residency program, and representative to the national Healthy People initiative. Dr. Chattopadhyay earned a dental degree with honors (Calcutta University, India); master's degrees in: Oral Pathology (Gujarat University, India) and Public Health – Epidemiology (Oklahoma University); and a residency training certificate in Dental Public Health (SUNY, Albany & New York State Department of Health). He is board certified by the American National Board of Public Health Examiners and by the American Board of Dental Public Health; and is a Fellow of the Faculty of Public Health of the Royal College of Physicians (London, UK). Dr. Chattopadhyay also earned a PhD in Epidemiology from the University of North Carolina at Chapel Hill with National Research Service Award funding, serving as an adjunct Assistant Professor in the Department of Dental Ecology in the School of Dentistry. He has also earned a diploma in journalism and a doctorate certificate in Family Medicine from India, and graduate certificates in international development and in public health outcomes from the University of North Carolina at Chapel Hill and a diploma in Global ethics from the University of Joensuu, Finland. At various times, he has taught Epidemiology, Oral Epidemiology, Public Health Biology, Research Methods and Dental Public Health at Universities of Kentucky; North Carolina; and Temple University. He is the author of chapters in several text books and was Guest Editor of the first-ever issue on Dental Public Health published in

Dental Clinics of North America. He has been an invited speaker in several meetings and conferences around the world. He serves on the Ethics Committee of the American Association for Dental Research, the Editorial Committee of the Journal of Dental Research and several other international dental and medical journals.

Vasiliki Chini is a molecular biologist with a degree from the Department of Biology, School of Science, University of Athens, obtained in 2002 and a PhD in molecular microbiology, achieved from the School of Medicine of the University of Patras, in 2007. She has long experience in molecular and microbiological techniques as she did research on the staphylococcal infections in hospitals and in community, studying the mechanisms of pathogenesis, of toxicity and of the resistance in antimicrobial agents in the Microbiology Department, School of Medicine, University of Patras, Greece from 2003 to 2007. She did a part of her PhD in the Centre National References des Staphylocoques, in Lyon, France, where she specialized in the bacterial molecular typing with sequencing. She also worked in the Virology Laboratory of the University of Patras. She worked for two years in Geno-Type Biotechnology, a private molecular diagnostic laboratory in Athens. Currently, she holds the position of the Head of Diagnostic Laboratory, in Shafallah Medical Genetics Center in Doha, Qatar, doing molecular diagnostic testing, as well as, research on inherited genetic disorders in children.

Georg Conrads (PhD) is Head of the Division of Oral Microbiology and Immunology at the Medical Faculty of the RWTH Aachen University, Aachen, Germany. He has been involved in research on the oral flora since 1992. In 1995, as postdoctoral fellow at the Eastman Dental Institute in London, he investigated the diversity of endodontopathic bacteria using molecular methods. After finishing his professorial thesis he spend 2000-2002 at the R.M. Alden Research Laboratory (Santa Monica, CA) with Ellie Goldstein and Diane Citron studying the taxonomy of anaerobes such as Fusobacterium and Porphyromonas as well as antimicrobial drugs for therapy in anaerobic infections. His main research interests are principals & methods for diagnosing infectious diseases in general and oral and odontogenic infections in particular (caries, periodontitis, actinomycosis, peri-implantitis) as well as oral probiotics and other new strategies for prevention & therapy of oral disorders. A new and promising subject under investigation is whole genome expression profiling of Streptococcus mutans with the ultimate goal for tracking highly active biofilm inhibitors.

Timo Dreiseidler received his medical as well as his dental education at the University of Bonn, Germany where he graduated in 2003 and 2007 respectively. In 2005 he obtained the Doctor of Human Medicine and in 2008 the Doctor of Dental Medicine. During the study of dentistry in the years from 2004-2007 he also worked as a research associate in the field of Cone-Beam technology at the CEASR research center in Bonn. Since 2007 Dr. Dr. Timo Dreiseidler works as assistant doctor at the Clinic for Cranio-Maxillofacial- and Plastic-Surgery, University to Cologne, Germany. He is frequent lecturer on international congresses on computer aided dentistry, craniomaxillo-facial surgers and implantology as well as author and co-author of some scientific papers and the book "Cone-beam Volumetric Imaging in Dental, Oral and Maxillofacial Medicine."

Nancy Hitschfeld received her BS and MS degrees in Computer Science from the University of Chile in 1984 and 1987, respectively, and the PhD degree in Technischen Wissenschaften from the Swiss Federal Institute of technology Zurich (ETH) in 1993. Currently, she is associate professor at the

Computer Science Department of the Engineering Faculty, University of Chile. Topics of her research include geometric modeling, 2- and 3-dimensional mesh generation, and object oriented design and programming.

Hans-Peter Horz completed his PhD in 2001 on studying the diversity of bacterial populations involved in the carbon and nitrogen cycles at the Max-Planck-Institute for Terrestrial Microbiology, Marburg. As postdoctoral fellow he investigated the impact of climate change on soil microorganisms at the Department of Biological Sciences, Stanford University, California from 2001 to 2003. Since then Hans-Peter Horz has been working at the Medical Faculty of the RWTH Aachen University, Aachen. At the Division of Oral Microbiology and Immunology his research is dedicated to the microbial ecology in human health and disease using the oral cavity as a model system. He is furthermore involved in the (time-critical) diagnosis of human infections at the Medical Faculty of the RWTH Aachen and develops molecular strategies for detection of uncultivable microorganisms in clinical samples. The completion of the Habilitation procedure is scheduled for April 2009.

Shen Hu received his Ph.D. in Bioanalytical Chemistry from Wuhan University, China, in 1996. Shortly after his graduation, he joined the College of Chemistry at the same university as Assistant Professor and, in 1998, he was promoted to Associate Professor. In 2004, Dr. Hu joined UCLA School of Dentistry as a Research Assistant Professor and, in 2008, he was elected tenure track Assistant Professor. Dr. Hu has published more than 65 scientific papers. His research interests and areas of expertise include head and neck cancer, Sjogren's syndrome, proteomics, salivary diagnostics and disease biomarker discovery.

Marios Kambouris is certified by the American Board of Medical Genetics in Clinical Molecular Genetics He finished his Ph.D in Medical & Molecular Genetics, at the Indiana University School of Medicine (USA). He served as an assistant Professor Adjunct, in the Department of Genetics, Yale University School of Medicine. He is Consultant for Biotechnology Services, in Zenican Consulting Limited, Cyprus. He established the GenoMed Biotechnology and Geno-Type Biotechnology in Greece both offering Predictive Genomics and DNA Diagnostic Services. He has an expertise in Clinical Genetics in diagnosing, and managing patients with genetic disorders, congenital malformations, dysmorphia andmental retardation, skeletal dysplasias growth abnormalities, and neurogenetic disorders at Henry Ford Hospital, Children's Hospital of Michigan and Riley Hospital for Children. He established and directed the Molecular Genetics & DNA Diagnostics laboratory at King Faisal Hospital & Research Center for eight years with extensive experience establishing, performing & interpreting DNA diagnostic testing, assessing and signing clinical and prenatal cases for hereditary diseases.

Christos Katsaros is Professor and Chair at the Department of Orthodontics and Dentofacial Orthopedics, University of Bern, Switzerland. He obtained his dental degree from the University of Thessaloniki, Greece, and he received his orthodontic training at the University of Saarland, Germany, where he also completed a Dr. med. dent. degree and a Ph.D. ("Habilitation"). Professor Katsaros worked also as a researcher at the Göteborg University, Sweden, where he completed a second Ph.D. ("Odont. Dr."). From 2002 to 2008 he served as a Professor of Orthodontics at the Department of Orthodontics and Oral Biology, Radboud University Nijmegen Medical Centre, Nijmegen, The Netherlands. His main research interests are craniofacial growth and cleft lip and palate. Since 2007 he serves as a Section

Editor Dentistry for the Cleft Palate Craniofacial Journal and he is a reviewer for several international scientific journals.

Robert B. Kerstein received his DMD degree in 1983, and his Prosthodontic Certificate in 1985, both from Tufts University School of Dental Medicine. From 1985 - 1998, he maintained an active appointment at Tufts as a clinical professor teaching fixed and removable Prosthodontics in the department of Restorative Dentistry, During those years Dr. Kerstein intensively studied computerized occlusal analysis where his research focused on the role that Occlusion and lengthy Disclusion Time plays in the etiology of Chronic Myofascial Pain Dysfunction Syndrome. Dr Kerstein's now 25 years of research with the T- Scan I -III Computerized Occlusal Analysis System, has led to his becoming the leading author and clinician in the field of Computerized Occlusal analysis. His findings have been published in the Journal of Prosthetic Dentistry, Practical Periodontics and Aesthetic Dentistry, Compendium for Continuing Education, Journal of Craniomandibular Practice, Quintessence International, General Dentistry, and Contemporary Esthetics. Additionally, he has lectured nationally and internationally regarding Prosthetic Dentistry, Anterior Guidance, Computerized Occlusal Analysis, and Disclusion Time Reduction. Dr. Kerstein maintains a successful private practice that is limited to Prosthodontics and Myofascial Pain Dysfunction in Boston, Massachusetts.

Panagiotis E. Lagouvardos graduated in 1974 from the dental school of Athens, and received his Doctor degree from the same school in 1985. Is an Associate Professor in Operative Dentistry at the dental school of the University of Athens, director of the preclinical education for undergraduate students in Operative Dentistry, and course director in Dental Informatics for dental students. Is the author of a book in "Dental Informatics", the editor in chief of the "Hellenic Dental Journal" and advisor to the Hellenic Dental Association in issues related to Dental Informatics.

Claudio Lobos was born in Antofagasta Chile. He followed his studies of computer engineering and master degree at the University of Chile. He is currently finishing his PhD at Joseph Fourier University at Grenoble France.

Markku Mikkonen, Lic. Dent., Specialist in Clinical Dentistry, is working as a Chief Dentist in the Social and Health Affairs department in the City of Lahti, Finland. Markku Mikkonen has been responsible for the development of GSM mobile phone appointment reservation in the City of Lahti, in cooperation with Quicklic Finland Oy. Mr Mikkonen is active in the Finnish Assocation for Dentists in Health Center. In addition, he gives specialized dentist training at the University of Helsinki.

Olivia Nackaerts obtained her Master's degree in Speech Therapy and Audiology Sciences in 2000. She obtained a postgraduate degree in Media and Information Sciences in 2001. At the Department of Periodontology, K.U.Leuven, she assisted in the organization of the "11th European Association for Osseointegration Congress" until 2003. From 2003, she started working at the Oral Imaging Center, K.U.Leuven. She was involved in the Osteodent project in the 5th European Commission Framework Programme. During 2007, she was working at Speech Therapy and Audiology, division Teaching Methodology and Practicals, while continuing her research at the Oral Imaging Center. In April 2009 she obtained her PhD degree in Medical Sciences. At present, she is involved in another European project co-ordinated by the University of Manchester, under the 7th Framework (Euratom), SedentexCT.

Yohan Payan received the Ph.D. degree in computer science and signal processing, from the Institut National Polytechnique of Grenoble, Grenoble, France, in 1996. Currently, he is researcher at the French National Research Institute (CNRS), La Tronche, France, in the TIMC laboratory, with interests that include biomechanics, computer-assisted surgery, signal processing, and neurosciences.

Pawel Pazera studied physics at the University of Neuchâtel, Switzerland and worked as a medical physicist. In 2003 he obtained a dental degree from the University of Bern, Switzerland, where he also completed a Dr. med. dent. degree and his postgraduate training in prosthodontics. Dr. Pazera obtained also a Master of Science degree in oral implantology at the Steinbeis University in Berlin. Since 2007 he follows the postgraduate program in orthodontics at the Department of Orthodontics and Dentofacial Orthopedics, University of Bern. His main research interests are in 3D-imaging.

Pauline Poinot is a food engineer who has continued her studies by a PhD in the Food Aroma Research Laboratory in ENITIAA. She works on a European Project (EU-Freshbake (Food-2006-36302)), in which she studies the impact of the formulation and the process on the aroma of bread. She has participated in the development of the "Munch-o-matic" by studying the mastication process on apples and the aroma profile of breads.

Carole Prost, Ph.D, is a senior lecturer and the leader of Food Aroma Research group. She has been working for 15 years in the research field of identification of food aroma quality markers, their pathway from precursors and safety, olfactometry analysis of numerous food products, influence of the mix of volatiles molecules on the odorous perception and aroma/food matrix interactions. She has participated in a number of international research projects in the area of "Food Quality and Safety". Supervisor for several Ph.D. students, she has a long experience in collaborating with the industry specialized in cereal baking, extrusion, smoking and aromatic valorisation and marine by-product processing.

Axel Rasche studied mathematics at the ETH Zurich and the Humboldt-University in Berlin. He is currently PhD student at the Max-Planck-Institute for Molecular Genetics in Berlin-Dahlem. His research topics are preprocessing of Affymetrix GeneChip arrays, statistical analysis of alternative splicing and data integration with a focus on type 2 diabetes mellitus.

Ari Serkkola (Doctor of Public Health, Licentiate of Social Sciences) works as a senior researcher at the Helsinki University of Technology Lahti Center. Mr Serkkola specializes in the multidisciplinary study of welfare services and related technology as well as electronic client communications. Ari Serkkola has written about 75 articles on subjects including electronic client communications in health care; development of processes; health anthropology; and innovation research. He also has many years' experience in development of health care services and of social and health programmes. He is a docent of health care information systems at Turku School of Economics.

Roland Strietzel was born in 21.10.1959 in Ottawa/Canada. Since 1.10.1997 he is the head of R & D dental alloys BEGO Bremer Goldschlägerei Wilhelm Herbst GmbH & Co. Dr. R Roland Strietzel received his bachelor of science in chemistry at Free University Berlin/Germany. The theme of his doctor thesis was "Determination of corrosion rates of dental alloys in artificial saliva". From 1.10.1987 until 31.6.1988 he has worked in the research program "Vi 33/7-2 artificial saliva for dental alloys" of the Deutsche Forschungsgemeinschaft. From 1.10.1988 to 30.9.1997 he has worked in the department of dental materials (Prof. Dr. J. Viohl) at the Free University Berlin/Germany. The private lecturer Dr. R Roland Strietzel received his postdoctoral lecture qualification (27.11.1998) in dental materials at Free University Berlin.

Reima Suomi is a professor of Information Systems Science at Turku School of Economics and Business Administration, Finland since 1994. He is a docent for the universities of Turku and Oulu, Finland. Years 1992-93 he spent as a "Vollamtlicher Dozent" in the University of St. Gallen, Switzerland, where he led a research project on business process re-engineering. Currently he concentrates on topics around management of telecommunications, including issues such as management of networks, electronic and mobile commerce, virtual organizations, telework and competitive advantage through telecommunication-based information systems. Different governance structures applied to the management of IS and are enabled by IS belong too to his research agenda, as well as application of information systems in health care. Reima Suomi has together over 300 publications, and has published in journals such as Information & Management, Information Services & Use, Technology Analysis & Strategic Management, The Journal of Strategic Information Systems, Behaviour & Information Technology, Journal of Management History and Information Resources Management Journal. For the academic year 2001-2002 he was a senior researcher "varttunut tutkija" for the academy of Finland. With Paul Jackson he has published the book "Virtual Organization and workplace development with Routhledge, London.

Toru Takeshita is an assistant professor of Department of Preventive Dentistry in Kyushu University Facutlty of Dental Science. He received his PhD degree in Dentistry from Kyushu University in 2009. The subject of his thesis is the study on the relationship between ecological proportions of indigenous bacterial populations in saliva and oral health. His current research focus is on the use of multivariate analysis of microbial community data in exploring specific pattern of oral microflora in relation to oral and systemic health or disease.

Bart Vandenberghe is dentist, master in medical imaging and PhD candidate at the University of Leuven. His doctoral research focuses on digitalization of 2D and 3D imaging modalities, and their influence on periodontal diagnosis. He has spent three years in the United States of America as research scholar at Temple University in Philadelphia (2005-2006) and at Tufts University in Boston (2007), to continue his academic research training. Shortly after, he was recruited by the University of Maryland, where he spent more than a year (2007-2008) in the department of Diagnostic Sciences and Pathology as Visiting Assistant Professor. Bart Vandenberghe was finalist for the Research Award of the International Dentomaxillofacial Radiology Association in 2007 in Beijing, China, and is reviewer for several international journals. Besides his academic endeavors, he organized a first dental mission for the Tierra Bomba Organization in 2007, Colombia. Currently, he is finalizing his PhD at the University of Leuven with a research grant in 3D Cone Beam imaging.

Yoshihisa Yamashita is currently a Chairman of Department of Preventive Dentistry in Kyushu University Facutlty of Dental Science. His current research focus is on the molecular genetics of oral microbes associated with oral diseases, dental caries and periodontitis and ecological analysis of oral flora concerning with both oral and systemic health. He has published extensively on oral microbes concerning with oral and systemic health and relationship oral health condition and systemic health. Prof.

Yamshita received his PhD degree in Dentistry from Kyushu Dental College in 1986 after undertaking his PhD studies in the Department of Orthodontics. After that, he engaged an assistant professor and an associate professor in Kyushu Dental College and Kyushu University School of Dentistry, and was appointed to be Chariman of Department of Oral Health Science, Nihon University School of Dentistry, Tokyo, Japan in 2000 and then moved in 2003 to Kyushu University Faculty of Dental Science as a Chairman of Department of Preventive Dentistry.

Index

E

F

G

H

I

J

K

L

M